W9-BRB-762

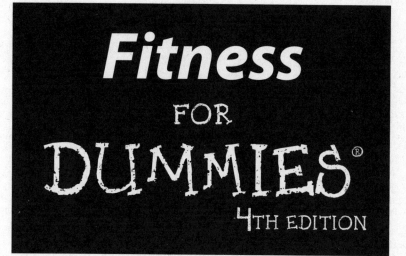

Fitness
FOR
DUMMIES®
4TH EDITION

by Suzanne Schlosberg and Liz Neporent, MA

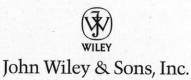

WILEY

John Wiley & Sons, Inc.

Fitness For Dummies,® 4th Edition

Published by
John Wiley & Sons, Inc.
111 River St.
Hoboken, NJ 07030-5774
www.wiley.com

Copyright © 2011 by John Wiley & Sons, Inc., Hoboken, New Jersey

Published by John Wiley & Sons, Inc., Hoboken, New Jersey

Published simultaneously in Canada

For general information on our other products and services, please contact our Customer Care Department within the U.S. at 877-762-2974, outside the U.S. at 317-572-3993, or fax 317-572-4002.

For technical support, please visit www.wiley.com/techsupport.

Wiley publishes in a variety of print and electronic formats and by print-on-demand. Some material included with standard print versions of this book may not be included in e-books or in print-on-demand. If this book refers to media such as a CD or DVD that is not included in the version you purchased, you may download this material at http://booksupport.wiley.com. For more information about Wiley products, visit www.wiley.com.

Library of Congress Control Number: 2010937829

ISBN 978-0-470-76759-7 (pbk); ISBN 978-0-470-94897-2 (ebk); ISBN 978-0-470-94898-9 (ebk); ISBN 978-0-470-94899-6 (ebk)

Manufactured in the United States of America

10 9 8 7 6 5 4

WILEY

About the Authors

Suzanne Schlosberg is a fitness, health, and parenting writer known for her humorous approach to lifestyle topics. A former senior editor of *Shape* magazine, she is the author or coauthor of ten books, including *Weight Training For Dummies, The Ultimate Workout Log, The Ultimate Diet Log, The Good Neighbor Cookbook,* and *The Active Woman's Pregnancy Log.* Her articles can be found on the Web sites of *Fit Pregnancy, Ladies' Home Journal, More, Parents,* and *Parenting,* among others, as well as her own Web site, www.suzanneschlosberg.com. An avid cyclist and totally mediocre Nordic skier, Suzanne lives in Bend, Oregon, with her husband and twin boys. She can be reached at suzanne@suzanneschlosberg.com.

Liz Neporent is a columnist and blogger for AOL Health and That's Fit, as well as a regular contributor to many other Web sites, publications, and media outlets. She cowrote *The Winner's Brain* with authors Jeff Brown and Mark Fenske. Liz brings a strong science background, fitness authority, and sense of fun to all her work. She holds a master's degree in exercise physiology from New York University and is certified by the American Council on Exercise, where she served on the board of directors for six years and now serves on the emeritus board and as a national spokesperson. She's a health consultant to Harvard Medical School in the publications division and is president of Wellness 360, a New York City-based wellness management and consulting company. She lives in New York City with her husband Jay and daughter Skylar. Follow her on twitter @lizzyfit or check out her Web site: www.w360.com.

Dedication

To all who are striving to improve their fitness.

Publisher's Acknowledgments

We're proud of this book; please send us your comments at http://dummies.custhelp.com. For other comments, please contact our Customer Care Department within the U.S. at 877-762-2974, outside the U.S. at 317-572-3993, or fax 317-572-4002.

Some of the people who helped bring this book to market include the following:

Acquisitions, Editorial, and Media Development

Senior Project Editor: Alissa Schwipps
  (Previous Edition: Elizabeth Kuball)

Acquisitions Editor: Tracy Boggier

Senior Copy Editor: Danielle Voirol

Copy Editor: Todd Lothery

Assistant Editor: David Lutton

Technical Editor: Carol Kennedy-Armbruster

Senior Editorial Manager: Jennifer Ehrlich

Editorial Assistants: Rachelle Amick, Jennette ElNaggar

Art Coordinator: Alicia B. South

Cover Photos: © istockphoto.com/Chris Bernard

Cartoons: Rich Tennant (www.the5thwave.com)

Composition Services

Senior Project Coordinator: Kristie Rees

Layout and Graphics: Lavonne Roberts, Christin Swinford

Proofreaders: Betty Kish, Lauren Mandelbaum

Indexer: Becky Hornyak

Photographer: Matt Bowen

Special Help
  Steve Kelly, Kaitlin McGlone

Special Thanks
  Robin Anderson, Shawn Cook (Cardinal Fitness at Windermere Place), S. R. Gunale, Swati Gunale, Vatsala Gunale, Deanna Holland, Brandon Hooks, Andrew Rezkalla, Jennifer Stewart, Kevin Stewart (www.stewartfitness.net)

Publishing and Editorial for Consumer Dummiest

  Kathleen Nebenhaus, Vice President and Executive Publisher

  David Palmer, Associate Publisher

  Kristin Ferguson-Wagstaffe, Product Development Director

Publishing for Technology Dummies

  Andy Cummings, Vice President and Publisher

Composition Services

  Debbie Stailey, Director of Composition Services

Contents at a Glance

Table of Contents

Part III: Building Muscle and Strengthening Bone 137

Introduction

· ·

So you want to get fit? You've come to the right place. Though we can't lace up your sneakers and lift you onto a moving treadmill, we can do the next best thing: explain the benefits and basics of exercise, cover the best workout programs and products, and give you some long-distance encouragement.

That's what we've been doing since the first edition of *Fitness For Dummies* was published back in the prehistoric mid-1990s, before you could tweet your bench-press stats or "friend" a fellow swimmer halfway around the globe. So much about fitness has changed since then — the equipment and training theories, the classes and gadgets. So once again, we've overhauled this book, adding chapters and substantially revamping others.

To understand how the field of fitness has been transformed, consider this: The first edition of *Fitness For Dummies* contained exactly four paragraphs about the Internet. Even in the 3rd edition, you couldn't find the word *podcast* or a mention of phone apps. But the book you're holding right now, the 4th edition, is loaded with tips on using the Web to get fit.

If you're a technophobe or just staunchly old-school, don't worry: Some of today's most popular fitness trends are among the most time-honored and low-tech. For example, kettlebells — cast-iron weights that were all the rage in Czarist Russia — have made a comeback. Yoga, dating back thousands of years, is more popular than ever; so is Pilates, developed more than a century ago. And one of today's trendiest and most useful workout gadgets, the physioball, is really just a glorified beach ball.

As always, the fitness field offers something for everyone, from gamers to grandmas — and heck, grandmas who are gamers. (Attention gamer grandmas: Check out Wii 10 Minute Solution: Knock-Out Body!) In *Fitness For Dummies*, 4th Edition, we strive to cover fitness from all angles.

About This Book

Fitness For Dummies, 4th Edition, updates you on all the latest — the good, the bad, the totally cool (free workout podcasts) and the totally weird (shoes shaped like feet). But our main mission remains the same as it was the first three times around: to get you jazzed to move, to make you a savvy consumer of fitness products and information, and to help you tackle your worries, whether you fear the chest-press machine or panic at the thought of attempting a spinning class.

Fitness For Dummies, 4th Edition, tells you the stuff you really want to know, such as:

- ✔ Will exercise really help me lose weight?
- ✔ Which weight-training exercises are best for beginners?
- ✔ What's the difference between yoga and Pilates?
- ✔ Is it safe to exercise in the third trimester of pregnancy or the ninth decade of life?
- ✔ Will diet soda help me lose weight?
- ✔ Can I really get in shape with a phone app or a Wii fitness game?
- ✔ Which brands of home exercise equipment are most reliable?
- ✔ How do I know whether I should join a gym or buy a DVD?
- ✔ Can I actually get a "Rock Solid Bod in 6 Weeks," like the Web sites say?

This book is basic enough for the fitness rookie to follow, but it's also intended for workout veterans who want to brush up on the latest fitness concepts, gadgets, and training techniques.

This is no textbook, so if a particular topic piques your interest, turn right to it; let the table of contents and index be your guides. Also, in every chapter we define terms and point you in the direction of any information that may help you.

Conventions Used in This Book

We use few conventions in this book because we want you to be able to pick it up and start anywhere. But two conventions to keep in mind are the following:

- ✔ New fitness jargon appears in italics, *like this,* along with a brief definition. Use these terms to impress your friends or the trainer you just hired using the guidelines in Chapter 20.
- ✔ Web sites appear in a special font, `like this`, to distinguish them from other text. Jump on over to your computer or smart phone and check them out.

What You're Not to Read

We intended for this book to be a pleasant and practical read so that you can quickly find and absorb the information you want. However, we sometimes couldn't help going a little bit deeper or relaying information that expands on the basics. You may find this information interesting, but you don't need it to understand what you came to that section to find.

When you see a sidebar (a gray-shaded box of text) or text flagged with the Technical Stuff icon, know that the information is optional. You can lead a full and happy life without giving it a glance. (But aren't you curious? A little?)

Foolish Assumptions

Before we could write this book, we had to make some assumptions about who you, the reader, might be. We assume that

- ✔ You're just beginning an exercise program, thinking about starting one, or returning to a healthier lifestyle after a few years in the recliner. Or you may have been working out for years and are looking for advice on how to reinvigorate your routine.

- ✔ You're interested in sorting out all the different options for fitness activities so you can decide which are best for you.

- ✔ You want to get the lowdown on all the latest fitness research, bargains, classes, equipment, and gear — anything that has to do with getting you into shape.

- ✔ You'd like to become more knowledgeable about exercise and fitness so you can avoid mistakes and injuries.

How This Book Is Organized

Fitness For Dummies, 4th Edition, is divided into seven parts, and the chapters within each part cover specific topics in detail. You can read each chapter or part without having to read what came before, although we may refer you to other sections for more information about certain topics. Here's a brief look at the seven parts.

Part 1: Getting Your Butt off the Couch

In this part, we give you the tools to start a fitness program. First, we explain the key components of fitness (did you know that being able to balance on one foot is as important as being able to walk a mile?) and offer tips on staying inspired to exercise so that it becomes a habit. Then, we help you evaluate your current fitness level with a series of fun tests; no worries — you can't flunk. We run down the basics of healthy eating so you can stay fueled for your workouts and fit into your jogging shorts. We also explain how to stay abreast of fitness developments through Web sites, blogs, TV, and other media and how to find reliable health and fitness information. Finally, we offer tips on keeping your muscles and joints injury-free and on treating aches and pains that do crop up.

Part 11: Going Cardio

This part is devoted to cardiovascular exercise — the kind of activity that strengthens your heart and lungs, burns lots of calories, lowers your stress level, and gives you the energy to chase down your cat for a bath. Walking, jogging, swimming, and cycling are a few examples. We explain terms such as *anaerobic* and *target heart-rate zone,* and we tell you how long, how often, and how hard you need to work out in order to slim down, live longer, or train for a 10K run. We also cover the most popular cardio-exercise options, both indoors and out, including essential gear, proper techniques, and tips for getting started.

Part 111: Building Muscle and Strengthening Bone

In this part we explain why everyone — whether you're 18 or 80, male or female — ought to strength-train. We give you the know-how to get started lifting weights, and we answer questions such as:

- What are the differences between weight machines, dumbbells, and barbells?
- What are *sets* and *reps,* and how much weight should I lift?
- Which exercises are most effective?
- What's a *deltoid,* and why should I care?

We also include a complete strength-training routine you can perform either at home or at the gym.

Part IV: Limbering Up with Flexibility, Balance, and Mind-Body Exercise

In this part we cover activities that typically don't involve buckets of sweat but are deceptively challenging and incredibly important, not to mention fun and relaxing. We're talking about stretching and balance training, as well as activities that usually incorporate both: yoga and Pilates. We show you numerous exercises you can do at home or in a class to make your body more flexible, graceful, and agile. These are all attributes that will serve you well when you work out or train for an event and as you get older and more prone to accidents and injuries.

Part V: Getting Fit in Health Clubs and Home Gyms

This part gives you the information you need to enter a gym with confidence. We explain how to choose a club that suits you, how to snag a membership bargain, and how to demonstrate stellar health-club etiquette. We also tell you how to get through an exercise class when you feel like you have two left feet that are tied together, and we update you on the latest in exercise classes, from Zumba to boot camp to IndoRow.

Fitness clubs and studios aren't for everyone, so in this part, we also help you choose the best home fitness equipment for your budget, your goals, and the size of your living room. We cover everything from space-age treadmills to $3 rubber exercise tubes and offer tips for designing your home gym so you'll actually use the stuff you buy.

We also help you find a qualified fitness trainer, if you're so inclined, as well as high-quality, low-cost, and motivating digital workouts, on DVDs and online.

Part VI: Exercising for All Ages and Stages

This part covers exercise from the beginning — we're talking in utero — all the way through the AARP years. Research has proven that prenatal exercise is not only safe for Mom but also gives babies a healthy start, lowering their risk for obesity and diabetes throughout life. This section fills you in on what kind of exercise program is ideal for moms-to-be. In light of the country's childhood-obesity epidemic, we include a chapter on getting kids of all ages, from toddlers to tweens, up and moving. For those of you entering your sixth decade and beyond, this part is for you, too. We show you how to get and stay fit so you can continue to stay active and look good in your jeans.

Part VII: The Part of Tens

Every *For Dummies* book has a Part of Tens. These chapters give you a different spin on some of the information already presented in the other parts, along with plenty of new stuff. For example, scattered throughout this book are many reasons to get and stay fit; in Chapter 25, you find a whole chapter of reasons. (Did you know that exercise lowers your risk of developing dementia?) And in Chapter 26, we tell you which fitness products we consider to be most worthy of your hard-earned dollars.

Icons Used in This Book

Icons are small pictures in the margins of this book that flag certain material for you. The following icons highlight information you want to pay special attention to.

This icon flags great strategies for getting in shape, such as testing your fitness every three to six months. We also use this icon to highlight money-saving tips — such as asking your health club to waive its initiation fee — and excellent fitness products, from treadmills to stretching devices to fitness games for your kid's Wii or Xbox.

When information is just too good to forget, this icon helps you remember. This is the stuff you want to jot down and attach with a magnet to your fridge.

We use the Myth Buster superhero to dispel popular fitness myths. For example, in Chapter 7, we explain that exercise doesn't have to hurt to be good for you. (In fact, the vast majority of the time, it shouldn't hurt at all.)

This icon warns you about hucksters who offer false promises, sell bogus products, or try to snare you with slimy sales tactics. We also use this icon to caution you about common exercise mistakes, such as neglecting to adjust the seat on an exercise machine.

We use this icon when we tell a story about our own adventures in fitness or recount the experiences of people we know. The anecdotes range from the wacky to the inspirational to the just plain helpful.

The Technical Stuff icon marks info that's interesting but not necessary to your understanding of fitness.

Where to Go from Here

You can dive into this book in two ways:

> ✔ **If you want a crash course in fitness, read the book cover to cover.** You'll get a thorough understanding of what it takes to get in shape, and you'll come across topics you may not have thought to look up, such as how to practice proper etiquette in the gym, how to judge the accuracy of fitness Web sites and blogs, and how often you need to buy new running shoes.

> ✔ **If you want to find out about a specific topic, you can flip to that section and get your answers right away.** Use the book as a reference every time you boldly enter uncharted territory, like a yoga class or a Web site that sells fitness DVDs.

Whatever your approach, enjoy your journey!

Part I
Getting Your Butt off the Couch

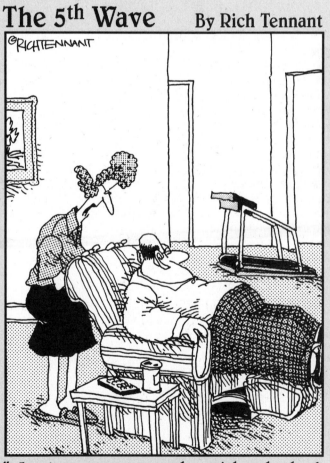

The 5th Wave   By Rich Tennant

@RICHTENNANT

"You know, anyone who wishes he had a remote control for his exercise equipment is missing the idea of exercise equipment."

In this part . . .

This part helps you get going on a fitness program, no matter what shape you're in. Chapter 1 explains what *fitness* really means and helps you devise a game plan. You find out how to set realistic goals, track your progress, and make exercise a habit. Chapter 2 explains the important first step toward getting in shape: testing your fitness. You can either do this on your own or hire a professional. Chapter 3 gives you the lowdown on healthy eating, including how to slim down without going hungry. Chapter 4 tells you how to become a savvy consumer of fitness media, including TV, Web sites, and blogs, so that you can distinguish accurate news reports from misleading fluff. In Chapter 5, we explain how to protect your muscles and joints from injury and what steps to take if you do sprain an ankle or strain a muscle.

Chapter 1

Establishing Your Plan of Attack

*I*f you're reading this chapter, you've decided to get fit. (Or like wannabe chefs whose action plan amounts to sitting on the couch watching cooking shows, you're pretending to get fit by reading this book!) Although transforming yourself from couch potato to fit, lean, exercise machine doesn't take a PhD in physiology, you'll have more success if you know what's in store.

This chapter explains what the term *fitness* really means, what's involved in becoming fit (no, you needn't quit your job and take up residence in a gym), how to get started, and how to stay motivated. We want to help make fitness a permanent and enjoyable part of your lifestyle (rather than some weird hobby, like UFO hunting, that you once took up for a month before moving on to something else).

Understanding What Fitness Means

Fitness, which some people refer to as wellness, has a lot of different meanings. You can be fit to run 5 miles, fit to hoist 200 pounds, fit to do a headstand in a yoga class or transform yourself into a pretzel. You can *look* fit — that is, lean — and not actually have much stamina, strength, flexibility, or balance. Or you can possess all those attributes but still consume doughnuts and soda for breakfast — not what we'd call a health-conscious diet. It's a rare human being who is a champ in all respects, and we don't expect that of anyone, including ourselves.

Individuals need to pick and choose which areas of fitness to focus on, the ones that make the most sense for the goals they have and the lives they lead. Still, it doesn't take that much effort to achieve a basic level of physical fitness in the five key areas: cardio, strength, flexibility, balance, and nutrition.

✔ **Cardio fitness:** Workouts that get your heart pumping and continuously work a lot of large muscles such as the arms, torso, and legs are known as *cardio* (short for *cardiovascular*) exercises. These activities, such as walking, cycling, and using an elliptical machine, improve your heart, lungs, blood vessels, stamina, and, to some extent, strength. Cardio workouts also burn plenty of calories, which can help you lose weight. Check out Chapters 6 through 9 for a primer on cardio exercise, both indoors and out.

✔ **Strength training:** Whereas some men focus on weight training to the exclusion of all other fitness activities (you may meet a buff bodybuilder who can't run a mile), some women shy away from lifting weights for fear of looking like that buff bodybuilder. In fact, for reasons we explain in Chapter 10, both men and women should incorporate some strength training into their fitness programs.

✔ **Flexibility:** Unlike cardio exercise and strength training, flexibility training — also known as stretching — doesn't get any glory in the fitness world unless you happen to be a gymnast or a dancer. Most people skip stretching altogether or do a few cursory toe touches and call it a day. That's because the benefits of stretching your muscles and joints aren't immediately obvious; being flexible doesn't make you slender or buff or able to outrun your teenager. So why bother? Because as you age, your joints become less mobile. Maintaining your flexibility through the exercises in Chapter 14, yoga (Chapter 16), or Pilates (Chapter 17) helps minimize your risk of falling and getting injured while allowing you to continue moving with grace and good posture even into old age.

✔ **Balance:** If flexibility is the forgotten stepchild of fitness, then balance is the ignored twice-removed third cousin. But like flexibility, balance is an aspect of fitness that's important when you're young and absolutely essential when you're not. A good sense of balance helps you move more fluidly and prevents unnecessary falls. Even if you have no aspirations to become a tightrope walker, doing the basic balance moves that we describe in Chapter 15 should be more than enough to help you maintain your sense of balance. Think your balance is already stellar? Take the balance tests described in that chapter and see how you rate.

✔ **Nutrition:** When you make wise food choices (ahem, that means nixing the peanut-butter cookie in favor of the whole-wheat toast with peanut butter), you have more energy to exercise, and you recover more quickly from your workouts. And of course, cleaning up your eating habits is the key to losing weight. But when you're faced with conflicting research reports and sneaky marketing tactics by food manufacturers, making good choices is tough. High protein or high carb? Do you really need eight glasses of water a day? How about a vitamin supplement? Chapter 3 guides you through the haze.

Setting Goals and Tracking Your Progress

You need to clarify why you want to improve your fitness. Maybe heart disease runs in your family, and you want to avoid carrying on that tradition. Maybe your kids, or grandkids, run you ragged. Maybe you're tired of spending money on new and bigger clothing every year. Whatever the reason, make sure you're doing this for yourself — not simply to please your doctor or to attempt to match your high-school-era Facebook photo.

Next, you need to set concrete fitness goals. In the following sections, we help you explore your current fitness level, set long- and short-term goals, and keep track of how you're achieving them.

Research shows that goal-setting works. In typical studies, scientists give one group of exercisers a specific goal, such as doing 60 sit-ups. Meanwhile, they tell a second group of exercisers simply, "Do your best." The exercisers with specific goals tend to have significantly more success than the "whatever" groups. This approach can work for you, too.

Assessing your current fitness level (yes, this class has tests)

To help you clarify what you want to work on — and to best determine how to reach your fitness goals — you first need to figure out where you are physically. We suggest undergoing a fitness evaluation that includes a full health/fitness history and other important measures, such as your resting heart rate, blood pressure, percentage of body fat, strength, and flexibility. We explain all these terms in Chapter 2.

Fitness tests can be done by a physician or a certified personal trainer. Or as we explain in Chapter 2, you can do many of them yourself. Don't worry: You can't fail these tests. Think of them as baseline measurements that help you decide where to put your emphasis and give you a basis for comparison a few months after you start working out.

Setting multiple goals and rewards

It's important to look at the big picture, setting long-term goals, while giving yourself smaller and more manageable stepping stones along the way. Having mini-goals makes your long-term goals seem more feasible. The following sections give you a look at the different types of goals you should set.

You give your golden retriever a doggy treat when he fetches the Frisbee, right? Be nice to yourself, too. Attach an appropriate reward to each of your goals. If you lift weights three days a week for a month or finish a 5K run, treat yourself to a massage. Sure, it's bribery, but it works. (By the way, triple-decker fudge cake isn't what we have in mind for a reward.)

You can get pretty creative with your rewards. We know a woman who put a coin in a jar for every mile she ran. When the jar was full, every few months, she counted the coins, totaled her miles, and had a little nest egg for splurging on new lipstick.

Long-term goals

Give yourself a goal for the next three to six months. Some people get really creative with their long-term goals.

Suzanne spoke to a woman in Ohio whose long-term goal was to walk to a friend's house — in Alabama. No, she didn't literally hoof it 697 miles. She charted the route on an auto-club map, and for every 20 minutes that she spent doing an aerobic exercise video, she gave herself credit for 1 mile. At the end of each week, she added up her "mileage" and used a yellow highlighter to mark the ground she covered on the map.

Make your long-term goals realistic. If you start your swimming program today, swimming the English Channel isn't a wise six-month goal. But don't be afraid to dream. Choose a goal that really sparks you, and you may be surprised by what you can accomplish.

Liz has a client who was 60 years old when he started training for a trek up Alaska's Mount McKinley. Liz eventually had the guy walking uphill for up to 90 minutes on the treadmill with a heavy pack and hiking boots. After six months of training, the man successfully completed his trek. He was the oldest one on the trip, but he wasn't the slowest.

If you're a beginner, we recommend setting moderately challenging yet still meaningful goals.

Short-term goals

Half a year is a long time to wait for feelings of success. In order to stay motivated, you need to feel a sense of accomplishment along the way. Set short-term goals for a few weeks to one month. Here are some examples:

- Take two spin classes a week for one month.
- Improve your 1-mile walk time by 20 seconds.
- Move up one weight plate on shoulder press in two weeks.
- Balance on one leg for a full minute without holding on to anything.

Immediate goals

Immediate goals refer to goals for each week, day, or workout. This way, when you walk into the gym, you don't waste any time figuring out which exercises to do. Here are examples of immediate goals:

- ✔ Spend a full 10 minutes stretching at the end of a workout.
- ✔ Do upper-body weight exercises and 20 minutes on the elliptical trainer.
- ✔ Run 2 miles.
- ✔ Bike a hilly 20-mile course.

Backup goals

You always need a Plan B in case something happens and you're not able to reach your primary goal as soon as you want to. By setting backup goals, you have a better chance of achieving something, and you don't feel like a failure if your long-term goal doesn't work out. Suppose your long-term goal is to complete a 10K run in the spring, but you sprain an ankle and have to stop running. If one of your backup goals is to strengthen your upper body, you can still keep on track while your ankle heals.

Putting it in writing

Setting goals and rewards is pretty easy; forgetting what they are is even easier. To keep yourself honest and psyched up, we suggest tracking your goals and accomplishments. Here are other ways to make a commitment and monitor your progress.

Making a goal sheet

Put your goals somewhere visible, and next to each goal, note the corresponding reward. Figure 1-1 shows a sample goal sheet that you can fill out each week. Underneath each heading, write down your goal and target date.

Suzanne knows a swimmer who writes his goals on his kickboard. Liz has a client who enters her workout goals into her computer's screen saver so that she sees them scrolling by every time she takes a break from typing.

Keeping a workout log

Tracking your workouts in a *workout log* (also called a *workout diary* or *training diary*) can help you get better results. You can look back at the end of each week and say, "Wow — look at what I did!" And you may be inspired to accomplish even more. A log also provides a reality check: You may think that you're working out four times a week only to flip through your log and discover that you've been overestimating your efforts.

Long-Term Goals	Long-Term Rewards
Backup Long-Term Goals	
Short-Term Goals	Short-Term Rewards
Weekly Goals	Weekly Rewards
Workout Goals	Daily Rewards

Figure 1-1:
Make a goal sheet like the one here (or photocopy this one).

TIP

Test your fitness regularly and track these numbers in your workout log so you can keep track of your progress over time. Exercise gives you intangible benefits like more energy and greater self-esteem, but it also helps to translate your progress into raw numbers: how many pounds you can bench-press, how many beats your resting heart rate has dropped, how fast you can run a mile.

For your first year that you work out regularly, you may want to get tested or test yourself every three months. (You make the most noticeable improvements when you first start exercising; then progress becomes less dramatic.) After that, we suggest getting tested every six months. If you don't want to spend the time or money on a whole battery of tests, ask a certified trainer to do the part you find most motivating, such as a body-fat test or blood-pressure reading. Or use the self-tests you find in Chapter 2. You can buy a log at a bookstore, use nifty computer software to monitor your progress, or use a Web-based tracking program.

Selecting Exercises That Are Right for You

When you shop for clothes, not every outfit you try on is right for you, but when you find the perfect one, doesn't it make you feel great? The same is true of exercise. Not every activity you try, whether it's a weight circuit, a kickboxing class, or a hike through the woods, will fit you like a custom-made suit. But when you find the workout that suits your current fitness level, your budget, and your personality, it's a fantastic feeling!

This book helps guide you through the myriad options so you can make that connection. If you're pregnant, for example, you'll want to flip to Chapter 22 to find out what activities are likely to suit you best. If you're over age 50 and just starting to think about getting in shape, then the information in Chapter 24 will get you started in the right direction. If you think you could get really get passionate about running, Chapter 9 will be a page-turner.

Along with sample exercises to interest virtually every type of exerciser, we offer leads on plenty of other resources to help expand your knowledge about fitness so you can find the best exercises for you — everything from selecting equipment to choosing the right Pilates class to finding the right workout group on Twitter. And if you want to seek the help of a personal trainer to set up a safe and effective routine, check out Chapter 20.

Staying Motivated to Make Exercise a Habit

What separates people who stick with exercise from those who fall off the wagon? Tracking your progress is an excellent way to keep yourself inspired. Following are several additional tips to help you get over the hump and stay jazzed. We discuss several of these topics in detail throughout the book, but we want you to keep them in mind from the start.

Getting inspiration from others

Sometimes the strongest motivation to stick with your workouts comes from other people. Here are some ways to get some support:

- ✔ **Work out with a buddy.** If you make a plan to meet up with a friend, you're a lot less likely to blow off your workouts. Plus, time flies when you're chit-chatting as you sweat.

    Liz knows a couple who decided to get in shape together. They took a class in healthy cooking, walked every morning together, and even pumped iron twice a week as a team. Each pushed and encouraged the other, and at the end of four months, both had lost more than 20 pounds. "Besides looking and feeling 1,000 percent better, it's done amazing things for our relationship," the wife says.

- ✔ **Join a group or a team.** For some people, exercising with a whole group of people — whether an informal group or an organized club or team — is even better than meeting up with a buddy. You have more people to socialize with, and if one person can't make it that day, the workout isn't derailed.

    Don't worry if you're the slowest one in the group; just do as much as you can handle. The group will likely push you to try harder and achieve things you never dreamed you could. Don't sweat it, either, if you feel like an outsider for a while; keep showing up, and eventually you'll be one of the gang. To find a group, check with local sporting goods and fitness-equipment stores.

- ✔ **Join an Internet fitness community.** Thanks to the Internet, you can gain inspiration from fitness buddies across the country — or even the world. There are now thousands of Web sites that bring together like-minded fitness buffs so they can discuss their training, share tips, and talk through challenges (see the nearby sidebar for details).

    Internet groups are especially helpful for home exercisers, who don't have the social benefit that you can get at a health club and may not have friends or family who exercise.

- ✔ **Read success stories.** The good ones offer not only inspiration but also specific and realistic advice. (Forget about those before-and-after ads in which a blubbery guy with a scowl on his face is miraculously transformed into a grinning hunk of muscle.) On AOL Health, for example, you may read about a woman who beat breast cancer and went on to run a marathon, or a woman who lost 100 pounds and is now a slim, trim fitness instructor. We especially like Internet success stories because you can post and read comments by other readers. Sometimes the posters have some amazing stories to tell.

Training for an event

Suzanne once interviewed an Olympic weight lifter who described himself as a "pretty lazy guy." "If I wasn't training for the Olympics," he said, "I probably wouldn't even work out."

Even if you don't aspire to hoist 424 pounds overhead before thousands of screaming fans, committing to an event can jump-start your workout program. The options are countless — a 5K walk, a 10K run, a mini-triathlon, a 100-mile bike ride. The minute you pay your entry fee, you have a whole new sense of purpose. And the feeling of accomplishment you get from completing your event is like nothing else.

Keeping it interesting

Boredom can be the enemy of any workout. Here are a couple of ways to stay engaged:

✔ **Keep yourself entertained.** Walk on the treadmill while listening to your favorite music on your iPod, and 30 minutes may fly by as if it's 10 minutes; accidentally leave that iPod at home, and those 30 minutes may seem like 3 hours. For many people, entertainment can mean the difference between sticking with exercise and skipping it. Some gyms now offer on-demand services, MP3 ports in each piece of cardio equipment, and more than 500 entertainment channels.

✔ **Mix up your workouts.** Some people thrive on routine. Suzanne used to ride her bike with a 67-year-old guy named Barry who had been cycling the exact same route on Saturdays for 41 years. Much to the frustration of his wife, Barry refused to take long vacations because he didn't want to miss his Saturday ride.

Most of us, however, need a bit of variety to stay motivated. For this reason, you may want to try *cross-training,* which simply means mixing up your workouts. You can vary your sport — running on Mondays, yoga on Tuesdays, hiking on Wednesdays, and so on. Or you can vary your pace and terrain — walking fast and flat one day, slow and hilly the next. Or you can try different equipment — using weight machines one session and dumbbells the next. In addition to relieving boredom, varying your workouts helps you avoid injuries from repetitive motions.

Dressing the part

You needn't become a fitness-clothing junkie, but buying snazzy new workout shorts or comfy new athletic shoes can get you fired up to exercise. Plus, you feel like a workout pro, and you let your fellow exercisers know you're one of them.

When Liz started indoor rock climbing, she'd show up in running shorts and a T-shirt. She noticed that all the good climbers wore tank tops and long sweat pants cut off at the bottom. Gradually, Liz conformed to the dress code and found out a few things. For one, the "in" crowd was more accepting of her because she looked serious about the sport. But more important, Liz realized that rock climbers dress that way for a reason: The long sweats protect you from bumps and bruises. Cutting off the elastic at the bottom lets you move your legs and feet more freely. And a sleeveless top makes moving your arms easier.

Staying realistic

Trying to do too much or setting your expectations too high can lead to a lot of frustration. Here are some ways to stay on track:

- ✔ **Pace yourself.** Don't buy every exercise DVD, listen to every podcast on the market, or try every weight machine in the gym the first day. You'll flame out fast. Always pace yourself so you live to fight the good fight another day.

- ✔ **Cut yourself some slack.** Recognize that everyone improves at a different pace. Getting inspiration from other people is great, but don't let anyone else's accomplishments diminish your own. Always keep in mind why you laced up your sneakers today and be proud that you've worked up to walking 3 miles every other day, even if your neighbor runs 10 miles a day. Fitness is something personal and unique to you.

And don't get down on yourself if you miss a few days — or even a few weeks — of exercise. If you fall off the wagon, just try again. You have the rest of your life to get this right.

Plugging in to online fitness communities

A Facebook or LinkedIn search for walking groups yields thousands of results. Refine your search for your location, age group, and fitness level, and chances are you'll still have more than 500 groups to choose from.

Liz especially loves the groups on Twitter. Where else can you get great advice and links packaged in a poetic 140 characters or less? Type in your search term, and you'll find others with the same search term in their name or profile. For example, if you type in "weight training," the search may return Twitter handles like Luv2weighttrain and weightlift4ever. It also gives you anyone who mentions a love of weight training in his or her profile.

If you don't feel like sifting through the results to weed out marketers and potential weirdos, search through a Twitter group-compilation site like www.twibes.com, twittgroups.com, or justtweetit.com. These sites also list instructions for how to communicate with your group through the use of tags and all the other strange little tricks you need to know in order to master any of these social networking sites.

Chapter 2

Testing Your Fitness

. . . .

In This Chapter

▶ Checking your health history to determine what's safe

▶ Measuring your heart rate, blood pressure, and body fat

▶ Evaluating your strength, flexibility, and balance

▶ Recording your results and finding out what they mean

. . . .

*W*e constantly hear people say, "I'm so out of shape. I need to lose weight." But that's like telling a travel agent, "I'm in Europe. I need to go to Africa." Your travel agent needs to know the specifics: Are you in Rome? Berlin? Madrid? Do you want to go to Cairo? Cape Town? The Kalahari Desert? Before you embark on a fitness program, you need to know your starting point with precision. A fitness evaluation gives you important departure information.

Don't panic. A fitness test isn't like your driver's license renewal exam: You can't flunk, and you don't have to stand in line for three hours listening to people rant about government bureaucracy. A fitness test simply gives you key information, such as your heart rate and body-fat percentage and how you rate in terms of strength, flexibility, and balance. Armed with these facts, you or your trainer can design an intelligent plan to get you to your fitness destination. And when you arrive, you'll have the numbers to prove just how far you've come.

In this chapter, we describe what to expect when a professional tests your fitness. We also explain how to evaluate your fitness on your own. If you do most of the testing yourself, consider getting certain aspects of your fitness assessed at a fitness center. As you complete the various tests, record your results in a log or on the chart near the end of this chapter.

Reviewing Your Health History

When you join a gym, one of the first things you should be asked to do is to fill out some sort of health-history questionnaire. That way, you and the staff can get an idea of your health limitations before you start exercising. In this section, we explain the kinds of questions you may be asked and help you evaluate yourself if a gym membership isn't in your future.

Talking to a tester at the gym

Your answers to health-history questions give a snapshot of your overall well-being, including your exercise and eating habits, your risk for developing cardiovascular disease, and any orthopedic limitations or medical conditions that you may have. Typical questions include: Do you have any chronic joint problems such as arthritis? Do you have a family history of heart disease? Are you currently taking any over-the-counter or prescription medications?

After you fill out your questionnaire, your tester should discuss the answers with you and ask for more information if necessary. If you're a smoker, for example, he may ask you how much you smoke.

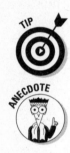

Respond honestly and thoroughly. Don't say that you run 5 miles a day if you haven't broken a sweat since high school — or if you intend to run every day but just haven't gotten around to it.

Liz once worked with a client who hid the fact that he had diabetes because he was ashamed to tell anyone. One day after a workout, he walked into the locker room, and several minutes later someone else came out screaming. The client had passed out on the floor. His blood sugar had crashed and he had gone into diabetic shock. A nurse was quickly summoned, and she probably saved his life. Afterward, he admitted it was far more embarrassing to be found lying naked on the bathroom floor than to reveal his medical issues.

Some gyms request that you be tested by a physician if a staff member feels you may have a medical problem. Don't groan; a request like this indicates that your gym is on the ball. Some health clubs just want your money. They may not require any testing — other than the test that determines whether you can sign your name on a credit-card slip. If that's the case, you need to take responsibility for getting tested.

Assessing your health history yourself

If you don't belong to a health club, ask yourself the following questions, which are designed to indicate your risk of developing heart disease. (These are from a questionnaire known as the Physical Activity Readiness Questionnaire, or PAR-Q):

- ✔ Has your doctor ever said that you have a heart condition *and* that you should only do physical activity recommended by a doctor?
- ✔ Do you feel pain in your chest when you do physical activity?
- ✔ In the past month, have you had chest pain when you were not doing physical activity?

- Do you lose your balance because of dizziness or do you ever lose consciousness?

- Do you have a bone or joint problem (for example, back, knee, or hip pain) that could be made worse by a change in your physical activity?

- Is your doctor currently prescribing drugs (for example, water pills) for your blood pressure or heart condition?

- Do you know of any other reason why you should not do physical activity?

If you answer yes to one or more of these questions, we recommend that you speak with your doctor by phone or in person before you start becoming much more physically active or before you go any further in the testing process. Tell your doctor about the questions you just answered and which questions you answered yes to. After this discussion, your doctor may give you the blessing to start on an exercise program so long as you start slowly and build up gradually. Or she may recommend restricting your activities based on your particular health issues. Talk with your doctor about the kinds of activities you want to participate in — and then follow that advice.

If you answered no honestly to *all* the preceding questions, you can be reasonably sure that you can safely start an exercise program, as long as you build up gradually and don't overdo it.

Vital Signs: Following Your Heart

Taking part in a fitness appraisal is an excellent way to determine your basic fitness so that you can plan the best way for you to live actively. We also highly recommend getting your heart rate and blood pressure evaluated before you start a workout program, even if you think you're perfectly healthy.

Determining your resting heart rate

Your *heart rate,* also known as your *pulse,* is the number of times your heart beats per minute. Your fitness evaluation should include a measure of your resting heart rate — your heart rate when you're sitting still.

To make sure your heart rate is accurate, measure it first thing in the morning for three consecutive days and find the average. If that isn't possible, at least try to take it at a time when you've been sitting quietly for at least 3 hours without having had any caffeine, and the boss hasn't yelled at you.

The simplest place to take your own pulse is at your wrist. Rest your middle and index fingertips (not your thumb) lightly on your opposite wrist, directly below the base of your thumb. Most people can see the faint bluish line of their radial artery; place your fingertips there. Count the beats for 1 minute. Or if you have a short attention span, count the beats for 30 seconds and multiply by 2. For a really, really short attention span, count the beats for 6 seconds and multiply by 10. The less time you count, the less accurate your measure will be, but at least you'll have a rough idea of where your resting heart rate stands. An easier and faster way to measure your pulse is to strap on a heart-rate monitor, an extremely useful gadget we describe in Chapter 6.

Ideally, your resting pulse should be between 60 and 90 beats per minute. It may be slower if you're fit or genetically predisposed to a low heart rate; it may be faster if you're nervous or have recently downed three double cappuccinos. In addition to caffeine, stress and certain medications can speed up your heart rate.

After a month or two of regular exercise, your resting heart rate usually drops. This means that your heart has become more efficient. It may need to beat only 80 times per minute to pump the same amount of blood (or more) than it used to pump in 90 beats. This is because your heart muscle gets stronger and is able to push out more blood per minute with less effort. In the long run, this saves wear and tear on your heart.

Knowing your blood pressure

Have a professional test your blood pressure. Home blood-pressure machines are getting more accurate, but they can be confusing to use, especially if you lack experience in reading and understanding blood pressure. That said, your doctor may recommend one for you or even use a type where you do the placement and she takes the reading over the phone or through a computer. If your doctor doesn't routinely take your BP at your next visit, ask a staff member to do it. Many trainers at the gym know how to take blood pressure, too.

Blood pressure is a measurement of how open your blood vessels are. Low numbers mean that your heart doesn't have to work very hard to pump the blood through your blood vessels. Here's how to interpret the numbers:

- ✔ **Ideal blood pressure:** Ideally, your blood pressure should read 115/75 or below, a lower standard than the old standby of 120/80. If it's slightly higher, don't get stressed (stress only increases blood pressure).

- ✔ **High blood pressure:** If your blood pressure is higher than 140/90, you're considered *hypertensive,* a fancy term for having high blood pressure. If your blood pressure is above 144/94, discuss this result with your doctor before you go any further.

In case you're wondering, the top number, called your *systolic blood pressure,* measures pressure as your heart ejects blood. The bottom number, your *diastolic blood pressure,* measures pressure when your heart relaxes and prepares for its next pump.

If you get a high blood-pressure reading, ask your tester to try again in just a few minutes or even on another visit. The numbers can be affected by many factors, such as illness, caffeine, nervousness, or racing into your test because you were late. But if you repeatedly get high readings, see a doctor.

Discovering how fit your heart is

Submax test is short for *submaximal test,* fitness jargon for a test that evaluates your heart rate when you're working at less than your maximum effort. Typically, this test takes you to about 75 to 85 percent of your maximum heart rate. (***Note:*** A *maximal test* — in which you go all-out — should be performed only by a physician or in the presence of a physician.)

Most reputable clubs perform submax tests. These tests are usually performed on a stationary bicycle, treadmill, or step bench. (If you're a runner, request a treadmill; if you're a cyclist, ask to be tested on a bike. You're best at what you practice most. Plus, you'll get a heart rate that's most accurate for training.) The test usually lasts about 15 minutes. During this time, you increase your intensity every 3 or 4 minutes while the tester monitors your heart rate and blood pressure. The test shouldn't be very hard. On a bike, the worst it should feel like is pedaling up a moderately steep hill for a few minutes.

If you don't belong to a health club, you can test your aerobic, or *cardio-respiratory,* fitness using a watch with a second hand and a course that's exactly 1 mile long:

1. **Warm up with a slow walk for 5 to 10 minutes, and then time yourself as you run or walk the mile as briskly as you can.**

   If a mile sounds like too much for you right now, do a half-mile or even walk around the block. Just choose a distance that you can measure again at a later date.

2. **Take your pulse for 60 seconds right before you stop, and make a mental note of the number. Also note your time as you complete your mile.**

3. **One minute after you finish the mile, take your pulse again.**

   See how far it has dropped from the pulse check you did right at the end of your walk.

4. **Record your results so that you can compare later tests to see how much more quickly you recover.**

Schedule a second fitness evaluation (or evaluate yourself again) in six weeks. Those first weeks of training can bring about some dramatic changes, and it's really motivating to see how well you've done. After that, changes tend to be steady but somewhat slower. Get tested again every three to six months. Certainly don't go longer than a year without reevaluating your progress. You don't want to waste time with a workout program that's not getting results.

Estimating Your Body-Fat Percentage

Although body-fat testing has its limits, your results can provide insight into how your fat-loss and exercise program is coming along. Sure, your scale can tell you that you lost 7 pounds. But a body-fat test can tell you that your 7-pound loss means that you lost approximately 10 pounds of fat and gained about 3 pounds of muscle, results that are probably more motivating.

Body-fat testing also can tell you if you have too *little* fat. Maybe you can never be too rich, but you definitely can be too thin. For women, super-low body fat — below about 16 percent — may lead to problems such as irregular menstrual periods, permanent bone loss, and a high rate of bone fractures.

This section describes different types of fat measurements and some common testing methods.

Getting the lowdown on fat measurements

During your fitness evaluation, your tester will probably weigh you. Just know that your weight is of limited value. When you hop on a scale, you discover the grand total weight of your bones, organs, blood, fat, muscle, and other tissues. This number can be misleading because muscle weighs more per square inch than fat. For instance, consider two men who stand 5'8" and weigh 190 pounds. One guy may be a lean bodybuilder who has a lot of muscle packed onto his frame. Another guy may be a couch potato whose gut hangs 4 inches over his belt buckle. Even a low weight doesn't necessarily indicate good health or fitness. It may simply mean that you have small bones and little muscle.

That's why fitness testers pay more attention to a few other fat-related numbers: body-fat percentage and waist measurements.

Body-fat percentage

More helpful than your body weight is your *body composition* — how much of your body is composed of fat and how much is composed of everything else. Your body composition is also called your body-fat percentage. If you score a 25 percent on a fat test, this means that 25 percent of your weight is composed of fat.

Like your weight, your body-fat percentage is not the entire snapshot of your health. True, cardiovascular disease, diabetes, and certain cancers are more prevalent among overweight people — men who have more than about 20 percent body fat and women who have more than about 30 percent body fat. However, some researchers believe that these health problems are not caused by the extra fat itself but rather by a lack of exercise and a poor diet. In other words, if you exercise regularly and eat well, extra body fat may not compromise your health, so consider your body-fat score in context with other health measures.

Waist circumference

A large body of evidence indicates that *where* you store your fat (around your tummy, to be specific) matters more than how much you have. That's why an additional number to consider is the circumference of your waist. Excess abdominal fat — the type that lies deep in your belly, engulfing your organs — is linked to increased risk for heart disease. Heavy thighs, on the other hand, do not appear to be related to health problems. In other words, a beer belly can cut years off your life; saddlebags merely make it more difficult to shop for jeans.

For an accurate result, wrap a tape measure around the smallest part of your waist and don't pull too tightly. Consult a physician if you're a man with a waist measurement greater than 40 inches or a woman with a waist measurement greater than 35 inches.

Measuring body fat

Keep in mind that every body-fat testing method has room for error. At a fitness convention, Suzanne had her body fat measured by two different methods — and appeared to have gained 11 percent body fat in a matter of 15 minutes. You may even get wildly different readings using the same test, depending on the skill of the tester or the condition of the equipment.

The only way to measure body fat with complete accuracy is to burn yourself up and take a carbon count of the ashes. Because that technique doesn't draw too many volunteers, scientists have developed a number of other methods. Here's a look at the ones you're most likely to come across.

Pinching an inch

The most common body-fat test uses the *skinfold caliper,* a gizmo that resembles a stun gun with salad tongs attached (see Figure 2-1). When your tester fires, the tongs pinch your skin, pulling your fat away from your muscles and bones. (You feel moderate discomfort, like when your great aunt pinches your cheek on the holidays.) Typically, the tester pinches three to seven different sites several times on your body, such as your abdomen, the back of your arm, and the back of your shoulder. The thickness of each pinch is plugged into a formula to determine your body-fat percentage. Your tester should pinch each site two or three times to verify the measurement.

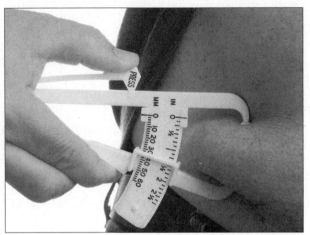

Figure 2-1:
Getting
pinched
with
calipers.

Many factors can cause inaccuracy with a caliper test. The tester may not pinch exactly the right spot, or he may not pull all the fat away from the bone. Or he may pinch too hard and accidentally include some of your muscle. Also, research suggests that certain formulas are more accurate for certain ethnic groups, age ranges, and fitness levels.

Experts give this test a margin of error of 4 points, meaning your actual body-fat percentage could be 4 points higher or lower than it actually is.

Be sure to get tested before your workout. When you exercise, blood travels to your skin to cool you down. This can cause your skin to swell, and you may test fatter than you really are. Plus, calipers can slip if your skin is wet from sweat.

If you want to try this method on your own, you can purchase calipers such as Accu-Measure. These calipers come with a decent booklet that explains how to test yourself and interpret the results. For better accuracy, you may want to have a friend perform the test on you.

Stepping on a body-fat scale or using a handheld tester

A common method of body-fat testing is called *bioelectrical impedance analysis* (BIA). These days, you do this test by stepping onto a scale or holding a gadget that looks like the steering wheel from a toddler's toy car. The device picks up a signal from your body and sends it into the device. The slower the signal, the more fat you have. This is because fat impedes or blocks the signal. The signal travels quickly through muscle because muscle is 70 percent water and water conducts electricity. Fat, on the other hand, is just 5 to 13 percent water.

Although simple, using a body-fat scale or handheld tester has its drawbacks, including, in some cases, a huge margin of error. Perhaps you're dehydrated, or perhaps the scale is having a bad day. Our advice is to step on the scale two or three times in a row to see how consistent the results are, and then draw your own conclusions.

Getting dunked: Underwater weighing

Underwater weighing is the most cumbersome method of body-fat testing, but it's also the most accurate method that's anywhere near affordable. You sit on a scale in a tank of warm water about the size of a Jacuzzi. (When Suzanne did this, she felt like a giant piece of tortellini floating in a big pot.) Then comes the unnerving part: You blow all the air out of your lungs and bend forward until you're completely submerged. If there's air trapped in your lungs, you score fatter than you really are. Knowing this fact makes you try really, really hard to blow out your air, which makes you feel like you're about to explode. You stay submerged for about five seconds while your underwater weight registers on a digital scale. The result is then plugged into a mathematical equation to determine your body fat.

This method of testing is based on the premise that muscle sinks and fat floats. The more fat you have, the more your body wants to float when dunked under water. The denser you are, the more you sink, and the more water your body displaces.

The margin of error for this test is 2 to 2.5 percent for young to middle-aged adults. The results are less accurate for children, older adults, and extremely lean people. This is because lean body tissue is made up of other things besides muscle. Bone, for example, isn't fully formed in children, and it may be somewhat porous in older adults and somewhat denser in super-fit people. You can get this test done at sophisticated sports-medicine clinics or labs for upwards of $300.

Sitting in a giant egg: The BOD POD

Underwater weighing has long been the standard for body-fat testing, but a sophisticated contraption called the *BOD POD* seems to rival it in accuracy, without forcing anyone to get wet. The BOD POD is a 5-foot-tall fiberglass chamber that looks like a giant egg with a tinted window. You sit in the chamber for two or three 50-second tests while computerized pressure sensors determine how much air your body displaces — in other words, how much space you take up. (Underwater weighing determines the same information, just in a way that's less convenient.)

Because the machine costs about as much as a luxury car, it's mostly used in research settings. However, BOD PODs occasionally visit health clubs, where members can pay about $50 for a test.

Getting scoped out by X-ray vision: DEXA

Another method to gauge body fat is dual-energy X-ray absorptiometry (DEXA or DXA). You lie on a bed while low doses of two different X-ray energies scan your body from head to toe. Not only does this method measure how much fat you have, but it also determines where the fat is located on your body, a more relevant health indicator. Originally developed to scan bone density, DEXA is available at hospitals and in doctors' offices; it usually requires a physician's referral. The test costs from $150 to $200.

Taking your measurements

A less-precise but helpful way to keep track of your body fat is to measure several parts of your body. You don't get a percentage, but you can use the numbers to keep track of inches lost (or gained, if you're trying to pack on muscle), which can be motivating in and of itself. If you're losing inches, chances are you're dropping body fat.

Some common places to measure include

- Across the middle of your chest
- The center of your upper arm
- The smallest part of your waist
- The widest part of your hips
- The widest part of your thigh
- The widest part of your ankle

In the case of your waist measurement, you can actually track something substantial about your health risks.

Calculating your body mass index

One method of estimating how "fat" you are is *body mass index* (BMI), a number derived from your height and weight. To determine your BMI, type "BMI calculator" into an Internet search engine and then enter your height and weight.

So what does your BMI mean? The National Institutes of Health has issued the BMI guidelines in Table 2-1.

Table 2-1	Understanding Your Body Mass Index
BMI	*Weight Status*
Less than 19	Underweight
19 to 24.9	Healthy
25 to 29.9	Overweight
30 or greater	Obese

People with a BMI of 25 or above are considered at higher risk for heart disease, stroke, hypertension, diabetes, gallbladder disease, cancer, and death. But these guidelines are controversial. Even members of the government panel that issued the guidelines believe that setting the low point for overweight at a BMI of 25 is somewhat arbitrary. Keep in mind that BMI, like body-fat percentage, is only one factor in assessing your health. Also know that BMI measurements for extremely muscular athletes and pregnant women are not very accurate.

If BMI has so many limitations, why are we including it in this book? Because it's the simplest way — no fees, no equipment, and no schlepping to the health club — of estimating whether you may be in the overweight ballpark. The BMI is a more accurate measure than scale weight because it tells you something about your weight in relation to your height.

Measuring Your Strength

Fear not: You won't be required to do one-arm push-ups or lift a barbell that weighs more than your dad. Strength tests, like the other tests that we describe in this chapter, are simply designed to give you a starting point. If you get started on a good weight-lifting program and stick to it, you're likely to see dramatic changes when you take another fitness test in two or three months.

Most health clubs don't take true strength measurements; in other words, they don't measure the absolute maximum amount of weight you're capable of lifting. Going for your "max" can be dangerous and can cause more than a little muscle soreness. Instead, gyms test your muscular endurance: how many times you can move a much lighter weight. You can do many of these tests at home. Having a friend count for you and make sure you're doing the exercise correctly is a help. Here are some common muscular-endurance measures.

Measuring your upper-body strength

Count how many push-ups you can do without stopping or losing good form. For this test, men do military push-ups, with their legs out straight and toes on the floor. Women do modified push-ups, with their knees bent and feet off the floor. Lower your entire body at once until your upper arms are parallel to the floor. Keep your abdominals pulled in to prevent your back from sagging.

Use Table 2-2 or Table 2-3 to find out how you stack up against other people of your age and gender.

Table 2-2	Push-Ups — Men			
Age:	**20–29**	**30–39**	**40–49**	**50–59**	**60+**
Excellent	55+	45+	40+	35+	30+
Good	45–54	35–44	30–39	25–34	20–29
Average	35–44	25–34	20–29	15–24	10–19
Fair	20–34	15–24	12–19	8–14	5–9
Low	0–19	0–14	0–11	0–7	0–4

Table 2-3	Push-Ups — Women			
Age:	**20–29**	**30–39**	**40–49**	**50–59**	**60+**
Excellent	49+	40+	35+	30+	20+
Good	34–48	25–39	20–34	15–29	5–19
Average	17–33	12–24	8–19	6–14	3–4
Fair	6–16	4–11	3–7	2–5	1–2
Low	0–5	0–3	0–2	0–1	0

Some health clubs also measure upper-body strength on a free-weight bench press or a chest-press machine. (In Chapter 12, we explain the difference between free weights and machines.) The amount of weight doesn't matter, as long as you use the same weight every time you get tested. You simply do as many repetitions as you can.

Testing your core strength

The strength of the core muscles, including your abdominals and lower back, is usually measured by a crunch test.

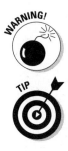

Crunches aren't the best exercise to strengthen and tone the core muscles, but the crunch test has been around a long time and it has well-documented results. Don't do this test if you have a history of lower-back problems.

To do the crunch test, place two pieces of masking tape about halfway down the length of a mat, one directly behind the other, about 2½ inches apart. Lie on your back on the mat with your arms at your sides and your fingertips touching the rear edge of the back piece of tape. Bend your knees and place your feet flat on the floor. Curl your head, neck, and shoulder blades upward, sliding your palms along the floor until your fingertips touch the front edge of the front piece of tape. Return to the starting position and keep going until you're too tired to continue or you can't reach the tape. Don't cheat by sliding your arms without moving your body or by moving only one side of your body. See Figure 2-2 for an example of the crunch test.

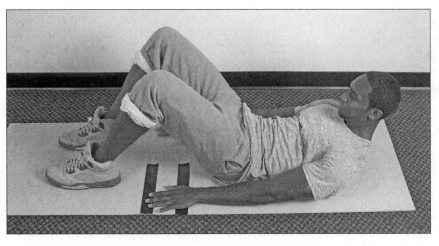

Figure 2-2:
The crunch
test.

Use Tables 2-4 and 2-5 to gauge the results of your crunch test.

Table 2-4	Crunch Test Results for Men		
Age	*Under 35*	*36–45*	*Over 45*
Excellent	60	50	40
Good	45	40	25
Marginal	30	25	15
Needs work	15	10	5

Table 2-5	Crunch Test Results for Women		
Age	*Under 35*	*36–45*	*Over 45*
Excellent	50	40	30
Good	40	25	15
Marginal	25	15	10
Needs work	10	6	4

One test we like is useful for measuring integrated core strength — that is, how strong your core muscles are when they work together to hold your body into position. Get a stopwatch and move into a plank position, as we describe in Chapter 13. Hold the plank as long as you can. Record the time. Note how much longer you can hold the position the next time you test yourself.

Measuring your lower-body strength

The strength of your lower-body muscles is often measured on a leg-extension machine, which targets your front-thigh muscles. (This machine is sort of like a big chair with a high back.) Some clubs test lower-body strength on other machines; others don't test your lower-body strength at all.

You can test the strength of your thigh and butt muscles at home by doing an exercise called a squat, described in Chapter 13. We suggest that if you're a woman, you do the squat as you hold a 5-pound dumbbell in each hand with your arms hanging down at your sides, and if you're a man, use 15-pound dumbbells. If you're a novice, skip the weight and place your hands on your hips.

This test has several standard norms, so just use your results as a basis of comparison for future evaluations. And keep in mind that other tests can give you other important pieces of information. For example, the sit-to-stand test in Chapter 15 is a good evaluation of real-world, "functional" strength and is especially useful in helping to evaluate the leg and core strength of older folks.

Stretchy Stuff: Checking Your Flexibility

How come gymnasts can wrap their legs around their shoulders while you have trouble touching your toes? Because gymnasts are more flexible than you are. *Flexibility* refers to how far you can move around a joint's axis (your range of motion) and how easily you can move it. Because your muscles attach to your bone and bones move around a joint's axis (therefore, muscles move the bones around a joint), flexibility also refers to the mobility of your muscles.

Flexibility tests sometimes feel like a cross between circus tryouts and an IQ test. The tester asks you to twist yourself into some strange positions, and you have to figure out what he's talking about. Then you have to see whether your body agrees to follow along.

One common test is the sit-and-reach, which measures the flexibility of your lower-back and rear-thigh (hamstring) muscles. You sit with your legs out straight and place your feet flat on the side of a special metal box. Keeping your legs straight, you lean forward and reach toward the box as far as you can. Along the top of the box, a scale in inches measures how far you reach forward. (We find it amusing that the special box costs $200. You can do this same test with the carton that the box comes in.)

Some clubs don't get that sophisticated with flexibility measurements; don't hold it against them. Estimating your flexibility instead of measuring it to the exact degree is okay. At least you find out which joints are tight, so you emphasize them when you stretch. For details about how to stretch properly, see Chapter 14.

Table 2-6 describes flexibility tests you can do at home. You may also encounter these tests during a health-club evaluation.

Table 2-6		Testing Your Flexibility		
The Test	*What to Do*	*You Have Good Flexibility If . . .*	*Your Flexibility Needs Work If . . .*	*Your Flexibility Needs a Lot of Work If . . .*
Rear thigh and lower back	Take off your shoes and stand with your feet together and your knees straight but not locked. Bend forward and reach for the floor.	You can touch the floor with little effort and no discomfort in your rear thighs or lower back.	You can just touch your toes with little or no discomfort.	You can't touch your toes, or you feel considerable pain when you try. You may be susceptible to lower-back problems.
Shoulder	Reach your right hand behind your back and your left hand across your back toward your right shoulder blade. Try to clasp your hands together behind your back.	You can clasp your hands together.	Your fingertips almost touch.	You aren't within an inch of touching your fingertips together. This means you're susceptible to shoulder and neck pain.
Calf and ankle	Sit on the floor with your legs straight out in front of you. Flex your foot so your toes move toward you.	Your toes move enough toward you so that they are beyond perpendicular to the floor.	Your toes bend so they are just in line with your ankles (exactly perpendicular to the floor).	You can barely bend your toes toward you. You may be susceptible to ankle injuries.

The Test	What to Do	You Have Good Flexibility If . . .	Your Flexibility Needs Work If . . .	Your Flexibility Needs a Lot of Work If . . .
Shin	Sitting in the same position as the calf-and-ankle test, point your toes and stretch them toward the floor.	Your toes touch or nearly touch the floor.	Your toes come to within an inch or so of the floor.	Your toes barely move toward the floor. You may be susceptible to shin splints (see definition, Chapter 5).
Top, front of hip; buttocks	Lie on your back and hug one knee to your chest; clasp your hands around your shin just below your knee. Keep the other leg straight.	Your straight leg rests on the floor directly in line with your hip, and you can easily hug your bent knee to your chest.	Your leg, when straight, rests along the floor but to the outside of your hip, and you can almost hug your knee to your chest.	Your straight leg doesn't touch the floor, and you can't bring your knee to within a few inches of your chest. You may be susceptible to upper-back and shoulder pain.
Upper back	Lie on your back with your legs out straight, and lift your arms straight up in the air. Now drop your arms back toward the floor, alongside your ears.	Your arms easily fall to the floor without your lower back arching up.	Your hands almost touch and your lower back remains in contact with the floor.	Your arms don't come within an inch of touching the floor, and your back arches up. You may be susceptible to upper-back and shoulder pain.

(continued)

Table 2-6 (continued)

The Test	What to Do	You Have Good Flexibility If . . .	Your Flexibility Needs Work If . . .	Your Flexibility Needs a Lot of Work If . . .
Front thigh	Lie on your stomach with one leg straight, and bend the other knee so that your heel moves toward your buttocks.	Your heel easily touches your buttocks.	Your heel comes close to but doesn't quite touch your buttocks.	Your heel doesn't come within a few inches of your buttocks. You may be susceptible to knee pain.

Checks and Balances: Standing on One Foot

More and more, trainers and even some physicians will have a look at your balance skills, especially if you're part of the over-50 crowd. Because good balance is one of the keys to preventing athletic injuries and falls in everyday life, assessing your balance is a good idea.

We recommend you add balance into your overall assessment. Balance is a fairly simple thing to evaluate on your own, but you also can have a pro help you. We include a thorough examination of balance skills, complete with some simple tests, in Chapter 15.

Recording Your Fitness Test Results

Need a place to store your score? Table 2-7 gives you spaces to jot down the results of the tests described in this chapter. Some of the results, like those for flexibility and balance, don't involve numbers, so you can use the boxes to make notes. You needn't note the results of every test you do, but if you want to and find you need more space, record your results in a notebook or formal workout log. For guidance on setting goals, see Chapter 1.

Table 2-7	**Your Fitness Test Results**			
Test	*Your Score (Test #1)*	*Your Score (Test #2)*	*Your Score (Test #3)*	*Goal*
Resting heart rate				
Resting blood pressure				
Aerobic endurance (Submax test)				
Body-fat percentage				
Measurements				
BMI				
Upper-body strength (Push-ups or presses)				
Core strength (Crunches or plank)				
Lower-body strength (Leg extensions or squats)				
Flexibility				
Balance				

Making Sense of Your Test Results

At the end of your fitness evaluation, your tester (who may, in fact, be you) should not simply say, "Well, your resting heart rate is 72, you did 23 sit-ups, and your body fat is 28 percent." You need to put these numbers in context. For example, how do your results stack up against other people who are your age and your gender, and even more important, which areas of your fitness need the most improvement?

Whether or not you have a professional helping you, use the results to build your exercise routine. Although your program should cover every aspect of fitness, it makes sense to give extra time to your weakest areas; after your evaluation, you'll no longer have to guess as to what those are. If you're working solo, flip to Chapters 7, 13, and 14 for guidance on structuring a program to meet your abilities and goals.

Document your test results in this book, on a piece of paper, or in a workout log (sort of like a report card). Save the results every time you test yourself so you can see how much you've improved. (In general, you want to retest after six weeks or so and then every three to six months thereafter.) One day, these results may mean more to you than your high school diploma.

Chapter 3

Watching What You Eat: Nutrition Basics

A while back, we came across a fitness book that proclaimed that a great exercise program can make up for a bad diet. Sounds great, but it just isn't so. If you scarf an extra muffin at the office, sure, you can burn off the calories on the treadmill — if you happen to have an extra hour to do so. On a daily basis, exercise isn't a realistic way to make up for overeating. In fact, this "earn and burn" notion is one reason scientists think that exercise alone isn't an especially effective weight-loss method.

Besides, weight control is hardly the only reason to watch what you eat. Making wise food choices keeps gas in your tank for your workouts, gives you the energy and concentration to get through your day, and helps your body ward off cancer, heart disease, osteoporosis, and plenty of other health conditions.

In this chapter, we present basic guidelines for nutritious eating. Adopting these common-sense strategies can help you maintain your weight, fuel your exercise program, and enhance your health while keeping your taste buds interested. (For a more in-depth discussion of nutrition, visit www.dummies.com for a wealth of health and nutrition books.)

Keeping an Eye on How Much You Eat

One big reason the collective American waistline has continued to expand is that we simply eat too much. Not too much salad or salmon but too much high-calorie fare with little or no nutritional value, like french fries and mega-burgers. We eat out more than we used to, and restaurant serving sizes have become two to five times heftier than they were in the 1970s. As a result, our calorie intake is out of whack with the number of calories we burn.

The number of calories you need to eat each day depends largely on your size and activity level. A ballpark figure is 1,800 for women and 2,200 for men. If you want exact numbers, search the Internet for "calorie needs calculator." Plug in your vital statistics and you'll get back a ballpark estimate of the number of calories a day you need to eat to either lose or maintain your current weight.

But you certainly don't need to count calories in order to eat less. Here are some simple strategies for downsizing your meals.

✔ **Pay attention to portions.** Did you know that a standard portion of shredded cheese is a quarter cup, about the size of a golf ball? Yet most Mexican restaurants sprinkle softball-sized mounds of cheese on their burritos. To learn how to identify reasonable portions, we recommend *The Portion Teller* by Lisa Young, PhD, RD. Action for Media Education (AME, nutritionandmedia.org) also has excellent resources, both visual and explanatory, on how to avoid portion distortion.

If you eat out a lot, consider the appetizer menu for a main meal selection, or when your meal arrives, immediately cut it in half and place the rest in a to-go bag. Many restaurant portions are double, triple, or even greater the size of a single serving.

✔ **Read labels and restaurant menu calorie counts.** All packaged foods indicate calorie counts, and there are now laws requiring large chain restaurants to list calorie counts on the menus. Pay attention! You needn't count every calorie you eat, but when you see that a large Dunkin' Donuts Vanilla Bean Coolatta drink has 860 calories — about half the daily calorie allotment for a woman — that should be a signal to say, "Nope!" Besides calories, be on the lookout for trans fat, saturated fat, and sodium content as well.

✔ **Don't confuse fat-free with calorie-free.** Many fat-free foods are plenty high in calories because they make up for the lost fat by adding sugar. One Reduced-Fat Chips Ahoy! cookie has 50 calories, and a regular Chips Ahoy! has 53. Not exactly major savings. The same is true of sugar-free foods; they are not a free pass to weight loss and are often pumped full of fat or chemicals to make up for the lack of natural sweetener.

✔ **Buy smaller packages.** Larger packages make us think it's normal to serve and eat more. In one study, people who were given jumbo jars of sauce and meat packages prepared 23 percent more food than those given medium-sized packages — and ate it all. If you buy large packages to save money, repackage the items into containers as soon as you get home.

✔ **Use smaller bowls, plates, and serving spoons.** Like big packages, big dishes skew your idea of what's normal and prompt you to eat more, as much as 57 percent more when it comes to large ice cream bowls and scoops.

✔ **Eat slowly.** Utter at least one complete sentence between bites. Many people eat so fast that they don't taste anything and then rush back for seconds. Give your body a chance to feel full. Eat half of what's on your plate and then take a ten-minute break and assess whether you're still hungry.

✔ **Cut out sweetened beverages — both regular and diet.** Americans consume 150 to 300 more calories per day than they did in the 1970s, and 50 percent of that increase has come from sweetened beverages such as sodas, sweetened teas, fruit drinks, and energy drinks.

Research suggests that the brain simply doesn't register liquid calories with appetite controls; when you drink a soda, you don't compensate by eating less food. Artificially sweetened beverages aren't a good substitute. In fact, research has found a 41 percent increase in risk of being overweight for every can or bottle of diet soda consumed daily. Diet soda may stimulate appetite; another theory is that people give themselves license to eat more when they drink diet soda. Stick primarily with water, nonfat milk, and unsweetened tea and coffee.

✔ **Go easy on the booze.** Alcohol stimulates your appetite and weakens your reserve. This combination can lead to some serious overeating. Instead of drinking before a meal, drink while you eat.

✔ **Eat regular meals.** Skipping meals sets you up for losing control and overeating. You're less likely to pig out if you avoid becoming a ravenous monster in the first place. That said, if you opt to take a "grazing" approach of six small meals a day, make the operative word *small*.

Although grazing is often touted as a helpful weight-loss strategy, there's little evidence to support it. And some experts feel that it may actually contribute to weight gain by disrupting the brain's ability to recognize hunger and satiety cues. Eating handful after handful of organic granola and taking frequent sips of a fruit smoothie will hit your waistline just as surely as a large meal or a binge.

Tracking your eating habits

How many grams of fiber have you eaten today? Seven? Seventeen? Thirty? How many daily fruit servings have you averaged this week? How about sodas or other sweetened drinks?

Research shows that most people have no clue how their eating habits stack up, and this lack of awareness holds them back from losing weight and improving their health. Tracking your eating habits, if only for a short while, keeps you honest and more mindful about your food choices and is a proven weight-loss method endorsed by the American Heart Association. A study of your log may explain why, after three months of dieting and exercising, your jeans still are snug; you may discover that you skip lunch at work and then compensate with a 500-calorie cookie and 400-calorie blended mocha at your coffee break.

We're not suggesting that you write down every morsel you eat on a daily basis for the rest of your life. But we do recommend that you keep a food and beverage diary for a few days every now and then as a reality check.

You can track your eating habits in a spiral notebook, an online food diary, or a formal paper log. A great (and free) online diary we like is FitDay (fitday.com), but there are certainly dozens of others. Not surprisingly, we also recommend *The Ultimate Diet Log*, cowritten by Suzanne Schlosberg and registered dietitian Cynthia Sass.

You can find information about the calories, fiber, and nutrients in each food and beverage you consume by reading labels and using online sources such as CalorieKing (www.calorieking.com) and Calorie Count (caloriecount.about.com). Do a search for "calorie counter" and see what pops up. Many online logs calculate and analyze this information for you in a neat series of graphs and charts.

We also recommend having a registered dietitian analyze your food log and offer tips on how to cut back on sugar or sneak more fiber into your diet.

Deciding What's for Dinner: Food, Real Food

Okay, this one sounds funny: Eat food. What else would you eat — cardboard? What we mean is stick to foods that look, feel, and sound like honest-to-goodness food, rather than, as food writer Michael Pollan puts it in his excellent book *Food Rules,* "edible food-like substances." Apples, squash, almonds, even home-baked oatmeal-raisin cookies — these are foods that your great-grandmother Hilda would have recognized. What would Hilda have made of the South Beach Diet Chocolate Peanut Butter Meal Replacement Bar, with its 57 ingredients, including soy protein isolate, maltitol syrup, oligofructose, and glycerin?

Sure, some processed foods contain plenty of vitamins, minerals, healthy fats, protein, and fiber. But many are loaded with unhealthy fats, sodium, sugar, artificial sweeteners, preservatives, and flavors whose health risks are unknown. And even those items that look nutritious on the label may not be all they're advertised to be. An energy bar with added vitamins and minerals doesn't have the phytochemicals and other disease-fighting substances that occur naturally in food.

We're not suggesting that you avoid processed foods altogether. Certainly, many breakfast cereals (the low-sugar varieties) and whole-grain breads are good choices. For most people, it's not exactly practical to go harvest their own wheat. But the shorter the ingredients list and the closer a food is to its original source, the healthier it's likely to be. You're a lot better off adding your own fruit, nuts, and a pinch of brown sugar to your steel-cut oatmeal than you are buying a presweetened oatmeal with miniscule bits of fruit.

Figuring Out Fat, Carbs, and Protein

The calories you eat and drink come from three nutrients: fat, carbohydrate, and protein. Depending on the nutrition fad du jour, any one of these nutrients may be on the "bad" list, but the truth is, to stay healthy and energized, you need a mix of all three. The following look at each of these important nutrients helps you make wise food choices.

Getting the real deal on fat

The "fat is bad" mantra has given people the wrong impression. In fact, some medical sources now refer to the lowfat fad as "the great American experiment in obesity." Some fat is actually good for you, whereas other types of fat clog arteries. The total amount of fat you eat doesn't seem to especially matter if you're eating healthy fats and not overeating. Certain Greek populations of the 1960s got as much as 40 percent of their calories from fat, primarily from olive oil, and their heart disease rates were 90 percent lower than those of Americans at the time. In the following sections, we take a look at the different types of fat.

The bad stuff: Saturated fat and trans fat

Saturated fat is found in animal products, such as beef, pork, chicken, milk, ice cream, and cheese. Trans fats — created through *hydrogenation,* a process that turns liquid oils into solids — is found in many chips, crackers, cookies, granola bars, and pastries. Both types of fats raise your risk of heart disease by clogging your arteries and boosting your body's natural production of cholesterol.

The most recent guidelines issued by the U.S. government call for even lower intakes of these fats than before: a maximum of 7 percent of calories from saturated fat (that's about 14 grams of saturated fat per day — 2 grams fewer than a Cheese Danish at Starbucks!) and 0.5 percent of calories from trans fats (essentially a call to avoid these fats altogether). So switch from whole milk to skim, replace butter with olive oil, and cut out fried foods. Trans fats are now banned from foods in many cities, and many major manufacturers have gotten the message and removed trans fats from their products. For example, most microwave popcorn used to be overflowing with the stuff, but now most brands contain little to none.

The good stuff: Unsaturated fats

Unsaturated fat is found in plant foods — avocados, olives and olive oil, canola and flaxseed oil, salmon and other fatty fish, nuts and natural nut butters. These fats help protect against heart disease by reducing levels of LDL cholesterol (the artery-clogging kind) without affecting HDL cholesterol (the kind that acts as a vacuum cleaner within your bloodstream). You don't want to go overboard with these fats because — like unhealthy fats — they have 9 calories per gram, but if you've been skimping, top your salad with sliced almonds or avocado, dip your apple in a little peanut butter, or top your breakfast cereal with crumbled pecans.

Particularly helpful are omega-3 fatty acids, polyunsaturated fats found primarily in fatty fish such as salmon, tuna, and sardines, and, to a lesser extent, in walnuts, flaxseeds, and a few other foods. Omega-3s appear to help lower the risk for heart disease, prostate cancer, stroke, depression, and macular degeneration, among other conditions.

Choosing your carbs carefully

No, carbs are not the root of all evil! In reality, carbohydrates are your body's main source of fuel, and exercisers need plenty of them. Nutritious foods such as fruits, veggies, whole grains, and beans are all high in carbs. Of course, so are white rice, Twinkies, and soda, so you need to be careful. Sports nutritionists recommend that between 50 percent and 70 percent of calories should come from nutritious carbohydrates, also known as complex carbs.

Picking whole grains over refined grains

Whole grains include whole wheat, brown rice, oatmeal, wild rice, bulgur, and quinoa. You can easily find whole-grain pastas, breads, and cereals in most supermarkets. Be sure to buy bread that is actually labeled *whole grain* or *whole wheat*. Don't be tricked by products labeled *multi-grain, stone-ground, 100% wheat, cracked wheat, 10-grain,* or *bran,* as they are usually not whole-grain products.

Whole grains are high in fiber, so they're digested and absorbed more slowly than refined grains, keeping you fuller longer than the carbs in cookies, crackers, and sodas. They also may keep blood-sugar levels down, triggering slower, smaller releases of insulin, and allowing the body to burn carbohydrate calories more efficiently over several hours rather than quickly storing them as body fat. Refined grains seem to do just the opposite, causing carbohydrate calories to be shuttled to the fat cells for storage.

Getting enough fiber

Most Americans eat just 12 to 17 grams of fiber per day — half of the 25 to 35 recommended. Fiber, found only in plant foods, is valuable for weight control because it's not digested. It comes in two varieties: soluble and insoluble. Soluble fiber, like the kind found in oats, nuts, and seeds, helps regulate blood sugar and cholesterol; insoluble fiber, found in fruits and veggies, moves bulk through the intestines, keeps you regular, and may reduce the risk of colon cancer.

Fiber-rich foods fill you up, but fiber itself doesn't provide calories because it doesn't get into your bloodstream. High-fiber foods tend to be low in calories, so you can pile your plate full of beans and veggies without packing on pounds.

Limiting added sugar

About 20 percent of the total calories in a typical American diet come from added sugars, including sweetened drinks, candy, cookies, yogurt, and pastries. Sugary foods tend to be really high in calories and quite low in nutritional value. We don't think it's realistic or necessary to cut out all sweet treats — it's important to satisfy cravings so that you don't go on binges. On the other hand, there's a massive amount of sugar in the food supply, and we suggest scrutinizing food labels to choose foods with minimal amounts of added sugar. Much of the sugar is hidden in foods you wouldn't suspect to have large doses of added sugar, including many pasta sauces, ketchup, crackers, and yogurts.

Read food labels carefully and find out where you're getting most of your refined sugar. Some name-brand breakfast cereals are more than 42 percent sugar. Flavored yogurts are loaded with sugar, too. Be aware that sugar goes by other aliases, including corn syrup, honey, maple syrup, maltodextrin, sucrose, and other words that end in *-ose*. Sugar is sugar.

When you do choose sweet treats, we recommend going for smaller doses of real sugar rather than artificial sweeteners. Though some sweeteners — Splenda, for example — seem to be perfectly safe, evidence suggests that artificial sweeteners don't actually help with weight loss. As we explain earlier in "Keeping an Eye on How Much You Eat," artificial sweeteners may actually be associated with weight gain. A good source to find out the latest on the safety of artificial sweeteners is the Web site of the nonprofit Center for Science in the Public Interest (`cspinet.org`).

Avoiding high-protein propaganda

Protein is crucial because it's made up of amino acids, which your body uses to build and repair your muscles, red blood cells, enzymes, and other tissues. Are you a protein overeater or undereater? Or are you right on target? The general rule of thumb for inactive people is to eat 0.4 grams per 1 pound of body weight. For example, a 180-pound couch potato multiplies 180 by 0.4. He needs about 72 grams of protein a day; a 130-pound person needs about 52 — the amount in one can of tuna (40 grams) plus two eggs (12 grams).

Exercisers need a bit more protein, although not nearly as much as many protein advertisements would lead you to believe. A recreational exerciser should aim for 0.5 to 0.75 grams of protein per pound of body weight. A competitive athlete may need as much as 0.9.

In general, about 15 to 20 percent of your total calories should come from protein, ideally more from combining a variety of plant foods (such as beans and nuts) to get complete proteins than from animal foods. Animal-based protein, especially fatty meats and whole dairy products, are loaded with artery-clogging fats, whereas plant-based proteins are rich in fiber. Fat-free and low-fat dairy products are a good choice. Eating a bit of protein at each meal may prevent you from overeating because, studies show, it can make you feel fuller for longer.

If you find that you're overshooting the mark on protein, cut back by using high-protein foods as a side dish rather than as your main course. Sprinkle ground turkey on your spaghetti or top your salad with strips of grilled chicken rather than planning your entire meal around a slab of steak. Switch to dairy foods like fat-free cottage cheese and fat-free plain yogurt. If you're a vegetarian, even a vegan, you have plenty of protein-rich choices.

Getting the Scoop on Supplements

Supplements are promoted everywhere these days — on infomercials, in health-food stores, and at health clubs. Whether they claim to build muscle, burn fat, or boost your metabolism, the vast majority of supplements aren't worth the cost of the plastic bottles they come in.

Are any supplements worth taking? Actually, yes. The American Medical Association, among other respected groups, recommends taking a daily multivitamin as an inexpensive health-insurance policy, and more and more, medical experts are recommending vitamin D supplements for individuals who don't get more than 15 minutes of sun exposure on most days of the year. Certainly a prenatal vitamin with folic acid is a good idea if you're a woman of childbearing age; studies show that women who take folic-acid supplements for a year or more before pregnancy have a 50 to 70 percent reduced risk of premature delivery.

However, no pill will compensate for a diet of Doritos and Pepsi. When you eat healthy foods, you get not only vitamins and minerals but also disease-fighting phytochemicals, plus protein, carbohydrates, fiber, and other nutrients.

You should always aim to get the vast majority of your vitamins and minerals from food and take the word *supplement* literally. Choose doses that don't go much beyond 100 percent of the U.S. RDA (recommended dietary allowance), and don't bother with super-potency megavitamins, which often contain more than ten times the U.S. RDA (and cost you bundles). Your body can absorb only so much of each nutrient; if you go overboard, most of the excess is just excreted when you go to the bathroom. As one doctor told us, "You'll have very expensive urine." Also, some vitamins are stored in your body, so megadoses can lead to dangerous outcomes.

Also, forget those designer vitamins hawked infomercial-style by has-been celebrities and former athletes. Generic drugstore brands are identical. Manufacturers have yet to come up with the magical combination of dosages to banish wrinkles or to make you live to 196.

Fueling Up

What you eat and drink before, during, and after your workouts can mean the difference between feeling like a million bucks and feeling like two bucks. Here are tips on using nutrition to perform your best.

Timing your meals

Eating regularly throughout the day is important, even on days when you don't exercise. Waiting for too long between meals can cause wide swings in your blood sugar levels, which in turn can zap your energy, disturb your concentration, and turn you into a crankpot. Plus, if you let yourself become ravenous, you're likely to overeat at your next meal, a pattern that can lead to weight gain.

So start your engines in the morning with a good breakfast — plenty of complex carbohydrates with an accent of protein and a dash of healthy fat. A good example: hot oatmeal with skim milk, half a banana, walnuts, and a glass of orange juice. Not an oatmeal eater? How about some scrambled eggs and toast? Then pay attention to your hunger cues, and when you feel your tummy get a little rumbly, it's time to eat.

Eating before you work out

Your mom may have told you not to go swimming until at least an hour after you eat, but we tell you the opposite: If your stomach can handle it, eat within an hour of your workout. (For some activities, such as running, you may need two or three hours between eating and working out.) We recommend a couple hundred calories of (primarily) complex carbohydrates, such as a bagel with some lowfat cream cheese or peanut butter, a couple pieces of fruit, and a slice of lowfat Swiss cheese. A little protein may help if you're going for a long workout lasting a few hours or more. You may be one of those people who simply can't handle eating before a workout; if that's the case, you'll find out quickly enough.

Snacking during your workout

During most workouts, you don't need to eat anything. But if you're going for a three-hour bike ride or a long afternoon hike, bring along snacks. Energy bars like PowerBars and Clif Bars are convenient choices because they easily slip into your pocket or fanny pack, but it's a lot cheaper to bring along real food, such as dried fruit and nuts or a peanut butter sandwich on whole grain, some turkey slices, or some good old Cheerios. Even though certain sports are associated with energy bars and so-called engineered foods, you don't have to give in to the marketing hype.

For workouts that last longer than about 75 minutes, sports drinks such as Gatorade and Cytomax are a good idea. They provide fluid as well as sodium and easily digestible energy. Water is sufficient for shorter workouts. Many people find their stomachs can't tolerate energy drinks no matter how far or long their workouts, so be sure to do a test run if you plan on sipping one during a race or extra long workout.

Refueling after your workout

Some people are under the impression that if they eat right after exercise, they somehow negate the benefits of their hard work. Just the opposite is true. If you eat within an hour of your workout, your body is more receptive to replenishing your energy stores. A postworkout snack that combines lots of carbs and some protein is ideal.

Drinking Plenty of Fluids

Staying hydrated isn't just important for when you work out. More than 75 percent of your body is made up of water — even bone is more than 20 percent water. Drinking enough fluids is important for blood flow and smooth digestion.

You've probably heard that you need to drink 8 glasses of water a day — 9 to 13 if you exercise. However, science is increasingly suggesting that this may be an overstatement. You get a fair amount of water from food, especially if you eat plenty of juicy fruits and veggies. And most doctors now agree that you should drink when you're thirsty. As with hunger, you should train your body to understand its internal thirst cues. You do need to drink more when you exercise on hot days than when you're sitting behind a desk enjoying your office's air conditioning.

When you exercise, it makes sense to carry water with you or be sure you have access to water at frequent intervals along your route. Plain old water is almost always your best choice. We recommend filtered tap water, which is up to 1,000 times less expensive than bottled water and does not add any plastic to your local landfill. Plus, drinking bottled water has no proven benefits.

You know that you're not drinking enough if your urine is dark and scanty rather than clear and plentiful. Keep in mind that vitamin supplements can make your urine dark or fluorescent yellow; in this case, volume is a better indicator.

Chapter 4

Educating Yourself

Getting fitness information online, through television, or in print can be a great way to stay abreast of the latest exercise techniques, gadgets, and controversies. But trying to keep up with fitness developments also can make your head spin faster than your legs can go on a spin bike. For one thing, more sources are available than ever before, including Web sites, blogs, podcasts, and online newsletters.

What's more, the sources often contradict each other. On one site, we read that "weight training will rev up your metabolism," burning 50 calories per pound of muscle; according to another site, "the effect of weight training on metabolism is minor," about 10 calories per pound of muscle. Both articles cited scientific research. Whom to believe? (For our take, see Chapter 10.)

In this era of intense media competition, sophisticated marketing techniques, significant competition for research grant money, and increasingly blurry lines between journalism and advertising, consumers need to view fitness information with a critical eye. Fortunately, the Internet has made it easy for media and science watchdogs to get the word out about misleading, biased, or fraudulent fitness information. Still, separating legit Web sites from Web sites set up purely for marketing purposes can be hard.

This chapter helps you evaluate media coverage as well as the scientific studies on which media stories, blogs, and other sources of information often are based. We help you discern reliable sources from quackery and puffery so that you're not changing your workout regimen or eating habits or buying new products every time you encounter a "startling new report."

Judging Fitness Media Reports

Because of the way news is generated and reported, media reports often are incomplete, misleading, or utterly false. Distortion may happen for numerous reasons — perhaps an expert passes along erroneous information, one small study is taken out of context, a media outlet is hungry for a big story, or a reporter had only an hour to decipher a 20-page study full of phrases like "deuterium oxide concentration was measured by using a fixed-filter single-beam infrared spectrophotometer." Some "articles" aren't journalistic articles at all; they're copied from press releases issued by manufacturers or universities promoting "breakthrough" studies from their scientists.

The following tips can help you find credible info and decide whether a media report on the latest exercise regimen should make you think, "Wow! I should try that" or "Hmm . . . sounds fishy."

Starting with reliable publications

One strategy for ferreting out the truth is visiting a Web site or blog devoted to critiquing health and fitness news reports. For example, `healthnews review.org` posts extensive reviews of online, print, and broadcast media reports. The site functions a bit like movie reviews, rating news stories on a scale of one to five stars. But instead of "I laughed! I cried! Five stars!" you may read, "Four stars! Accurate and informative" or "Cute wordsmithing but not enough data or context." The site often posts reviews of competing articles on the same topic so you can see how the *Wall Street Journal*'s coverage of a study compares with MSNBC.com's coverage of the same research.

Nonprofit organizations that do not accept advertising, such as Consumer Reports (`www.consumerreports.org`) and the nutrition-focused Center for Science in the Public Interest (`cspinet.org`), tend to report on products and research in a trustworthy manner. AOL Health generally does a good job reporting on fitness and health. Also, `www.health.harvard.edu`, `www.mayoclinic.org`, and `my.clevelandclinic.org/default.aspx` are written by the health and medical professionals who work at these highly respected organizations. We also like `www.medpagetoday.com`, which is aimed primarily at physicians. All these outlets offer free e-mail newsletters.

A few other sites, like `www.sciencedaily.com`, `eurekalert.org`, and `livescience.com`, post press releases about studies that have been vetted by a team of knowledgeable professionals. You can also check out the sites of fitness organizations:

✔ **ACE:** The official site of the American Council on Exercise (www.
acefitness.org) posts many of its own studies, a roundup of peer-
reviewed studies, and other fine content for free; this site offers a
phenomenal exercise video library that is expanded on a regular basis.

✔ **ACSM:** The official site of the American College of Sports Medicine
(www.acsm.org) posts, among other valuable resources, its positions
on virtually every aspect of fitness. This is where you'll find its official
recommendations on how much strength training you should do or
which type of workouts pregnant women should avoid, along with the
detailed explanations of the science behind the recommendations.

✔ **NASM and NSCA:** The National Academy of Sports Medicine (www.
nasm.org) and the National Strength and Conditioning Association
(www.nsca-lift.org) are among other respected fitness organizations that have excellent Web sites.

For nutrition information, we recommend the American Dietetic Association
(www.eatright.org). Besides tons of resources, they also offer a registered-
dietitian finder, a search that can be refined to your area of interest (for
instance, weight loss or sports performance). Established health organizations, such as the American Cancer Society (www.cancer.org), American
Heart Association (www.americanheart.org), and the American Diabetes
Association (www.diabetes.org), also have a tremendous amount of
reputable, scientifically vetted resources available, as well as phone hotlines
or e-mail addresses for asking a professional a question. The sites of the
National Institutes of Health (nih.gov), the Centers for Disease Control and
Prevention (cdc.gov), and the U.S. Department of Agriculture (usda.gov)
also have a wealth of diet and fitness information — your tax dollars at work!

Watching out for sensational headlines

For starters, dismiss headlines that seem way too good to be true, such as
"Drop 9 lbs. in 7 Days with New Diet," which is the fitness equivalent of "Elvis
lives." Of course, sometimes, reputable media outlets run misleading headlines
to draw in readers.

Liz once wrote an article on which leg exercises were most effective when
tested in the lab and was slightly miffed to see it posted under the headline,
"The miniskirt is back — are your legs ready?" The editor explained to her
that the headline grabbed people's attention and lured more readers to the
site than something like, "EMG analysis finds single leg squatting movements
superior for gluteus maximum development." She was right: No matter what
made them click through to the article, readers were treated to reliable,
accurate information.

Considering credentials and biases

Media reports usually quote "experts." Sometimes these people are steeped in credentials and expertise and have no financial stake in the outcome of a research study or the effectiveness of an exercise device. Other times, they're people with no credentials who are simply trying to profit.

For example, we read an article about heart-rate monitors that quoted the executive assistant to the president of a heart-rate monitor manufacturer. "Anyone who is concerned about their fitness or athletic competition . . . can benefit from using a heart-rate monitor," said the assistant. We agree, but the information doesn't have a heckuva lot of credibility coming from someone who not only stands to gain financially but also isn't a credentialed trainer, coach, or physiologist.

If an article is reporting on a scientific study, the report typically will quote the researcher who conducted the study. This expert is more likely to be legit if he is a professor at Harvard University Medical School or on staff at the National Institutes of Health rather than affiliated with some mysterious, private institute in Uzbekistan. Some private companies and foundations do valid research, but many organizations with impressive-sounding names, like Sportlife Exercise Health Sciences Institute, are just facades for companies promoting their products. If the study is published in a well-respected peer-reviewed journal, the source is more likely to be trustworthy.

Many professors receive funding from pharmaceutical or other product manufacturers, so a fancy title alone isn't going to guarantee the expert has no financial stake in the outcome. Researchers are required to indicate the source of their funding when studies are published, but often this fact doesn't make it into the media reports. (However, most peer-reviewed journals and reputable outlets point out affiliations upfront.) This doesn't necessarily mean the research is flawed, but you need to know quite a bit more about the study before you can judge the product. (See "Evaluating Scientific Research," later in this chapter, for tips on judging the studies themselves.)

When gauging the legitimacy of a report, check that the person who conducted the study is quoted and that the story includes a second opinion — a quote from an expert who was not involved in that research and has no vested interest in the product or advice being touted.

Making sure there's a source

Just as unreliable as a biased expert or flawed study is no source at all. Sometimes statements are repeated often enough that they become conventional wisdom, even though they have no basis in fact. Take the notion that you need eight glasses of water a day to stay healthy and hydrated. Ever wonder where that one comes from? One small study done decades ago on Army trainees in the desert. There is literally no other source to substantiate this claim, yet it's now accepted health folklore that has been appropriated by the bottled-water industry as gospel. In truth, some people need more, and some people need less.

Remembering that advertisers can influence content

The editorial and advertising departments of media companies are supposed to be like church and state: completely separate. In reality, health and fitness media outlets sometimes censor or alter their stories to favor the companies that buy advertisements from them.

Product reviews are a good example. We know many magazine and Web site writers and bloggers who have been asked by their editors to sugarcoat gear reviews because of advertising pressures. One writer told us, "With certain shoes, we had to search for aspects that weren't negative and emphasize those. Like if a shoe was incredibly stiff, we'd write some innocuous copy about how the shoe had a good lacing system."

Look out for *advertorials,* paid ads designed to look like articles, with layouts, fonts, and photos similar to the Web site or magazine's editorial style so that readers have to work hard to make the distinction. They're the written version of infomercials. A prominent women's magazine, for example, ran an advertorial on home exercise equipment, complete with a "reporter's" byline and a ratings system. Surprise — all the products received the largest number of stars possible! If you look hard enough, you can see the word *advertisement* at the top or bottom of the page, but sometimes the type is so small it's easy to miss.

In an even more egregious example of the crumbling wall between editorial and advertising, a newspaper that lacked the budget to hire a health reporter allowed a local hospital to provide content for its health and fitness page, featuring stories — always flattering! — about its physicians and programs. Though a disclaimer was displayed at the top of the page, the stories were written in newspaper style and looked like articles written by staff members.

What's more, a recent report found that small, struggling newspapers increasingly are asking for money before they agree to write reviews of products. Liz experienced this disturbing phenomenon with a health and fitness charity event she volunteers for. One local newspaper refused to include anything about the event or print any health advice by the not-for-profit unless it paid up.

Being wary of celebrity endorsements

Sometimes paid celebrities are quoted in major media outlets endorsing products or medications, and the sponsorship isn't mentioned, either because the reporters don't know or overlook the fact in order to snag a high-profile interview. In a *New York Times* article about high-tech mouth guards designed to increase athletic performance, an elite triathlete was quoted recommending one of these mouthpieces. What the article failed to mention — until an "editor's note" was added after publication — was that the manufacturer was paying the triathlete to endorse the product.

When a celebrity gives media interviews about a disease or plugs a medical treatment or fitness regimen, chances are that person is getting paid, especially if he or she says, "I feel it's a miracle." Be wary, too, of articles that offer fitness advice from celebrities; being a movie star doesn't make you an exercise expert. Actors may have the best of intentions and really believe what they're saying, but unless they've received a degree in nutrition between Oscars and Emmys, best to let the experts weigh in.

Putting limited stock in personal stories

Like stories about celebrities, anecdotes about regular people draw you into a story. Heck, we include lots of personal stories in this book. Just keep in mind that one person's experience is not "evidence" of anything, except perhaps that the person enjoys the spotlight. Personal stories are subjective and not reliable sources of information. One person may lose weight with exercise but no dietary changes, but that doesn't mean the majority of people will be able to pull this off.

Asking whether a study is newsworthy

The "news" business is, by nature, looking for something new to report. But just because a scientific study or fitness product is new doesn't mean it is useful or even different from what came before. Look for the media report to explain how this "revolutionary breakthrough" fits in with previous developments. Reports of a "seismic shift" typically raise a red flag.

If the hook for a new report is a new study, notice whether the study has been published in a *peer-reviewed* journal — in other words, whether it was scrutinized by independent experts before publication. Many studies are presented at scientific conferences before they're accepted for publication. Media outlets often attend these conferences looking for news and hype very preliminary reports as if they were published studies. Many of these studies never actually make it to publication.

Watching for outdated information

You may think of the Internet as the most up-to-date of all media, but in an attempt to get Web sites up and running quickly — and to appear loaded with "content" — many sites are cluttered with ancient material. When you do a search, articles surface from ages ago, not necessarily in order from most to least current. Check the original publication dates — if you can find them — and search again for updates. However, sites often don't include the date of publication.

Evaluating Scientific Research

Yes, you can read studies yourself! Most published research is available to the public via PubMed (www.pubmed.gov), an online library funded by the National Institutes of Health. Often, only the *abstract* (summary) is available free of charge, but sometimes the complete article, known as the *full text,* is free as well. Though you do have to wade through a massive amount of scientific jargon, you may learn something that would otherwise be obscured by media coverage.

Following are approaches to take when you encounter scientific research. We include this info not to make you disbelieve the results of every study you read, but rather to urge you to maintain a healthy skepticism.

Paying attention to the experiment

Here are some things to pay attention to when you read about how researchers conducted the experiment:

✔ **Controls:** Look for controls, or comparison groups. One magazine article we came across touted the benefits of a powdered food replacement. As evidence, the article cited a study of 28 overweight women who cut their daily calories by taking the powder twice a day instead of eating food; the subjects also exercised three times a week. After two months, the article stated, "an astounding 100 percent" of the women lost weight and felt better. Astounding? Any overweight person who cuts calories and exercises regularly is going to see results after two months. For the study to have any validity, the researchers should have compared the group taking the powder with a control group of similar subjects who ate the same number of calories and followed the same exercise program but didn't use the product.

In many instances the most accurate method is a *double-blind* study, where neither the subjects nor the researcher know who is taking the real treatment and who is taking a placebo. However, some experiments can't be designed in this way.

✔ **Choice of subjects:** Don't make too much of animal studies. The way an obese mouse responds to a diet drug may not be the same way you respond.

✔ **Number of subjects:** A study performed on a dozen people can't tell you much of anything, but this doesn't stop manufacturers from hyping research conducted with a sample size no larger than your morning workout group. The makers of an anticellulite pill launched a massive national campaign publicizing an Italian study that purported to show that their pill worked. But the study was conducted on only ten women.

✔ **Length of the study.** A four-week study doesn't tell you whether a weight-loss pill or exercise regimen is safe or effective. Maybe a pill stops working after two months or a year.

Noting that results can be manipulated

Sometimes researchers play games with the study design, statistics, charts, and graphs in order to wind up with a conclusion that they or their sponsors set out to "prove." Studies may be manipulated because the researchers have vested financial interest. For example, a tobacco study done by R. J. Reynolds or a rating of treadmill brands done by a treadmill manufacturer should fall under the category of things that make you go "Hmm."

Sometimes, scientists toy around with data for reasons that have nothing to do with money. Perhaps they've staked a career on a particular theory or they know that a more exciting result will boost their career. In an investigative report titled "Why Most Published Research Findings Are False," John P. A. Ioannidis, MD, a scientist affiliated with a Greek medical school as well as Tufts University School of Medicine in Boston, wrote, "Many otherwise seemingly independent, university-based studies may be conducted for no other reason than to give physicians and researchers qualifications for promotion or tenure. Such nonfinancial conflicts may also lead to distorted reported results and interpretations." The article is available online for free (search for it under the title and author's name), and we urge you to read it.

Every once in a while, studies are tainted not by bias but rather by outright fraud. A few years back, obesity expert Eric Poehlman, a tenured faculty member at the University of Vermont, was sentenced to jail for falsifying data in a federal grant application. He admitted to fabricating years' worth of scientific data on obesity, menopause, and aging — data he used to get nearly $3 million in federal grants from government agencies. Ten scientific papers he'd been involved with had to be corrected or retracted.

Looking at who conducted the study

Once when Liz was writing a story on a popular supplement, she spoke to the company president, who claimed to have all sorts of scientific research to back up the claims made on the packaging. It turned out the research was performed in the company's own laboratories without outside comment, publication, or peer review. Liz was told that the company did not allow outside entities to test their products because they were "ill-equipped" and "did not understand how to evaluate the products." The supplement may or may not work, but it seems to us if a product is truly effective, a company should not fear having it tested by outsiders.

One way to get to the bottom of things is to read blogs that specialize in critiquing scientific health and fitness research, such as junkfoodscience. blogspot.com.

Checking the math

You often read that a certain habit "doubles" the risk of death or "increases the risk of disease by 50 percent." These figures can be misleading. In a study that followed 115,000 nurses for 16 years, researchers found that gaining 11 to 18 pounds in middle age raised the nurses' heart disease risk by 25 percent. But the number of deaths in the study was so small that a 25 percent increase would mean the difference between 10 deaths in 10,000 people and 12 or 13 deaths in 10,000.

Not assuming cause and effect

A recent study found that men who walked briskly 30 minutes a day, four days a week, were 65 percent less likely to experience sexual dysfunction than inactive men. But this result doesn't necessarily mean that exercise leads to better sex. It could be that because the exercisers are healthy, they're able to exercise more and have better sexual health.

Putting a study in context

Think of any individual study as one piece in a giant, complete puzzle. The scientific community can take decades and hundreds of studies to reach a consensus, and even when it does, that consensus may change years later.

When you read the discussion section of any studies, you find that researchers often explain their findings in context with the rest of the related science, and they discuss the possible shortfalls of their own study design. Comments like these suggest the authors are critical thinkers who believe in what they have found but acknowledge that more work needs to be done in the field.

Trusting Credible Coverage

So many media reports and scientific studies can be misleading or downright false that you may be wondering: Can I believe *anything* I read about health and fitness? Actually, yes.

A lot of interesting information is coming out every day, and much of it is accurate, well-reported, and performed by honest and dedicated scientists. Also, many health reporters and bloggers are sincere and hardworking — Liz and Suzanne count themselves among them. We may not get it right every time, but we do our best to make sure that we present information accurately and in the correct context. The majority of health writers we know aim to do the same and largely succeed.

What's more, when you come across fitness media reports and health and fitness research, trust your instincts. The body is an amazing tool, and no matter how much research is conducted, what works for one person is likely to be different for people of other makes and models. Trusting your gut is important, so don't wait for something to be published before you believe it. The combination of listening to your body, finding reliable sources, and reading good research will take you far.

Chapter 5

This Doesn't Have to Happen to You: Avoiding Common Injuries

*W*hen you start an exercise program, injuries are probably the last thing on your mind. Chances are you imagine parading around your fancy new biceps and bounding up mountains like an Austrian yodeler. You don't envision yourself laid up in bed with an ice pack on your groin muscle.

But the reality is that injuries happen because people *don't* think about them. That's why we include this chapter early in the book. We want you to know, right off, how to avoid getting hurt and how to recognize the early signs of an injury so that minor muscle aches and pains don't turn into major problems that sideline you (and turn you into a video-game addict) for six months. In this chapter, we also help you distinguish run-of-the-mill soreness from a bona fide injury and advise you on how to treat the most common exercise-related ailments.

We especially urge anyone over age 10 to read this chapter. Yes, 10 is young — so young that most people that age are still running around without a second thought to muscles, tendons, ligaments, and joints. If you're older than that now — and you probably are — this chapter contains information that is essential for you to know, because your body is considerably less springy and more vulnerable to injuries than a child's.

Reducing Your Risk of Injury

 Short of residing in a plastic bubble, you can't cut your risk of injury to zero. (And actually, living in a bubble is likely to give you back problems from limited opportunities to stretch your legs.) However, if you heed the following tips and are lucky enough to avoid being run over by a wayward skier or beaned by a softball, you're likely to keep your muscles, joints, ligaments, and tendons pretty darned happy throughout life:

- **Use appropriate, good-quality equipment.** We're talking about shoes that fit your particular foot, a bike that's the right height, a seamless shirt that wicks away moisture to prevent chafing and irritation. The best equipment need not be the most expensive. Just buy exactly what you need. (See the sidebar "Know your feet" for tips on shoe selection.)

- **Warm up.** Easing your body into a workout prepares your muscles and your mind to get in the game, preempting unwelcome surprises. As we explain in Chapter 6, a warm-up does not involve reaching over and touching your toes but rather engaging in easy movement like a brisk walk.

- **Use proper technique.** Don't yank on your neck when you do a crunch. Don't drop your butt to the floor when you do a squat. You get the idea.

- **Progress gradually.** If you haven't broken a sweat since middle-school gym class, don't inaugurate your training program with a 90-minute interval session. (Remember the fable about the tortoise and the hare? Well, what they don't tell you is that the hare lost because he was sidelined for three days with sore ankles.)

- **Listen to your body.** Pay attention to every ache and pain. Is your body telling you that you've pushed yourself harder than usual or harder than you should have? What you hear may not be music to your ears, but it will help you adjust your program to suit where you are right now.

Know your feet

We talk a lot about buying the proper athletic shoes to avoid injury. But you can't always trust the salesperson at your local shoe shop to help you select the best shoe for your foot. Before you shop, you need to know a little something about your feet. For example: Are you flat-footed or blessed with a natural arch?

To test this, wet your foot and then step onto a piece of paper. If your entire foot is visible in the footprint, you have a flat foot. If there is a slight c shape in the print where your arch should be, you have a medium arch; the bigger the c, the higher your arch. If all that's visible is the front of your foot and the back of your heel, then you have a really high-arched foot.

Owners of high-arched feet should run from shoes that offer little or no arch support because these people already have so much pressure placed on the balls of their feet. People with low-arched or flat feet need shoes with firm, durable heels with lots of overall cushioning. This is especially helpful for taking the pressure off of your knees if you *pronate*—ride the inside edge of your foot when you step down. Most shoes have descriptions on the tags that describe what type of feet and training they're good for. Many Web sites also have shoe finders: You plug information about your feet and training into a questionnaire, and suggestions for shoes pop out. Also, many specialty stores have knowledgeable salespeople who can evaluate your feet and help you select a good shoe for you.

Recognizing When You're Injured

Sometimes, no matter how careful you are, exercise hurts. If you never lift anything heavier than a bag of potato chips and then start lifting dumbbells, even light ones, you're going to feel some soreness. That type of pain usually isn't anything to worry about. But if you wake up the morning after a weight-lifting session and feel like your arm has been shredded by a meat grinder, that's a different story. That's "bad" pain. You can consider yourself injured.

Normal pain is achy, dull, and very general. Usually, you feel it throughout an entire muscle or over a large area of your body. Bad pain tends to be sharp and specific. It typically hurts when you do certain movements, like bending your knee or lifting your arm overhead. It's important to recognize this type of pain and act accordingly.

A while back, Suzanne ignored the shoulder pain that flared up after she performed certain chest exercises. Eventually, the pain got so bad that she couldn't lift a pitcher of water without wincing. Suzanne was forced to take off three entire months from upper-body weight training while her tendon healed. This made her grouchy and set her way back fitness-wise but taught her a good lesson.

Identifying Common Exercise Injuries and Ways to Avoid Them

Among restaurant cooks, common injuries include cut fingers and scalded skin. When motorcycle racers get hurt, they're usually dealing with broken collarbones and dislocated shoulders. People who engage in fitness activities have their own set of injuries to contend with. You don't see a lot of sliced thumbs or fractured clavicles among power walkers and Pilates practitioners, but here's a rundown of the hazards that you may encounter.

Inside information: Surveying injuries to muscles, bone, and more

When you're working out, different tissue types are at risk of injury, including muscles, tendons, ligaments, bones, and skin. In the following sections, we cover injuries ranging from pulled muscles to blisters.

Strains: Pulling muscles

When you *strain* a muscle (commonly called a *pulled muscle*), you overstretch or tear the *tendon* (the tough, cord-like end of the muscle that attaches to the bone). Strains happen when you push yourself harder than normal, like when you decide to race your co-workers to the bus stop.

Two of the most commonly strained muscles are the hamstrings (rear thigh muscles) and groin (inner-thigh) muscles (see Chapter 11 for pictures of and more information about these muscles):

- ✔ **Strained hamstring:** You know you've strained your hamstring if a sharp pain shoots up the back of your thigh when you straighten your leg. If you watch the running sprints during the Olympics, you inevitably see this injury. A runner will be sprinting for all she's worth and then suddenly grimace and come to a screeching halt. It's almost always the hamstring that goes. In fact, if you're close enough to her when it happens, you may even hear a loud pop.

- ✔ **Groin pull:** You have a groin pull if a stabbing pain prevents you from lifting your leg in toward your other leg or out to the side. In both cases, you may feel a lump or a knot where the muscle has tightened up.

Treating strains

Stop the offending activity for a few days until the muscle repairs itself. Otherwise, you may be headed for a full-blown tear and end up sidelined for months instead of days. To speed up the healing process, apply ice to the injured area for the first 24 to 48 hours. (See the "Treating Sports Injuries with RICE, RICE, Baby" section in this chapter for icing tips.) Gentle — emphasis on *gentle* — massage may help work out muscle kinks.

Preventing a recurrence

To prevent another pulled muscle, ease into a workout by starting slowly and gradually increasing your pace. Carefully stretch your muscles every day, always *after* your thorough warm-up, and increase your exercise program on a gradual basis. Make sure your shoes aren't too big or wide.

Sprains: Injuring joints

A *sprain* refers to a torn or overstretched *ligament* (the connective tissue that joins two bones together). You can sprain a joint — like when you turn your ankle while stepping off a curb — but you can't sprain a muscle. Sprains occur most commonly at the ankle. You often hear a loud pop with this sort of injury. Usually you're left with a bruise and swelling, and you can't place any of your weight on the injured foot without pain.

Treating sprains

The treatment for a sprained ankle is to keep your shoe on for as long as possible (this keeps the ankle from swelling) and then follow the RICE formula (see the section "Treating Sports Injuries with RICE, RICE, Baby" later in this chapter).

Preventing a recurrence

Even though it's your ligament that's at risk for a sprain, strengthening the nearby muscle will prevent the injury. For example, adding calf exercises to your weight routine keeps your ankles firmly heading in the right direction and less susceptible to the occasional misstep.

Stress fractures: Gradually breaking bones

The first large group of modern-day athletes to experience stress fractures were soldiers in World War II. The Army took out-of-shape civilians, placed heavy packs on their backs, and sent them off to march for miles in heavy combat boots. Soon the rookies complained about foot pain, but because nothing showed up on X-rays, doctors assumed they were faking it. Often, a second X-ray was taken several weeks later, revealing a fuzziness along the bone. *Bone callus* (a buildup of bone material) was forming; the healing process had started.

Today, long-distance runners, hikers, backpackers, and in-line skaters are the most common sufferers of stress fractures. *Stress fractures* are typically not one but a series of microfractures or hairline breaks that run along the bone.

You don't usually have a telltale snap or pop that occurs in other breaks. More often, you wake up one day with pain radiating down the top of one or two of your toes to the center of your foot or along your shinbone. You may feel pain when you walk. You may even notice redness or swelling on top of your foot. When you press your finger on that spot, you feel a stabbing pain that immediately grabs your attention. The front of the shin is also a likely place for a fracture accompanied by the trademark pinpoint of pain.

Treating stress fractures

Don't try to treat this kind of pain yourself. It definitely warrants a visit to your orthopedist or podiatrist, who will X-ray your foot to make sure that your injury is a stress fracture. The doctor will probably prescribe anti-inflammatory medication, ice, and elevation and will implore you to stay off your feet. In extreme cases, she may even put you in a soft or hard cast.

If you think you have a stress fracture, stop exercising immediately. We can't tell you how many times marathoners in agonizing foot pain at mile nine go on to finish the race anyway. When you continue to run on a stress fracture, you transform a minor injury into one that can take months to heal.

Preventing a recurrence

Don't overdo it! If you've had a layoff from a stress fracture, don't start back with 90 minutes of pounding, and build rest into your routine. And here again, weight training (along with a diet rich in calcium and vitamin D) helps maintain strong bones. After a layoff start back gradually and build back up slowly. Consider incorporating low- and no-impact workouts like swimming and water running to help your body heal.

Chafing: Getting rubbed raw

Your legs feel great, and you've barely broken a sweat, yet you can't continue your bike ride because your butt is rubbed raw. You have what's essentially a case of adult diaper rash, an irritation that can crop up anywhere your clothing touches your skin and is known as *chafing*. It's particularly common in hot weather, when heavy sweating contributes to the problem. But you also see it in the winter if you wear clothing that doesn't breathe properly; the sweat pools between the skin and the first layer, creating the perfect storm of moisture, rubbing, and sensitive skin. Every sport has special hot spots to watch. The bra line, underarms, and sock line are the most common among runners. But you can also get chafed if your tights, shorts, or shirt rub against your skin as you move. Only streakers are immune.

You can also develop a similar condition, *blisters* (a small buildup of water or blood under your skin), when your feet rub against the seams in your shoes, slide around in too-loose shoes, or feel friction against too-tight or bunched-up socks. Small, deep blisters and large blisters not only are painful, but they can keep you off your feet and off your training routine for days at a time.

Treating chafing

Clean your chafed area with soap and water or hydrogen peroxide, let it dry, and then apply a liquid bandage. After the liquid has dried, goop the area heavily and evenly with petroleum jelly. Or use a product like Lanacane Anti-Chafing Gel, an all-purpose skin lubricant that lasts longer than petroleum jelly and won't come off until you wash with soap and water. (Check online for this and other similar products.) Long-distance cyclists slather their butts with udder balm, an ointment made for cows but helpful for reducing chafing in humans. It feels kind of icky, but it usually does the trick.

Preventing a recurrence

Your feet are the most common and painful site of blistering. You may not give much thought to the lowly sock you put on before you slip on your $85 athletic shoes, but often that thin layer of fabric is all that stands between you and a monster blister. We prefer thin socks to thick ones and socks that aren't too loose; you don't want extra fabric bunching up and causing friction. Look for seamless brands. They may cost a few cents more but you'll recoup those pennies by replenishing your antichafing gel supply less often.

The same theory applies to all other clothing: Go for proper fit, as few seams as possible, and materials that don't irritate. Dry-fit products are sold by many leading sports clothing manufacturers. This is one example of a material that helps prevent sweat from pooling and causing chafing. Softer fabrics that include at least some cotton tend to be the kindest to your skin, but it's a matter of personal preference. A good sports bra is also essential for comfort when exercising. Also, be sure to slather your hotspots with lubricant.

We know one runner who used to get a severe case of irritation on his nipples. He solved this with the strategic placement of bandages. Not very macho, but then, neither were the two spots of blood leaking through his shirt.

Looking at injuries by body part

In the following sections, we cover types of injuries that are specific to certain parts of the body, from the heel on up.

The back of the heel: Achilles tendonitis

Achilles was the mighty Greek warrior whose mother dipped him into the waters of the River Styx to make him invulnerable, missing just one spot: the point on the back of his heel where she held him. This area, where the *Achilles tendon* connects to the heel, is a weak spot for just about anyone who happens to stand or move in an upright position, especially runners, walkers, in-line skaters, cyclists, and tennis players. When the Achilles tendon becomes swollen, sore, or inflamed, you have *Achilles tendonitis*.

Treating Achilles tendonitis

Your old friend ice can reduce swelling and relieve pain (see the "Treating Sports Injuries with RICE, RICE, Baby" section for details). If you wear high heels, wean yourself from them and switch to flats. Heels can contribute to Achilles tendonitis by keeping your calves in a contracted (shortened) position for hours on end, which shortens the tendon; you then have to stretch out the tendon again to go barefoot or wear flats.

For chronic Achilles inflammation, the remedy that works best is something many die-hard exercisers don't want to hear: Stop exercising. Give your Achilles tendon a few days off to rest and repair. Ice the spot, but don't do any stretching or strengthening exercises that put pressure on your heel. (You can swim but only if you feel no pain.) If your Achilles problem persists, see an orthopedist or a podiatrist. You may need more-aggressive remedies.

Preventing a recurrence

The most common culprit in Achilles tendonitis is a calf muscle that's too short and tight, so a regular stretching program that focuses on your foot, calf, and hamstring muscles (see Chapter 14) goes a long way toward preventing the problem.

Shin splints

Shin splints is a catch-all term for shin pain, usually caused by a slight separation between the shin muscles and the bone. Depending on how severe your splints are, the pain ranges from a dull, intermittent ache to unrelenting agony that, according to some people, rivals labor pain. You can develop shin splints from doing more exercise than your body is ready to handle or simply from introducing a new aspect to your training, such as wearing a new pair of shoes, running downhill, or running on the beach when you normally run on asphalt.

Treating shin splints

Back off on exercise for a few days, and use ice to reduce inflammation and dull the pain. For shin splints, we recommend the ice massage method described in the "Treating Sports Injuries with RICE, RICE, Baby" section. Also, gently but deeply massaging the area several times a day can help.

Preventing a recurrence

When you're free of pain from shin splints, start back up gradually; don't increase your exercise time or distance by more than 10 percent a week. To strengthen your shin muscles so that they work more in harmony with your calves, the muscles that operate in opposition to them, try this simple exercise: Stand on the floor or with your heels on the edge of a stair (holding on to a rail for balance), with your weight distributed evenly over the entire length of your foot, and lift and lower your toes and the balls of your feet (like you're tapping your toes to the beat of music) 20 to 30 times. Ask a trainer to show you some other shin exercises. Stretching the calf muscles (see Chapter 14) also helps prevent injury to the shin and ankle.

We know one guy who solved his chronic shin-splint problem overnight by buying a pair of shoes with a slightly wider heel. A podiatrist or sports-medicine specialist (or even a well-informed running store associate) can help you find the solution that suits your style. If all else fails, your podiatrist may make a special pair of inserts, called *orthotics,* to properly position your feet in your shoes.

Knee pain

On the surface, the knee seems to be a wonderfully uncomplicated mechanism with a pretty simple job description: to bend and straighten your leg. In reality, knee function is controlled by more muscles, tendons, ligaments, and cartilage than any other joint in your body. That's one reason it's often the first joint to break down. The other is that the knees are involved in virtually every sport or activity, making it one of the most common joints to suffer injury.

Knee pain comes in more varieties than ice cream. It can be caused by a tear in a ligament, a tendon, a muscle, or a piece of *cartilage,* the cushioning that prevents two bones from rubbing against each other. You may feel a slight, dull ache in the front of the kneecap, or your pain may be so severe that you can't straighten or bend it without screaming. Either way, you should get checked out by a professional.

Though we can't diagnose your specific ailment, we can tell you this: Knee pain is often the result of doing too much of the same movement over and over again. Typically, you can't trace it to a specific incident; it's more likely the result of one bike-a-thon or walk-a-thon too many. It's also affected or caused by a lack of stability and strength in supporting musculature of the hips and thighs.

Treating knee pain

If you feel knee pain coming on, cut back on your exercise routine or switch to an activity that doesn't aggravate the situation. Some people with knee problems from running can bicycle with no pain whatsoever, and vice versa.

Ice is always a good choice, too. But don't mess around here. If pain persists, recurs frequently, or is caused by a single incident, get thee to a doctor ASAP.

Preventing a recurrence

Cross-training is a good way to avoid knee pain. By varying your exercise activities — running one day, cycling the next — you use different muscles, or at least you use the same muscles in different ways. You can still injure your knees with a cross-training regimen, so be careful not to overdo it. Be sure to include squats, lunges, and similar exercises in your weight-training routine as well. Some athletes, especially runners, shy away from weight training because they worry that they will bulk up (they won't) or that lifting weights will cause injuries (the opposite is true). Maintaining strong leg muscles keeps your knees tracking properly. You may also consider changing surfaces, although that can sometimes exacerbate the problems. Consider rotating through several pairs of shoes or at least replacing a pair of shoes that are fried; this can sometimes make a knee issue disappear overnight.

Back pain

Nearly 80 percent of people utter the words "Oh, my aching back," at some point in their adult lives. Although regular workouts (especially core exercises that work the abdominals and lower back) can do a lot to help prevent back pain, fitness activities also can cause back problems, particularly if you do a lot of pounding or use improper form when you run or cycle. You also can wrench your back by failing to bend your legs when you lift a weight off the rack.

Of course, you can throw out your back by doing completely nonathletic activities, such as — well, anything. Always use proper form (lifting and bending with your legs, not your back) when lifting and carrying anything.

Back pain comes in lots of forms. It can be a nagging stiffness that makes tying your shoes a difficult proposition or a chronic, debilitating pain that keeps you curled up in bed for weeks at a time.

Treating back pain

In many instances of back pain, the worst thing you can do is just stay in bed. This weakens the very muscles that need to be loosened up and strengthened (and lack of activity may have led to the back pain in the first place). Another time-honored treatment, the heating pad, makes many back conditions worse by further inflaming the nerves.

So what helps back pain heal? Time, for one thing. Many cases of back pain disappear within four weeks without any treatment. If that doesn't work, see a professional. Most experts believe that the majority of back pain is muscular in nature and can be treated successfully with nonsurgical procedures, such as practicing good posture, exercise, massage, physical therapy, and chiropractic. (To find a good chiropractor, get a recommendation from a friend, or better yet, from a medical doctor.)

For an episode you're having right now, ice and gentle movement are probably your best bet for back-pain relief. Also try lying on the floor with your knees bent and calves and feet resting on a chair (if it isn't too painful to get yourself into that position). Gently rock back and forth in a tiny, easy movement; this simulates a gentle massage that many physical therapists say can help ease back pain.

Some experts recommend seeing a *physiatrist,* a medical doctor who rehabilitates the disabled and is more likely to prescribe exercise than medication or surgery. If you experience severe back pain that prevents you from performing normal activities, see your physician first to rule out any underlying medical causes, such as kidney infections or intestinal disorders.

Don't ignore the symptoms, like Liz's husband, Jay, once did. One night Jay woke up in the middle of the night to get some ice but got so dizzy from his back pain that he fainted. When he hit the floor, Liz woke up and found him lying in the hallway, blood dripping from his mouth. Liz thought he had been shot. For the next two days, Jay was confined to bed because he couldn't walk. His cut lip didn't feel too good, either.

Preventing a recurrence

Swimming, walking, and yoga seem to be the best activities for limbering up tight back muscles. Core strengthening exercises supervised by a physical therapist or trainer experienced in dealing with back pain can give you long-term immunity from further recurrence of back pain. For a helpful back stretch, see Chapter 14.

Also, be careful about the shoes you wear. Lay off the high heels, and make sure your shoes fit properly and don't have too much wear and tear. Consider how you sleep as well. A bed that is too hard or too soft may be the root of chronic back pain — like Goldilocks, you need one that is just right. Ditto for pillows. And speaking of pillows, sleeping with a pillow between your knees also can help diminish and prevent back pain.

Tennis elbow

You don't need to be a tennis player to experience tenderness on the bony bump on the outside of your elbow or an aching sensation whenever you straighten your arm or pick up an object. In fact, *tennis elbow* (inflammation of the tendons in your elbow) can be caused by carrying a gym bag or briefcase with a straight arm or by lifting weights or any heavy object with improper form.

Treating tennis elbow

If you feel pain in your elbow, stop the offending activity. Ice can help, and you can buy a brace or slip-on wrap at the drugstore to help support your elbow. Your doctor may even suggest that you wear the brace while you sleep to keep up continuous compression on your elbow joint.

Preventing a recurrence

Strengthen your wrists (forearms) and your triceps, the muscles at the back of your arm (see Chapter 11 for more information on triceps muscles; see Chapter 13 for a triceps-building exercise). Strong wrists are particularly important because most elbow pain is caused by swollen tendons that originate in the wrists and end in the elbow.

When you lift weights take care not to lock your elbows. This is a common mistake, and the people who do it often fail to make the connection between their elbow pain and their sloppy form. Also avoid quick, jerky movements that involve snapping the elbows open or closed suddenly. For instance, when you are doing biceps curls, don't let gravity simply throw your arm back to the straight position.

Try doing strengthening exercises with hand weights: With your elbow cocked and your palm down, repeatedly bend your wrist, stopping if you feel any pain. Stretch the muscles in and around the elbow before beginning a potentially stressful activity by grasping the top part of your fingers and gently but firmly pulling them back toward your body, while keeping your arm fully extended and your palm facing outward.

The shoulder: Rotator-cuff injuries

What's the capital of Belgium? If you can't raise your hand to answer that question, you may have a rotator-cuff tear. Throwing a ball, digging, shoveling snow, and lifting your arm to the side may also be painful. (By the way, the answer is Brussels.)

The *rotator cuff* is a group of four muscles that surround and protect your shoulder joint (see Chapter 11 for details about the muscles in your body). They're particularly delicate and susceptible to injury. They can tear if your arm is violently pulled or twisted or if you fall with your arm outstretched. But the most likely scenario is damage from repetitive movements such as throwing a ball, playing a racquet sport, and improperly lifting weights. Which movements cause pain depends on which rotator-cuff muscle you damage and how badly you injure it. Rotator-cuff tears are often the reason for the early retirement of baseball and softball players.

Treating rotator-cuff injuries

Rotator-cuff injuries usually are treated with ice and compression (see the "Treating Sports Injuries with RICE, RICE, Baby" section later in this chapter), plus strength-training exercises using very light weights or exercise tubes. Do weight-training exercises properly, or ask a trainer to check your form. Reeducate yourself on throwing, golf or racquet sport form, or swim stroke technique — make sure to involve your entire body rather than just your arm and shoulder. In some cases, the rotator cuff is too far torn to strengthen through exercise, and the damaged muscle needs surgical repair or physical therapy to heal.

Preventing a recurrence

After your rotator cuff is damaged, you're typically at increased risk for reinjury, so be sure to keep your shoulders strong. They need to be flexible, too, but avoid overstretching these muscles, as this can leave the rotator cuff less stable. You may have to limit certain activities, such as swimming or throwing. At the very least, go back to basics and review technique to ensure you are not using your shoulder and rotator-cuff muscles improperly.

Neck pain

You may not realize how useful your neck is until you can't move it, like when the guy standing next to you asks a question, and answering him requires a three-quarter turn of your body.

Just about anything can cause neck pain — you may sleep on your neck in a funny way or spend too much time cradling the phone on your shoulder. But neck pain is often caused by fitness activities. We're talking about poor weight-lifting technique, poor posture in boot camp class, and letting your head and shoulders droop forward when you walk.

Neck pain usually signals tightness in the muscles of your neck, upper back, and/or shoulders. When you press a finger into the area between your shoulder and your neck and there's very little give or springiness, you have tight neck muscles.

Treating neck pain

If you experience neck pain after a traumatic incident, such as getting whacked on the head with a soccer ball, check with your doctor immediately. Also consult a physician if you have constant or recurring neck pain.

Gentle stretching of the neck muscles is a good remedy for nontraumatic neck pain. See Chapter 14 for details. Gentle massage is also useful for freeing up knotty neck muscles. You can give yourself a massage, but somehow that isn't as satisfying as enlisting a friend, significant other, or professional therapist.

Ice, usually an injury-friendly treatment, isn't always the best choice for neck pain. If you're stiff to begin with, applying ice may cause you to tense up even more. If your trouble is a stiff neck, moist heat in the form of a warm washcloth, shower massage, or whirlpool may be the way to go.

Preventing a recurrence

Good exercise technique is the best way to avoid neck strain. Stretching after your workouts, while watching TV, or while sitting at your desk can help, too. Generally practicing good posture makes a big difference as well.

Treating Sports Injuries with RICE, RICE, Baby

If your doctor or trainer prescribes RICE for an injury, he isn't suggesting some New Age nutritional treatment. He's referring to the common way to treat sports injuries: Rest, Ice, Compression, and Elevation. Usually, this treatment is all you need to get back on your feet, particularly if you do it diligently for the first 48 hours after an injury. Here's how it works:

✔ **Rest:** Stop doing activities that aggravate your injury. If you sprain your ankle, don't try to "walk it off." Rest can often mean the difference between an injury that heals fast and one that nags you for months.

Don't use your injury as an excuse to quit exercising altogether. Simply choose an activity that doesn't hurt. If you pull a hamstring, you don't have to stop upper-body weight training. Swimming is also often a great activity when injured, unless, of course, your injury is swimming-related.

✔ **Ice:** Apply ice for 15 to 20 minutes, three or four times a day, for as long as you feel pain. Ice reduces swelling and deadens pain by constricting blood flow into the injured area. Contrary to popular belief, ice is not useless after the first day. You can apply ice with a pack, a plastic bag full of cubes, or a package of frozen corn.

Don't allow the ice to rest directly on your skin; otherwise, you're inviting a whole new list of problems, such as ice burns. Instead, put a thin, damp washcloth between your skin and the ice.

One of our favorite icing techniques is ice massage. Fill a paper cup three-fourths full of water and stick it in the freezer. When the water freezes, peel the cup down so you have what resembles an ice cream cone of ice. Use this to massage the injured area in a circular motion for as long as you can take it, usually four or five minutes. Ice massage penetrates more deeply into your muscles than passively throwing an ice pack over the injured area. Be sure to keep the ice moving.

✔ **Compression:** Put pressure on the injured area to keep the swelling down. Wrap a damp elastic bandage around the injury, or buy a special knee, elbow, or wrist wrap or brace. Wrap tightly enough that you feel some tension but not so firmly that you cut off your circulation or feel numbness.

✔ **Elevation:** Elevating your injured body part reduces swelling by allowing fluids and waste products to drain from the area, much like water runs downstream. (Waste products are the bits of broken blood cells and other inflammatory agents hanging around the injury.) If your ankle is injured, you don't need to raise it so high that it's perpendicular to the ground. Propping it up on a couple of fluffy pillows will do. Elevation works best when used in conjunction with the rest of the RICE treatment.

Part II
Going Cardio

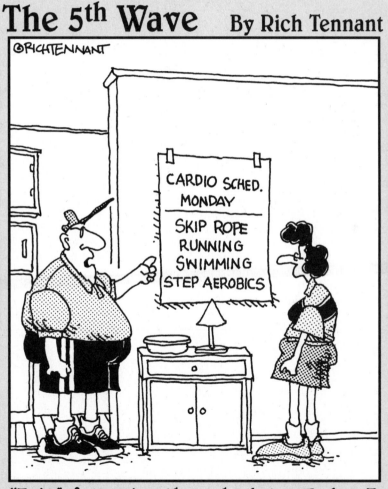

The 5th Wave   By Rich Tennant

"I AM following the schedule! Today I skipped the rope, then I skipped the running, then I skipped the swimming."

In this part . . .

We tell you everything you need to know about *cardiovascular* exercise, also known as *cardio*. In Chapter 6, we give you a crash course on cardio basics, including how to know whether you're pushing yourself hard enough or maybe even overdoing it. In Chapter 7, we help you design a cardio workout program suited to your goals and fitness level. Chapter 8 explains how to use indoor cardio equipment such as elliptical trainers, treadmills, rowers, and other fun machines. Chapter 9 covers tips and equipment for popular outdoor cardio activities — such as walking, running, in-line skating, cycling, and swimming — along with winter cardio activities, such as snowshoeing and cross-country skiing.

Chapter 6

Cardio Crash Course: Getting the Right Intensity

*I*f you hang around people who exercise, you're going to hear the word *cardio* or *aerobics* pretty often. Someone may say, "I do cardio four days a week," or, "My gym has awesome cardio equipment." *Aerobics* — a term coined in the 1960s by fitness pioneer Dr. Kenneth Cooper — refers to *cardiovascular exercise,* the kind that strengthens your heart and lungs and burns lots of calories.

In Chapter 25, we list all kinds of reasons to pursue this sort of exercise — everything from lowering your risk of dementia and diabetes to trimming that spare tire to experiencing the glory of a personal best in a 10k run. This chapter explains what it takes to reap those benefits — in other words, what type of exercise counts as cardio. We introduce you to terms such as *aerobic, anaerobic,* and *target heart rate zone.* After you understand the basic concepts involved in cardio exercise, use the plans in Chapter 7 to design a cardio workout program based on your goals.

Note: After you read this chapter, you may be very excited about all the information and want to put it — and your feet — into action. On the other hand, with all this talk of maximum heart rate, anaerobic threshold, and heart-rate monitors, you may wonder whether cardio exercise is just too darned complicated to bother with. Trust us: It's not! We provide all this information so that you understand the basics of how to determine your exercise intensity and set goals for your program. As we show you in Chapter 7, all this science is pretty simple to put into action.

Comparing Aerobic and Anaerobic Exercise

Aerobic exercise is any continuous, repetitive activity that you do long enough and hard enough to challenge your heart and lungs. To get this effect, you generally need to use your large muscles, including your butt, legs, back, and chest. Walking, bicycling, swimming, and climbing stairs count as aerobic exercise.

Movements that use your smaller muscles, like those leading into your wrists and hands, don't burn as many calories. Channel surfing with your remote control can certainly be repetitive, sustained, and intense — particularly when performed by certain husbands we know — but it burns very few calories.

Aerobic means "with air." When you exercise aerobically, your body needs an extra supply of oxygen, which your lungs extract from the air. Think of oxygen as the gasoline in your car: When you're idling at a stoplight, you don't need as much fuel as when you're zooming across Montana on Interstate 90. During your aerobic workouts, your body continuously delivers oxygen to your muscles.

However, if you push yourself hard enough, eventually you switch gears into using less oxygen: Your lungs can no longer suck in enough oxygen to keep up with your muscles' demand for it. But you don't collapse, at least not in the first 3 minutes. Instead, you begin to rely on your body's limited capacity to keep going without oxygen. During this time, your individual muscles are exercising *anaerobically,* or without air.

Anaerobic exercise refers to high-intensity exercise like all-out sprinting or very heavy weight lifting. After about 90 seconds, you begin gasping for air, and you usually can't sustain this activity for more than 3 minutes. That's when your body forces you to stop. You may still use large muscle groups, but you do so for only a short burst of time, and then you need to take a break before starting the next burst. Running a 30-minute loop around the neighborhood is aerobic, whereas doing all-out sprints around the track with a 2-minute break between them is anaerobic. Both count as cardio because they challenge your heart and lungs and burn lots of calories. You also may do hybrid activities referred to as "stop-and-go" sports, such as basketball, soccer, and tennis. These activities involve long periods of slow, sustained movement with some short bursts of high-intensity activity mixed in.

Understanding the Importance of Warming Up and Cooling Down

Automobiles are built to go from 0 to 60 miles per hour in mere seconds and to stop practically on a dime if necessary; humans aren't. With any type of physical activity, whether it's walking, playing basketball, or cross-country skiing, you need to ease into it with a warm-up and ease out of it with a cool-down. (Weight-training workouts also require a warm-up, as we explain in Chapter 13, although they typically don't require a cardio cool-down.)

Warming up

A *warm-up* simply means 3 to 15 minutes of an activity performed at a very easy pace. Ideally, a warm-up should be a slower version of the main event so it works the same muscles and gets blood flowing to all the right places. For example, runners may start out with a brisk walk or a slow run. If you're going on a hilly bike ride, you may want to start with at least a few miles on flat terrain. Be aware that stretching is not a good warm-up activity (see Chapter 14).

People who are out of shape need to warm up the longest. Their bodies take longer to get into the exercise groove because their muscles aren't used to working hard. If you're a beginner, any exercise is high-intensity exercise. As you get more fit, your body adapts and becomes more efficient, thereby warming up more quickly.

Many people skip their warm-up because they're in a hurry. Cranking up the elliptical machine or hitting the weights right away seems like a more efficient use of time. Bad idea. Skimp on your warm-up, and you're a lot more likely to injure yourself. Besides, when you ease into your workout, you enjoy it a lot more. A trainer we know says, "If you don't have time to warm up, you don't have time to work out!"

What exactly does warming up do for you? Well, for one thing, a warm-up warms you up — literally. It increases the temperature in your muscles and in the tissues that connect muscle to bone (tendons) and bone to bone (ligaments). Warmer muscles and joints are more pliable and, therefore, less likely to tear. Warming up also helps redirect your blood flow from places such as your stomach and spleen to the muscles that you're using to exercise. This blood flow gives you more stamina by providing your muscles with more nutrients and oxygen. In other words, you tire more quickly if you don't warm up because this redirection of blood flow takes time.

Finally, warming up allows your heart rate to increase at a safe, gradual pace. If you don't warm up, your heart rate will shoot up too quickly, and you'll have trouble getting your breathing under control.

Cooling down

After your workout, don't stop suddenly and make a dash for the shower or plop on the couch. (If you've ever done this, you've probably exited the shower with a hot red face or dripped sweat all over the couch.) Ease out of your workout just as you eased into it, by walking, jogging, or cycling lightly. If you've been using a stationary bike at Level 5 for 20 minutes, you can cool down by dropping to Level 3 for a couple minutes, then to Level 2, and so on. This *cool-down* should last 5 to 10 minutes — longer if you've done an especially lengthy or hard workout.

The purpose of the cool-down is the reverse of the warm-up. At this point, your heart is jumping and blood is pumping furiously through your muscles. You want your body to redirect the blood flow back to normal before you rush back to the office. You also want your body temperature to decrease before you hop into a hot or cold shower; otherwise, you risk fainting. Cooling down prevents your blood from pooling in one place, such as your legs.

When you suddenly stop exercising, your blood can quickly collect, which can lead to dizziness, nausea, and fainting. If you're really out of shape or at high risk for heart disease, skipping a cool-down can place undue stress on your heart.

Using Simple Methods to Gauge Your Level of Effort

To reap the benefits of cardio exercise, how much huffing and puffing do you need to do? Not as much as you probably think. Sure, you don't burn many calories from walking on the treadmill at the same pace that you stroll down the grocery store aisles; they don't call it *working out* for nothing. On the other hand, exercising too hard can lead to injury and make you more susceptible to colds and infections; plus, you may get so burned out that you want to set fire to your stationary bike. Also, the faster you go, the less time you can keep up the exercise. Depending on what you're trying to accomplish, you may gain just as much, if not more, from slowing things down and going farther.

To get fit and stay healthy, you need to find the middle ground: a moderate, or aerobic, pace. You can find this middle ground in a number of different ways. Some methods of gauging your intensity are extremely simple, and some require a foray into arithmetic. This section looks at the two most basic ways to monitor your intensity.

The talk test

The simplest way to monitor how hard you're working is to talk. You should be able to carry on a conversation while you're exercising. If you're so out of breath that you can't even string together the words "Help me, Mommy!" you need to slow down. On the other hand, if you're able to belt out tunes at the top of your lungs, that's a pretty big clue you need to pick up the pace. Basically, you should feel like you're working but not so hard that you feel like your lungs are about to explode.

Perceived exertion

If you're the type of person who needs more precision in life than the talk test offers, you may like the so-called *perceived exertion* method of gauging intensity. This method uses a numerical scale, typically from 1 to 10, that corresponds to how hard you feel you're working — the rate at which you perceive that you're exerting yourself.

An activity rated 1 on a perceived exertion scale would be something that you feel you could do forever, like sit in bed and watch the Olympics. A 10 represents all-out effort, like the last few feet of an uphill sprint, about 20 seconds before your legs buckle. Your typical workout intensity should fall somewhere between 5 and 8. To decide on a number, pay attention to how hard you're breathing, how fast your heart is beating, how much you're sweating, and how tired your legs feel — anything that contributes to the effort of sustaining the exercise.

The purpose of putting a numerical value on exercise is not to make your life more complicated but rather to help you maintain a proper workout intensity. For example, suppose you run 2 miles around your neighborhood, and it feels like an 8. If after a few weeks running those 2 miles feels like a 4, you know it's time to pick up the pace. Initially, you may want to have a perceived exertion chart in front of you. Many gyms post these charts on the walls, and you can easily create one at home. After a few workouts, you can use a mental chart. Table 6-1 shows a sample perceived exertion chart.

Table 6-1	Perceived Exertion
Scale	*Description*
10 Maximum effort	It's nearly impossible to continue. You're completely out of breath, your heart is pounding, you're sweating profusely, and you're unable to talk.
9 Very hard effort	It's very challenging, though not impossible, to maintain activity. You're breathing hard, your heart is pounding, you're sweating a lot, and you can barely talk.
7–8 Vigorous effort	You're on the edge of your comfort zone. You're short of breath, your heart is beating hard, and you're sweating, but you're able to speak short sentences.
4–6 Moderate effort	It feels like you can keep moving for quite a while without having to stop. You can have short conversations even though you're breathing heavily, your heart is beating fast, and you're sweating.
2–3 Light effort	It feels like you can keep moving with very little effort for a long time. Your heart rate is somewhat elevated and you may be sweating lightly, but you can breathe easily and hold a conversation.
1 Very light effort	You're doing something that requires virtually no physical effort — sedentary activities such as watching TV, riding in a car, or working on a computer.

Measuring Your Heart Rate

The talk test and the perceived exertion chart (see the preceding sections) are both valid ways to make sure that you're exercising at the right pace. But there's a numerical way for those of you that like concrete numbers: measuring your *pulse*, or *heart rate*, the number of times that your heart beats per minute. You can determine this number either by wearing a gadget called a *heart-rate monitor* or by using your fingers and counting the beats manually. This section discusses both methods and also explains why you want to measure your heart rate and how to determine your own target heart-rate zone.

Looking at what heart rate tells you

Keeping track of your heart rate, by whatever method, sounds like an incredibly advanced thing to do — something way beyond a beginner's needs. But especially when you're just starting out, heart-rate monitoring is immensely effective. Here are three reasons to follow your heart rate:

✔ **You find out whether you're working too hard.** When you're just starting to exercise, you may not have a good sense of how hard to push yourself. And with all that "no pain, no gain" propaganda, you may be exerting yourself more than is good for you. For example, running 9-minute miles on a hot, humid afternoon takes a lot more effort than running at the same pace on a cool, overcast morning. If you rely only on your stopwatch, you may push yourself to run 9-minute miles in the heat, when that pace may put excess stress on your body. If you pace yourself according to your heart rate instead, you know when you need to back off.

The same goes for when you're tired. Without checking your heart rate, you may force yourself to walk up an 8-percent grade at 4 miles per hour, when on that particular day, your body isn't up to the task. If you monitor your pulse, you may find that, in order to keep up with Level 4 on the bike, you have to exceed the high end of your training zone — a signal to drop down a notch or two.

✔ **You have another way to track your progress.** When you start exercising on a regular basis, your cardio respiratory system gradually becomes more efficient. Suppose when you started, Level 1 on the exercise bike used to get your heart up to about 140 beats per minute; now, two months later, your heart rate is 125 beats per minute. This drop means that you need to step up the difficulty of your workout.

Another way to see how much your fitness level is improving is to watch how fast your heart rate drops after a workout. Measure your heart rate immediately upon finishing your exercise session and then one minute later. The better shape you're in, the faster your heart rate drops. Ideally, your heart rate should plunge at least 20 beats in the first minute. People in really good shape drop 40 beats or more. Keep track of this measure (we discuss fitness logs in Chapters 1 and 26). You'll see a gradual improvement over a period of weeks and months. (**Note:** Taking prescription or over-the-counter medication may affect the way your heart and blood pressure respond to exercise. Check with your doctor about this.)

Yet another measure of your progress is your *resting heart rate,* the number of times your heart beats per minute when you're just sitting around. We discuss resting heart rate in Chapter 2.

✔ **You see how well you've recovered from your last workout.** You can use your resting heart rate to follow your recovery from day to day. Keep your monitor by your bed and strap it on first thing in the morning. Or take your pulse manually. If your heart rate is 10 beats higher than usual, you probably haven't recovered from yesterday's workout. Consider easing up or taking a day off.

Understanding your target zone

How do you know what heart rate to aim for? There's no magic number. Rather, there's a whole range of acceptable numbers, commonly called your *target heart-rate zone.* This range is the middle ground between slacking off and knocking yourself out. Typically, your *target zone* (as it's called for short) is between 50 and 85 percent of your *maximum heart rate,* the maximum number of times your heart should beat in a minute without dangerously overexerting yourself.

The top end of your target zone — somewhere between 80 and 90 percent of your maximum heart rate — is the point at which your body switches from using oxygen as its primary source of energy to using stored sugar. The point is referred to as your *anaerobic threshold.* Lactic acid builds up in the blood vessels of your muscles during especially high-intensity (or very long bouts of) exercise. As soon as more lactic acid builds up in your muscles than they can flush out, you begin to feel a burning sensation. Your muscles start to slow down, and moving becomes difficult. Fortunately, after you slow back down or stop, lactic acid clears your system within minutes (it's not responsible for the soreness you feel for several days after a hard workout session).

When you're in poor physical shape, your body isn't very efficient at taking in and utilizing oxygen and food sources, so you hit your anaerobic threshold while exercising at relatively low levels of exercise. As you become more fit, you're able to go farther and faster yet still supply oxygen to your muscles. If a couch potato tries to run an 8-minute-mile pace, he's going to go anaerobic pretty darned fast. An elite runner can run an entire marathon at about a 5-minute-mile pace and stay primarily aerobic.

At the low end of your zone, you're barely breaking a sweat; at the high end, you're dripping like a Kentucky Derby winner. If you're a beginner, stick to the lower end so you can move along comfortably for longer periods of time and with less chance of injury. As you get fitter, you may want to do some of your training in the middle and upper end of your zone. In Chapter 8, we offer examples of ways to mix up your training.

Finding your maximum and target heart rates

So how do you know what your maximum heart rate is? Well, we don't recommend running as hard as you can until you keel over and then counting your heartbeats for one minute. A safer and more accurate way is to have your max measured by a professional such as a physician or exercise specialist. (See Chapter 2 for details on exercise testing.) You can also use a number of mathematical formulas to estimate your max.

The best way to understand your max is to have it tested by a personal trainer or a doctor. The tester puts you through your paces on a cardio machine, usually a treadmill, and either makes you work as hard as you can, taking the highest heart rate you can sustain, or takes you to some percentage of your true maximum heart rate, as we describe in Chapter 2. The tester then uses a mathematical formula to get a decent prediction of what your max is.

The Karvonen method for target heart rate

One of the problems with the standard formula for finding your target heart rate is that it takes only your age into consideration. This is a valid consideration because your recommended maximum heart rate declines as you age. However, the following formula, called the Karvonen method, is somewhat more accurate because it also factors in your *resting heart rate,* the number of times your heart beats when you're sitting still. Typically, as you become more fit, your heart rate drops.

The Karvonen method requires a bit more math, but don't let that intimidate you. In this example, we use the case of a 40-year-old man who has a resting heart rate of 60 beats per minute and who wants to work at between 50 percent and 85 percent of his maximum heart rate. Grab your calculator and follow these instructions:

1. **Subtract your age from 220 to find the estimated maximum heart rate.**

   $$220 - 40 = 180$$

2. **Subtract your resting heart rate from your estimated maximum.**

   $$180 - 60 = 120.$$

3. **Multiply the number you arrived at in Step 2 by 50 percent. Then add your resting heart rate back in to find the low end of the target zone.**

   $$120 \times 0.50 = 60$$

   $$60 + 60 = 120$$

   The low end of the man's target zone is 120.

4. **Multiply the estimated maximum from Step 2 by 85 percent. Then add your resting heart rate back in to find the high end of the target zone.**

   $$120 \times 0.85 = 102$$

   $$102 + 60 = 162$$

   The high end of the man's target zone is 162.

Okay, now you can compare the results of this formula with those of the traditional formula. Using the age-related formula, this 40-year-old's target zone is 90 to 153 beats. But when you factor in his resting heart rate, this allows him to work up to 162 beats per minute. And he knows that if he drops below 102 beats, he probably needs to pick up the pace.

Using that easy formula to find your max, find your *target heart rate* by calculating 50 percent and 85 percent of your maximum. For instance, for a 40-year-old man, his maximum is 220 − 40 = 180. Take 50 percent of that to get the low end of his target zone: $180 \times 0.50 = 90$. If his heart beats fewer than 90 times per minute, he knows he's not pushing hard enough. Take 85 percent of the max to find the high end of his target zone ($180 \times 0.85 = 153$). If his heart beats faster than 153 beats per minute, he needs to slow down.

Measuring your pulse

Okay, say you've figured out your target heart-rate zone (see the preceding section). How do you know whether you're in the zone? In other words, how do you know how fast your heart is beating at any given moment? You can check your heart rate in two ways: using a heart-rate monitor or taking your pulse manually.

Using a heart-rate monitor

The most accurate way to determine your heart rate at any given moment is to wear a heart-rate monitor. The most accurate type of monitor is the chest-strap variety, which operates on the same principle as a medical electrocardiogram (ECG). You hook an inch-wide strap around your chest. This strap acts as an electrode to measure the electrical activity of your heart. This information is then translated into a number, which is transmitted via radio signals to a wrist receiver that looks like a watch with a large face. All you have to do is look at your wrist, and you instantly know how many times your heart is beating that moment, whether it's 92 or 164.

This is much more convenient than taking your pulse manually (see the next section) because you don't need to stop exercising or take the time to count anything. Yes, this convenience will cost you, but a basic model is only about $30. See Chapter 26 for details on buying a heart-rate monitor.

Most of the cardio equipment in fitness facilities are heart-rate-monitor compatible. The machines pick up the signal from the monitor around your chest, and your heart rate pops up on the display console, so you don't have to wear the wrist watch. Some machines have heart monitor grips as well; however, these generally can't be used while running or doing high-intensity exercise.

Chest monitors are very accurate, but some are subject to interference from electromagnetic waves like those given off by some treadmills and stair-climbers. Exercising next to someone else who's wearing a monitor may also scramble signals, a sort of electronic equivalent of getting your braces locked with someone else's when you're kissing. You may need at least 4 feet between users for monitors to function properly, although several companies now offer models with a special device to eliminate interference.

Taking your pulse manually

If you aren't wearing a heart-rate monitor, a manual pulse check can give you some useful information about how hard you're working and what to do with the rest of your workout. (We explain how to find your pulse in Chapter 2.)

Feel the steady pounding of blood flowing through your arteries. When you're fairly comfortable with the rhythm, count how many beats you feel in 15 seconds. Then multiply this number by 4 — voilà, your heart rate.

During your workout, take your pulse about every 15 minutes (or do some sort of intensity check) and focus on what you're counting. Otherwise, you may end up counting the number of steps you take on the treadmill rather than the number of pulses in your wrist. You may want to slow down while you take your pulse. True, this is disruptive to your workout, but it's not nearly as disruptive as getting launched off the treadmill.

Chapter 7

Creating a Cardio Program

· ·

In This Chapter

▶ Following cardio plans for good health, weight loss, and peak fitness

▶ Trying fun training techniques and workout plans

▶ Knowing how many calories you're burning

▶ Deciding when to take a day off

· ·

*U*nless you're a professional athlete, you probably don't have unlimited time, energy, or motivation to work out. So you may be wondering: Just how much of this cardio business do I need to do? You may have heard what seem to be conflicting answers to this question from various important-sounding organizations, such as the U.S. Department of Health and Human Services, the World Health Organization, the American College of Sports Medicine, and the U.S. Surgeon General. Perhaps you've heard one authority recommend 30 minutes of exercise a day, while another authority recommends 150 minutes a week. Which recommendation is correct?

The answer is *both*. If you read the fine print on these guidelines, it's clear that some of the recommendations pertain to health benefits and others pertain to weight loss. The bottom line: How often, how long, and how intensely you need to work your heart and lungs depends on your goals. If you're mainly aiming to feel better and lower your risk of developing health problems, you can get away with less huffing and puffing than if you want to fit back into your skinny jeans. If your ambitions rise to, say, trouncing your office nemesis in a 10k running race, you need to work harder still.

In this chapter, we help you develop a cardio plan, depending on whether your goal is to lose weight, improve your health, or get in the best shape of your life. We also discuss training methods, such as interval training, and provide you with a couple of 6-week programs. Finally, we discuss burning calories and knowing when to rest.

Following a Cardio Plan

In the next three sections, we offer cardio guidelines for improving your health, losing weight, and finding out how much you really rock.

Doing cardio for good health

Not everyone has designs on losing weight or hiking the Appalachian Trail. Lowering your odds of developing diabetes, heart disease, and other serious, chronic conditions is a mighty fine goal. Here's how to achieve it.

How long your workouts should last

If your goal is to feel better and live longer, a little aerobic exercise goes a remarkably long way. The U.S. Surgeon General recommends that "people of all ages include a minimum of 30 minutes of physical activity of moderate intensity (such as brisk walking) on most, if not all, days of the week." Research shows that a daily half-hour of exercise is enough to boost your stamina and lower your risk of developing chronic diseases and health conditions (see Chapter 25).

The people who gain the most from aerobic exercise are those who go from being completely slothful to only marginally slothful — not the ones who go from being fit to super fit. The people in the bottom 20 percent of the population, fitness-wise, are 65 percent more likely to die from heart attack, stroke, diabetes, or cancer than the highly fit people in the top 20 percent. However, when those couch potatoes move up just one notch on the fitness scale, by simply adding a daily 30-minute walk, they're only 10 percent more likely to die from these causes than super-fit people.

Here's more good news: Although the recommendation is 30 minutes, nowhere is it written — in the U.S. Constitution, the Bible, or the California Penal Code — that in order to benefit from aerobic exercise, you need to do it for 30 *consecutive* minutes. Studies show that doing three 10-minute bouts of aerobic exercise has about the same health benefits as doing one half-hour continuous session. And in fact, emerging evidence suggests that the "exercise snacking" method may have advantages. Frequent bursts of calorie burn throughout the day may give continual, temporary boosts to your metabolism, and some evidence shows it may help your body burn more fat, especially if some of those mini-sessions are done at a high intensity. (For more details about exercise for weight loss, see "Doing cardio for weight loss.")

How often you should do cardio for good health

For good health, health authorities recommend getting some physical activity "most, if not all, days of the week." Technically speaking, four counts as "most," but we recommend five or six days. If you haven't exercised since the first time skinny jeans were in style, you may want to start with three days a week and build up to more.

How hard you need to push for good health

Being active is the key, even if you don't always reach your target zone (we explain this term in Chapter 6). However, to realize the maximum health benefits — significantly lowering your heart-disease risk, for example — it's wise to work out in your target zone the majority of the time. Plus, even if you have modest goals, you may want to crank up your intensity just to keep things interesting.

Realize that, when you're a beginner, any exercise you do is high-intensity exercise. As you get fitter, you need to adapt your routine to match your increasing strength and lung power.

When Liz's mom started working out, she couldn't complete 10 minutes on the treadmill at 2 mph. After three months, she was able to do 20 minutes at 4 mph — an improvement that in the beginning would have seemed inconceivable.

Doing cardio for weight loss

If your goal is permanent loss of fat (stored energy), the "cardio plan for good health" doesn't cut it. You simply won't burn enough calories to make a significant impact. Here's an overview of what you need to do to slim down. For anyone serious about losing weight, we suggest consulting a registered dietitian and certified fitness trainer to come up with a plan best suited to your specific goals and schedule.

How long your workouts should last for weight loss

A dose of reality: If you want to lose weight, you should aim for at least 60 minutes of daily cardio activity/exercise. And in fact, research shows that an hour of daily activity may only be enough to avoid gaining weight. To actually shed pounds, you may need to exercise even more, in conjunction with making dietary changes. But you don't need to do your 60 minutes of sweating in one dose.

Here's why it takes so much exercise to lose weight: To drop a pound of fat, you need to create a 3,500-calorie deficit; in other words, you need to burn off 3,500 more calories than you eat. A 30-minute power walk on flat ground burns about 120 calories, the same number of calories in less than half a Snickers bar. (See the section "Estimating How Many Calories You're Burning" later in this chapter.) To burn off a whole Snickers bar by walking, you'd have to hoof it for more than an hour at a moderate pace. To burn off 1 pound of fat in one week, without altering your diet, you'd have to walk for more than 2 hours a day!

Don't worry — we're not suggesting that you exercise 2 hours every day! In fact, we think the best way to lose fat is to create a calorie deficit by burning calories through exercise and cutting calories you eat. For example, over the course of a week, you can cut 250 calories per day — by nixing that Snickers bar, for example — and burn an extra 250 calories a day by taking a one-hour walk or a half-hour jog. (For lots of ideas on improving your diet, see Chapter 3.)

But keep in mind that all these numbers are theoretical. In real life, it's difficult to account for individual differences in metabolism, how your body responds to exercise, or how exercise affects your appetite. (Some scientists speculate that women get hungrier after exercise than men, though other evidence suggests that both men and women experience less hunger after a high-intensity workout.)

Many exercisers throw caution to the wind and eat up all the calories they just burned, figuring they've been virtuous by working out, so they deserve a treat. That's a mistake.

Although diet is probably the most important factor for the average person when it comes to weight loss, we caution you not to run away from the treadmill just yet. Every calorie you burn brings you closer to the calorie deficit needed for weight loss, and exercise has untold temporary benefits for your metabolism. Though studies are mixed on exercise as a weight-loss tool, they're very clear that it's essential for weight maintenance; in other words, if you manage to get thin, you had better keep exercising if you want to stay that way. Consider: More than 90 percent of participants in the National Weight Control Registry, a database of people who have lost more than 30 pounds and kept it off for at least five years, say they exercise vigorously on a regular basis, though only 1 percent say they lost weight by exercise alone.

How often you need to do cardio for weight loss

Three days a week isn't likely to get you back to your wedding weight. To make a dent in your excess poundage, you probably need to do five or six cardio workouts a week.

Skinny genes?

Genetics plays a large role in weight loss, as research on twins confirms. In a classic study published in the *New England Journal of Medicine*, researchers sequestered 12 sets of identical male twins for 100 days. Six days a week, the twins were fed 1,000 more calories per day than they needed to maintain their weight; other than walking for 30 minutes daily, the subjects did virtually no physical activity.

At the end of the study, each subject had consumed enough extra calories, theoretically, to gain about 24 pounds. But that's not what happened: Some men gained as little as 9.5 pounds, whereas others gained as much as 29 pounds. The difference in weight gain between the various twin pairs was three times greater than the average difference *within* the pairs.

How hard you need to push for weight loss

We suggest that you work out in your target zone most of the time, including one or two workouts a week at the upper end of the zone (see Chapter 6 for info on your target zone). But keep in mind: If you're pretty darned "deconditioned," even exercising at 50 percent of your maximum heart rate burns calories and therefore helps with weight loss.

You may have heard that exercising at a slow pace is more effective for fat loss than working out more intensely. In fact, many cardio machines have "fat burning" programs that keep you at a slow pace. But this is misleading. As it turns out, the concept of a fat-burning zone is no more real than the twilight zone.

During low-intensity aerobic exercise, your body does use fat as its primary fuel source. As you get closer to your breaking point, your body starts using a smaller percentage of fat and a larger percentage of carbohydrates, another fuel source. However, picking up the pace, or just moving more throughout the day, allows you to burn more total calories, as well as more fat calories.

Here's how: If you go in-line skating for 30 minutes at a leisurely roll, you may burn about 100 calories — about 80 percent of them from fat (so that's 80 fat calories). But if you spend the same amount of time skating with a vengeance over a hilly course, you may burn 300 calories — 30 percent of them from fat (that's 90 fat calories). So at the fast pace, you burn more than double the calories and 10 more fat calories.

Also, recent studies offer tantalizing evidence in favor of busting a gut, especially following a regimen known as *interval training,* alternating short bursts of high-intensity exercise with low-intensity recovery bouts. For example, Australian researchers led two groups of women through stationary bike workouts three days a week. One group alternated 8-second, all-out sprints with effortless, 12-second recovery periods for 20 minutes; the other cruised at a conversational pace for 40 minutes. After 15 weeks, despite an equivalent calorie burn, only the sprinters lost fat — on average, 5.5 pounds of body fat, including 3 pounds of belly fat. The sprinters who were overweight fared best, dropping on average 8½ pounds of blubber.

These researchers believe that interval training is especially helpful for fat loss because the recovery periods enable you to crank it up that much higher, increasing the *afterburn,* the small, temporary post-exercise metabolism boost. Also, high-intensity exercise (like a fun boot camp) seems to trigger a flood of hormones, such as growth hormone and adrenaline, that makes fat more readily available for energy. It's also possible that pushing super hard suppresses appetite. We include sample interval workouts later in this chapter. Other studies suggest that continuous high-intensity exercise may be more effective for burning belly fat than continuous low-intensity exercise.

Still, pushing yourself hard is not something anyone should do on a daily basis, no matter how fit you are or how motivated you are to lose weight. High-intensity exercise carries more injury risk and brings more fatigue; there's no point in killing yourself if you can sustain the fast pace for only a few minutes. If you go slower, you'll be able to exercise a lot longer and therefore burn more calories.

Doing cardio to maximize your fitness

When you get the hang of this exercise thing, you may find that you want more of a challenge. Instead of being satisfied with a boost in energy and a lower cholesterol level, you may want to test yourself in a 5k run or a weeklong hiking tour of Canada.

We know a funeral director from Minnesota who smoked 2½ packs of cigarettes a day and one day realized that if he didn't get his act together, he was going to become one of his own customers. So he quit smoking, took up bicycling, and at age 51 cycled 3,230 miles across the United States. "I've never felt this good in my life," Bernie said upon finishing. "To be able to pedal my butt up a hill without any shortness of breath — that's exhilarating." (How can you get in shape like Bernie?)

How long your workouts should last for maximum fitness

Depending on your sport and your goal, you probably need to mix in at least a couple long workouts — more than an hour — per week. Just make sure you don't increase your total weekly time spent exercising by more than 10 percent a week; otherwise, your risk of injury shoots pretty high. So if you walk 150 minutes one week, walk no more than 165 minutes the next.

In other words, it's not a great idea to do three 30-minute workouts one week and then jump to three 45-minute workouts the next. It's more sensible to increase the time of just one of your workouts to 25 minutes and keep the others at 20.

How often you need to do cardio for maximum fitness

If you want to maximize fitness, five days of cardio a week is a good goal to shoot for. Everyone who does exercise of moderate intensity or higher should take at least one day of complete rest. You can achieve excellent fitness taking two days off a week from cardio (you may still be strength training on those days, or you may choose to take complete days off), so if that's what fits best into your schedule or feels best on your body, don't sweat it, so to speak. In the "Knowing When to Give It a Rest" section later in this chapter, we explain how to tell whether you need more rest.

How hard you need to push for maximum fitness

Even when you're training to get in your best shape ever, you don't want to go all-out every day. In fact, only serious athletes peaking for an event should ever go all-out — and even then, only once or twice a week. Your target zone (see Chapter 6) includes a large range of intensity levels. On some days, stay near the bottom of the range and go for a longer workout; on other days, push harder and go for a shorter workout. Try any or all of the training techniques and workouts we describe in the next section.

The bottom line about training for maximum fitness: Increase your training gradually — don't go longer, more often, and harder all at once. Otherwise, you really increase your chances of injuring yourself. If you really want to ramp up your fitness, we suggest hiring a trainer or sports coach to develop an individualized program for you.

Fun Ways to Dial Up Your Fitness and Burn More Calories

At any fitness level, you can play games to challenge your body and keep your mind interested while you do it. This section discusses training techniques that you can try after about a month or two of training at 50 to 60 percent of your maximum heart rate and provides sample workouts to implement these techniques. (In the next section, we show you what a sample week of exercise may look like for beginners and intermediates.) The less conditioning you start with, the more cautious you should be.

Interval training

With *interval training,* you alternate short, fairly intense spurts of exercise
with periods of relatively easy exercise. For example, say you're out bicycling.
After warming up for 15 minutes or so, you may try cycling all-out for 30
seconds and follow this with a few minutes of easy pedaling until your heart
rate slows down a little, to about 120 or fewer beats per minute. Then you
do another tough 30-second interval, and so on. In essence, you're switching
between the low and high ends of your target zone.

When you first try interval training, keep the high-intensity periods short —
15 to 30 seconds. Follow these periods with at least three times as much active
rest (so, 45 to 90 seconds). *Active rest* means that you keep moving between
intervals instead of stopping dead. So after you do that 30-second bike sprint,
pedal slowly for about 90 seconds. You may need even more recovery than
that, especially if you're a beginner. As you become more accustomed to
higher levels, you can increase the length of the high-intensity intervals as you
decrease the length of the low-intensity intervals. Eventually, you can aim for a
1:1 hard-to-easy ratio, measuring intervals in terms of time or distance.

Here are a couple of interval workouts to try. In Tables 7-1 and 7-2, THZ
stands for *target heart-rate zone* (see Chapter 6). The charts call for walking
and running, but you can substitute any other type of cardio exercise.

Table 7-1		Beginner Interval Workout	
Workout Segment	*Duration*	*Activity*	*Pace*
Warm-up	5 minutes	Walk	Easy pace (low end of THZ)
Interval 1	2 minutes	Walk	Brisk pace (high end of THZ)
Interval 2	2 minutes	Walk	Moderate pace (middle of THZ)
Repeat intervals 1 and 2 three to five times for a total of 12 to 20 minutes.			
Cool-down	5 minutes	Walk	Easy pace

Table 7-2		Intermediate Interval Workout	
Workout Segment	*Duration*	*Activity*	*Pace*
Warm-up	5 minutes	Walk	Easy pace (low end of THZ)
Interval 1	3 minutes	Run	Brisk pace (high end of THZ)
Interval 2	2 minutes	Walk	Moderate pace (middle of THZ)
Repeat intervals 1 and 2 three to five times for a total of 15 to 25 minutes.			
Cool-down	5 minutes	Walk	Easy pace

Fartlek: Racing to the next landmark

Fartlek is basically interval training without an exact measure of time or distance. This charming word means "speed play" in Swedish. You just do your intervals whenever you feel like it. You may try sprinting to every other telephone pole. Or set your sights on that horse standing in the field down the road and pick up your pace until you reach him. Your fast and slow periods vary with your energy level and motivation.

Uphill battles

You can add hills to walking, biking, running, or skating workouts. You have to work harder when you come to a hill, but ultimately you're rewarded with extra strength and stamina. As a bonus, going uphill can burn twice as many calories as exercising on flat land. One fun drill is to do "hill repeats," a workout regimen that involves — you guessed it — conquering the same hill repeatedly. Here's a good, basic workout to try:

1. **Find a long, fairly steep hill that takes you 90 seconds to 2 minutes to run up at a moderate pace.**

2. **Warm up for 5 minutes at an easy pace on flat terrain, and then sprint to the top of the hill at between 80 and 90 percent of your best effort.**

3. **When you reach the top, turn around and jog down slowly, zigging and zagging across the hill.**

4. **Repeat this sequence four to eight times.**

5. **Cool down for 5 minutes at an easy pace on the flat.**

Here's a trick to make hill workouts seem easier: Pick a landmark that's partway up the hill, such as a bush or mailbox. Pretend that you have a rope in your hands and cast it over your landmark. Now picture pulling yourself up the hill with your imaginary rope. When you reach your landmark, cast your rope on something farther up the hill and keep doing this until you reach the top.

Another fun type of hill repeat is to walk, run, or cycle uphill for a predetermined amount of time — say, 3 minutes. When your stopwatch hits 3 minutes, you stop and go back down at a super easy pace. Notice how far you've gone, remembering the particular tree or sign you've reached. Go up the hill four times, and each time, aim to make it farther up the hill.

Tempo workouts

Tempo workouts help you move faster. During a tempo drill, you move at a pace that you consider challenging but not brutal, keeping that pace for 4 to 10 minutes. Do that a couple of times each workout. In between, exercise at your normal pace. If you're new to tempo training, begin with short tempos and gradually increase their length. Anyone training for a local road race or a bike-a-thon will find tempo work helpful. Tempo differs from intervals in that the hard intervals are longer but not quite as intense.

Here's a sample tempo workout for cycling. You can follow this pattern with any kind of cardio exercise.

1. **Cycle at a very easy pace on flat terrain for about 5 minutes.**

2. **Ratchet up the intensity to between 65 and 85 percent of your maximum effort, holding this pace for 6 minutes.**

3. **Back off the pace for 2 minutes.**

4. **Repeat the moderate- or high-intensity cycles twice more.**

5. **Cool down by cycling at a very easy pace.**

Lifestyle movement

You don't need to make a formal appointment with Dr. Exercise to burn calories or do good things for your body. In fact, many experts think that incorporating more movement into your daily life gets you better results than regular exercise sessions, and that the best results may come from pairing more daily movement with regular workouts. When you think about how little the average person now moves on a daily basis, this makes sense. With the advent of modern "conveniences" such as leaf blowers, snowblowers, remote controls, self-propelled vacuum cleaners, and the like, we've essentially engineered movement out of our lives.

Some studies show that the average American now spends more than half his day with his tush firmly rooted in the seat of a chair. Consider what would happen if you kicked that chair aside for just two hours and decided to stand instead. Standing burns only about 115 calories an hour, but the calorie burn while sitting is downright paltry — only about 80 calories an hour. The extra 70 calories a day you can burn while giving up your seat on the train or standing while you watch your kid play soccer can add up to nearly 500 calories a week. (You burn even more if you pace up and down the sidelines.) That's 26,000 calories a year, or the equivalent of 7 pounds lost, or at least not gained. And again — that's without pressing the "on" button of the treadmill.

You can bump up the calorie burn even more by pacing while on the phone, walking up the escalator instead of just going along for the ride, parking at the far end of the parking lot — all those standard suggestions you may never have paid attention to in the past but that really do make a difference. Also consider washing your own car, volunteering for Habitat for Humanity, retrieving the tennis ball someone hit over the fence, and other opportunities to burn calories without changing into your workout clothes. We're not suggesting for a minute that you give up, cut back on, or avoid starting an honest-to-goodness exercise program, but we're real believers that leading a more active lifestyle is mighty good for your heart, muscles, and waistline. If you lack the motivation to, say, walk into Starbucks for your latte rather than use the drive-through window, strap on a pedometer and watch your motivation soar. (See the sidebar "Making every step count" for more information about pedometers.)

Putting It All Together: Sample 6-Week Exercise Programs

In the preceding sections, we give you several different cardio workouts to choose from. But you still may wonder which workouts to do on which days. Here are two sample cardio training plans lasting 6 weeks.

Sample beginner program

This 6-week program is a great intro to cardio if you haven't done much formal physical activity but you're confident that you can walk briskly for at least 20 minutes without feeling winded, dizzy, or sick. This is a walking program, but you can substitute any cardio activity if you prefer, as long as you strive for the intensity levels suggested. Be sure to warm up and cool down for 2 to 5 minutes.

Table 7-3 describes Week 1 of the beginner program, and the bulleted list that follows explains what to do in the following weeks. In the table, THZ stands for *target heart-rate zone* (see Chapter 6).

Table 7-3		Week 1 of a Beginner Cardio Program	
Day	*Workout*	*Description*	*Variations*
Day 1	Moderate Walk	20-minute walk at a moderate pace (mid THZ)	You can split this into two 10-minute walks
Day 2	Moderate Walk	20-minute walk at a moderate pace (mid THZ)	You can split this into two 10-minute walks
Day 3	Interval Walk	Alternate 2 minutes of fast-paced walking (high end of THZ) with 2 minutes of moderate-paced walking (mid THZ); repeat for a total of 3–5 interval cycles or 12–20 minutes	
Day 4	REST		
Day 5	Moderate Walk	20-minute walk at a moderate pace (mid THZ)	You can split this into two 10-minute walks
Day 6	Moderate Walk	20-minute walk at a moderate pace (mid THZ)	You can split this into two 10-minute walks
Day 7	REST		

Here's how to modify the program in the subsequent weeks:

- **Week 2:** Increase each of the Moderate Walk workouts (Days 1, 2, 5, and 6) to 24 minutes.

- **Week 3:** Increase the Interval Walk workout (Day 3) by a total of 4 minutes: Add one 2-minute fast-paced interval and 2 minutes of moderate recovery.

- **Week 4:** Increase each of the Moderate Walk workouts (Days 1, 2, 5, and 6) to 28 minutes.

- **Week 5:** Increase the Interval Walk (Day 3) by 4 minutes.

- **Week 6:** Substitute one of the Moderate Walk workouts with an Interval Walk workout so you're now doing two Interval Walks per week.

Sample intermediate program

This 6-week program is for you if you can already jog at an easy pace for 5 continuous minutes without feeling winded, dizzy, or sick and you can easily walk for 30 continuous minutes. This is a walk/run program, but you can substitute any cardio activity as long as you strive for the suggested intensity levels (for info on intensity, see Chapter 6). Be sure to warm up and cool down for 2 to 5 minutes.

Table 7-4 shows Week 1 of the program, and the bulleted list that follows explains how to modify the plan in Weeks 2 through 5.

Table 7-4	Week 1 of an Intermediate Cardio Program		
Day	*Workout*	*Description*	*Variations*
Day 1	Moderate Run/Walk	Alternate 5 minutes of running at a moderate pace (mid THZ) with 2 minutes of walking at an easy pace (low end of THZ) for 2–4 interval cycles	
Day 2	Moderate Walk	30 minutes walk at a moderate pace (mid THZ)	You can split this into three 10-minute walks
Day 3	Moderate Run/Walk	Alternate 5 minutes of running at a moderate pace (mid THZ) with 2 minutes of walking at an easy pace (low end of THZ) for 2–4 interval cycles	
Day 4	REST		
Day 5	Moderate Walk	30 minutes walk at a moderate pace (mid THZ)	You can split this into three 10-minute walks
Day 6	Interval Run	Alternate 2 minutes of running at a high-intensity pace (high end of THZ) with 2 minutes of running at an easy pace for 3–5 interval cycles	
Day 7	REST		

Here's how to modify the program in the subsequent weeks:

- **Week 2:** Increase each of the Moderate Walk workouts (Days 2 and 5) to 34 minutes.
- **Week 3:** Increase each of the Moderate Run/Walk workouts (Days 1 and 3) by 7 minutes each.
- **Week 4:** Increase the Interval Run workout (Day 6) to 34 minutes.
- **Week 5:** Increase each of the Moderate Walk workouts (Days 2 and 5) to 38 minutes.
- **Week 6:** Substitute one of the Moderate Walk workouts (Day 2 or 5) with a Moderate Run workout in which you run at an easy-to-moderate pace for 30 minutes (or break it up into three 10-minute runs).

Estimating How Many Calories You're Burning

We're guessing that no matter what your fitness level or goals, you're curious to know how many calories you burn in a given workout. The truth is all calorie counts are a rough estimate. Unless you're hooked up to a special machine that measures your oxygen and heart-rate levels via gas mask and blood tests, you need to accept the numbers here — and the numbers you find elsewhere — as an estimate. If you eat a 250-calorie piece of cake, you may or may not officially burn it off when your treadmill readout hits 250. And although spot checks show that the calorie counts of foods are often understated, keep in mind that the calorie burn of exercise is often overstated.

Table 7-5 may serve as a reality check to some of the claims you see in advertisements for exercise machines — claims such as, "Maximize your workout and burn over 1,000 calories per hour!" That claim may happen to be true — if you crank up the machine to the highest level and have bionic legs. If you're a beginner, you'll last about 30 seconds at that pace, at which point you'll have burned 8.3 calories, and the paramedics will pick you up off the floor and haul your wilted body away on a stretcher.

There's a better approach to calorie burning: Choose an activity that you can sustain for a good while — say, at least 10 or 15 minutes. Sure, running burns more calories than walking, but if running wipes you out after a half mile or bothers your knees, you're better off walking.

Table 7-5 gives calorie estimates for a number of popular aerobic activities. The number of calories you actually burn depends on the intensity of your workout, your weight, your muscle mass, and your metabolism. In general, a beginner is capable of burning 4 or 5 calories per minute of exercise, and a very fit person can burn 10 to 12 calories per minute.

The table includes a few stop-and-go sports such as tennis and basketball. Activities like these are not aerobic in the truest sense, but they can still give you a great workout and contribute to good health and weight loss. The numbers in this chart apply to a 150-pound person. (If you weigh less, you'll burn a little less; if you weigh more, you'll burn a little more.)

Table 7-5	Calories Burned during Popular Activities			
Activity	*15 min.*	*30 min.*	*45 min.*	*60 min.*
Aerobic dance	171	342	513	684
Basketball	141	282	432	564
Bicycling				
12 mph	142	283	425	566
15 mph	177	354	531	708
18 mph	213	425	638	850
Boxing	165	330	495	660
Circuit weight training	189	378	576	756
Golf (carrying clubs)	87	174	261	348
In-line skating	150	300	450	600
Jumping rope, 60–80 skips/min.	143	286	429	572
Karate, tae kwon do	180	360	540	720
Kayaking	75	150	225	300
Racquetball	114	228	342	456
Rowing machine	104	208	310	415
Running				
10-minute miles	183	365	548	731
8-minute miles	223	446	670	893
Ski machine	141	282	423	564
Skiing, cross-country	146	291	437	583
Skiing, downhill	105	210	315	420
Swimming				
Freestyle, 35 yds./min.	124	248	371	497
Freestyle, 50 yds./min.	131	261	392	523
Tennis, singles	116	232	348	464
Tennis, doubles	43	85	128	170
Walking				
20-minute miles, flat	60	120	180	240
20-minute miles, hills	81	162	243	324
15-minute miles, flat	73	146	219	292
15-minute miles, hills	102	206	279	412
Water aerobics	70	140	210	280

Knowing When to Give It a Rest

For most people, exercising too much is about as big a problem as saving too much money. However, some beginners — in their zeal to make up for 20 years of neglecting their bodies — vow to exercise every day for the next 20 years. This is not a good idea. If you're trying to get fit, your workouts are only part of the equation; rest is just as important.

Aim for a balance between hard days and easy days. If you do an intense interval day on Monday, do an easy workout Tuesday. If you do two tough days in a row, your legs may feel like someone inserted lead pipes in them while you were sleeping. Everyone who is exercising at a moderate or high intensity should rest at least one day a week. (Just don't let that one day off slip into three years.) And when we say take a rest day, we mean no planned exercise. ***Remember:*** An easy day does not count as a rest day, although we believe it is a good idea to get plenty of low-intensity "lifestyle activity" in your day, such as standing and strolling.

In addition to taking a day or two off each week from formal exercise, you may also want to take an easy week every month or two. So if you usually jog 15 miles a week, cut back to 7 just for the week. Drastic cutbacks can help remotivate you and give your body the vacation it may need.

There's no magic formula to determine exactly how much rest is best for your goals and fitness level. But here's a good rule: If you're doing everything right, you should be able to wake up in the morning and say, "I know my workout's going to be really good," rather than, "How the heck am I gonna drag my butt to the gym?"

Exercisers of all levels are susceptible to overtraining. For an elite athlete, overtraining may be running 80 miles in a week; for a beginner, running 8 miles may be too much. Here are some signs that you've overdone it:

- ✔ Your resting heart rate sounds like a jackhammer drilling through concrete. In other words, if your heart rate is way above what it normally is — say, about 10 beats — take it very easy or take a day or two off. (For details about your resting heart rate, see Chapter 2.)

- ✔ You feel chronically sore or weak. If you lift a ketchup bottle and it feels like a 10-pound dumbbell, stay home.

- ✔ You get chronic colds and infections.

- ✔ You're not sleeping well.

- ✔ You're irritable, anxious, or depressed. It's not a good sign if you lock your keys in your car and smash the window to retrieve them instead of calling the auto club.

- ✔ You can't concentrate or you feel disoriented. If you make a left-hand turn signal while you're on a stationary bike, it's time for a rest.

Making every step count

Looking for inspiration to take the stairs instead of the elevator? Clip on a *pedometer,* a beeper-sized gizmo that research shows can dramatically boost your motivation to move.

Many of us perceive ourselves as active when in reality we're just busy, multitasking from our desk rather than walking across the hall to speak with a co-worker. A few days wearing a pedometer will show you just where you stand (or sit, as the case may be).

The typical American adult takes 5,900 to 6,900 steps a day, a range just above the sedentary mark of 5,000 steps. In stark contrast, traditional Amish women take 14,000 steps daily, and Amish men take 18,000. Not surprisingly, obesity is virtually unheard of among the Amish.

We're not suggesting you need to match the horse-and-buggy crowd. But start by shooting for 7,500 steps a day, then increase your daily steps to 10,000, and ultimately try to take at least 12,500 steps a day.

Research suggests that setting your daily exercise goal in terms of steps, rather than miles or minutes, makes the target seem more achievable and can increase your daily step count by 2,000 to 4,000 steps. Having that little reminder at your hip may suddenly inspire you to mow the lawn yourself instead of waiting for your spouse to do it.

Pedometers, available on countless fitness-product Web sites for $20 to $30, are a real fitness bargain.

Chapter 8

Using Cardio Machines

. . . .

In This Chapter

▶ Using a treadmill, elliptical trainer, stationary bike, stair-climber, or rowing machine

▶ Fighting boredom in your cardio workout

▶ Knowing whether to trust calorie counters on cardio machines

. . . .

*W*alk into a health club or fitness-equipment store, and you're likely to encounter rows of high-tech contraptions that appear to be part video game, part escalator, and part lawn mower. Don't be alarmed. The consoles of these machines may resemble the control panel of a Mars Explorer, but with a little help, a rookie can easily master the flashing red dots and beeping green arrows. Be thankful for all this technology because it can make exercising in the great indoors entertaining. For all your sweat, the screen offers you instant gratification — the number of miles that you walk, steps that you climb, minutes that you cycle, and calories that you burn.

Cardiovascular machines tend to come and go. Since the first edition of this book, we've seen the rise and fall of various riders, gliders, and skaters. So we're not going run down every crazy invention that's made its way onto an infomercial. Instead, this chapter covers the proven machines, such as treadmills, ellipticals, bikes, stair-climbers, and rowers. We tell you how to position your body on each machine so that you burn the most calories and avoid injury. Plus, we offer tips on taking the drudgery out of exercising in place.

Most exercisers have a favorite cardio machine and one that they probably can't stand. Some people find the treadmill invigorating; others consider it more tedious than peeling potatoes. We suggest you try all the machines at your gym or at an equipment store before you buy one. No single cardio machine is better than the rest. What matters most is how often you use the thing.

Treadmill

Treadmills are the motorized equivalent of walking or running in place. You simply keep up with a belt that's moving under your feet (see Figure 8-1). Treadmill workouts burn about the same number of calories as walking or running outdoors. The only exception seems to be running uphill. When you incline the treadmill to simulate running up a grade, it's somewhat easier than running up real-life hills that are equally steep. But walking uphill on a treadmill achieves virtually the same calorie burn as walking uphill outdoors.

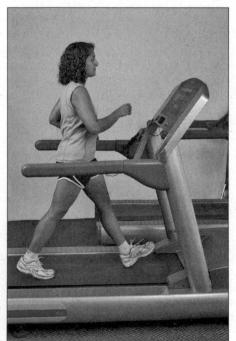

Figure 8-1: Treadmills are a great indoor cardio alternative.

You may see a newer type of treadmill at your gym, one that's wider and shorter than a traditional model. It's called an *incline trainer*. These treadmills typically go only to about 5 miles per hour in speed, but they incline a lot — up to a 40-percent grade, the equivalent of a very steep hiking trail. Incline trainers are a terrific training tool for those who want a tough workout but don't feel like pushing their speed. They're also great for people who want to burn a lot of calories, train for hiking and walking, chisel their leg muscles, or just want something new. We love incline trainers, but if you have bad knees or your back can't handle the stress of walking up hills, proceed with caution. Know that you don't have to pump the hill up to the full incline to get a great workout, and realize that incline trainers are strictly for walking, not jogging or running.

Who will like it

Treadmills are especially popular in crowded cities, where you need to be part cutting horse, part smog filter to run or walk through the streets. Treadmills are great for beginners because they require little coordination to use, and they're good for times where it may not be safe to run alone. Plus, treadmills can move at a slow enough pace to accommodate even the most out-of-shape exercisers. People with back pain, bad knees, or weak ankles often find treadmills kinder to their joints than concrete or cement.

Today's treadmills are springier and more shock-absorbing than ever. Many have added flashy new features, such as Internet hookups, which let you race against people from all over the world or simply stroll through a relaxing beach scene. Many also store and analyze your personal data on a chip that you can pop into your computer or via a direct link-up to a special Web site. Of course, treadmills also offer basic features such as a heart-rate monitor and speed, incline, time, and distance controls. In Chapter 19, we suggest features to look for when you shop for a home treadmill.

Why the treadmill may not be your thing

You need a very strong or very blank mind to do long workouts on a treadmill. Most people find more than a half hour on this machine mind-numbing, even while listening to their favorite music on their iPod or zoning out to one of the more than 500 cable channels you can now watch through the built-in TV screen. If you crave the wind whipping through your hair and scenery flashing by, reserve the treadmills for emergency cardio situations only. Running also places more impact on your joints than most other indoor cardiovascular activities and may not be a favorite if you have a bad lower back, achy knees, or weak ankles.

Treadmill user tips

Treadmills are among the easiest cardio machines to use. Still, treadmill users are not immune to poor posture. And if you're not paying attention, you can stumble. On occasion you may see someone slide off the treadmill like a can of beans on a supermarket conveyor belt. Here are some tips to make sure this doesn't happen to you:

> ✔ **Start slowly.** Most treadmills have safety features that prevent them from starting out at breakneck speeds or stop them immediately if you stumble, but don't take chances. Always place one foot on either side of the belt as you turn on the machine, and step on the belt only after you determine that it's moving at the slow set-up speed, usually between 1 and 2 miles per hour.

✔ **Don't rely on the handrails.** Holding on for balance as you figure out how to use the machine is okay, but let go as soon as you feel comfortable. You move more naturally if you swing your arms freely. You're working at too high a level if you have to imitate a water-skier — in other words, if you hold onto the front rails and lean back. This is a common phenomenon among people who incline the treadmill, and this position is bad news for your elbows and for the machine. Plus, you're not fooling anyone; you're burning far fewer calories than the readout indicates. However, if you have balance issues, go ahead and grasp the handrails lightly so that you feel steady and secure.

✔ **Look forward.** When you're in the middle of a workout and someone calls your name, don't turn around to answer. This piece of advice may seem obvious now, but wait until it happens to you.

✔ **Expect to feel disoriented.** The first few times you use a treadmill, you may feel dizzy when you step off. Your body is just wondering why the ground suddenly stopped moving. Don't worry. Most people only experience this vertigo once or twice.

✔ **Never go barefoot.** Always wear a good pair of walking or running shoes for your treadmill workout.

✔ **Don't read on the treadmill.** You risk losing your balance and stumbling off the side or back.

Elliptical Trainer

Just when we thought that all good cardio machines had been invented, along came the elliptical trainer. Ellipticals have two large, fat foot pedals. Your feet follow a path that's sort of a stretched-out oval known as an ellipse (hence, the name *elliptical* trainer) — see Figure 8-2. The motion feels like a mix between fast walking, stair-climbing, and cross-country skiing. There are now variations on the movement; the Cybex Arc Trainer, for instance, has more of a swinging motion. Some models also have arm poles where you pump your arms as you move your feet, and some of these have heart-rate monitors built in. The popularity of the elliptical now rivals that of the treadmill; in some gyms, you see a line for the elliptical and some unused treadmills.

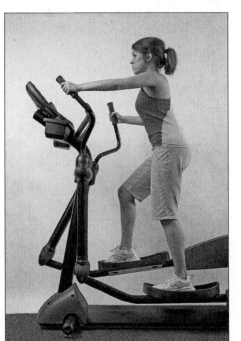

Figure 8-2:
Elliptical trainers feel like a mix between fast walking, stair-climbing, and cross-country skiing.

Who will like it

Runners who need a day off from the pounding gravitate toward this machine like moviegoers to the concession stand. It's also popular with walkers looking for a more spirited workout and pregnant walkers or runners who find the motion much easier on their joints than pounding the pavement or treadmill belt.

Suzanne, who used to find the elliptical motion awkward, became the machine's biggest fan when she got pregnant with twins; she discovered it was the only cardio machine she could use without feeling as big as a pregnant elephant. The elliptical trainer is also popular among people who are bored with stair-climbing or find stair-climbing hard on their knees.

Why the elliptical may not be your thing

If you're in shape, it takes a lot more wherewithal to push yourself on the elliptical than on some other machines. People with Achilles problems and knee problems don't always do well on this machine. And some people experience toe numbness after a few minutes. You may be able to avoid this by wearing thinner socks and lighter, more flexible shoes.

Elliptical-trainer user tips

Elliptical trainers can take a bit of getting used to, but they don't require great skill. You'll be up and running — well, elliptical-ing — in no time by following these tips:

- **Limit backward pedaling.** Contrary to popular belief, pedaling backward does *not* work your buttocks more than pedaling forward (and it may even be hard on your knees). Both motions emphasize the front thigh muscles, so do it once in a while but not for any prolonged amount of time.

- **Use the machine's versatile features.** To adjust the intensity of your workout, you can pedal faster, raise the incline, increase the resistance, or any combination.

- **Don't lock your knees.** Keep a slight bend in your knees, keeping the motion smooth.

- **Remind yourself to stand up straight.** Although the elliptical trainer lends itself to better technique than the stair-climber, you can still commit postural violations such as leaning too far forward and hugging the console.

Stationary Bicycle

Bikes come in three varieties: upright, studio, and recumbent. Upright bikes roughly simulate a regular bike, only you don't go anywhere. Studio bikes, more commonly called Spin bikes, are upright bikes that more closely resemble road bikes, with a flywheel, a skinnier seat, similar pedal and seat positions, and an absence of electronic gadgetry (see Figure 8-3). Recumbent bikes have bucket seats so you pedal out in front of you. No type is superior; which one you like best is a matter of preference. The recumbent does offer more back support and may be more comfortable for people with lower-back pain but may not be ideal if you're in the later stages of pregnancy or sporting an extra-large tummy. Avid road cyclists tend to feel more at home on a Spin bike, the type used in indoor cycling classes, also called *spinning classes.* Many gyms also include a Spin bike or two among the high-tech cardio machines.

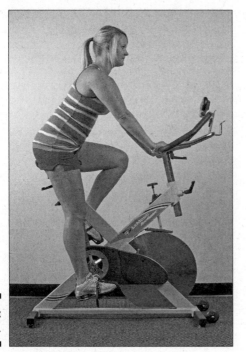

Figure 8-3:
A Spin bike.

Who will like it

Bikes are great for toning your thighs (and recumbents are especially good for your butt), and they give your knees a break while offering a terrific cardiovascular workout. Bikes also suit anyone who wants to read while working out. Holding a book or magazine in place on a stair-climber or elliptical is tougher, and it's impossible on a rowing machine.

Why the bike may not be your thing

Some hard-core cyclists complain that even Spin bikes aren't similar enough to outdoor bikes, though cyclists who live in snowy climates tend to complain about this less. In general, stationary bikes don't offer as much calorie burn as a treadmill or elliptical unless you work really, really hard. Different bike brands offer very different positioning. You may like some bike brands more than others.

Stationary-bike user tips

Bikes give you less opportunity to use atrocious form than do most other machines. Still, there's room for injury or discomfort. Here are some tips to help you avoid both:

✔ **Adjust the seat.** When the pedal is at the lowest position, your leg should be almost, but not quite, straight. Your knees shouldn't feel crunched when they're at the top of the pedal stroke. With a recumbent bike, you adjust the seat forward and back, rather than up and down, but the principles are the same. Spin bikes typically also have a seat adjustment that pushes the seat farther forward or back, and two handlebar adjustments so you can lean forward and grip the bars without compromising good form.

✔ **Get to know the display panel.** For instance, notice how many levels the bike has. Some bikes feature 12 levels; others have 40. So if you just hop on and press Level 6, you'll get two very different workouts. Also, pay attention to your *cadence* — that is, how many revolutions per minute (rpm) you're cycling. Varying your cadence is a good idea. You may want to hum along at 80 rpm for 5 minutes and then do 30-second intervals at 100 rpm using the same tension level.

✔ **Adjust the pedal straps so that your feet feel snug — but don't let the straps cut off your circulation.** Riding a bike with the foot straps is much more comfortable and efficient than pedaling without them. Don't remove the pedal straps from your bike; this forces the next person to waste time putting them back on.

✔ **Don't pedal with just your toes.** Otherwise, you may bring on foot and calf cramps. Instead, press from the ball of your foot and through your heel as you pump downward on the pedal, and pull up with the top of your foot on the upstroke.

✔ **Don't hunch over.** Rounding your back is the way to develop back and neck pain. Don't get your upper body into the effort, either. Instead, keep your chest up, shoulders back and down, ears in line with your shoulders, and belly button drawn in. Unlike some other machines, stationary bikes don't offer a total-body workout; don't try to achieve one. If you have to rock wildly from side to side, grit your teeth, or clench the handlebars, you need to lighten your load.

✔ **Make sure the bike is sturdy.** At one New York City gym, a guy was pedaling furiously when the frame collapsed and the bike shot forward and out the second story window — with the guy still seated. Ironically, he landed on a bike rack below. This being New York, the doorman said, "Hey buddy, you can't park that thing here." Actually, we made the last part up, but the rest of the story was reported on the news. Although the guy was hospitalized, he walked away more or less unscathed.

Stair-Climber

The most common type of stair-climber you now see is a rolling staircase, which looks sort of like a department store escalator to nowhere (see Figure 8-4). You used to see a lot more of the pedal-stepper variety, which involves standing on two pedals and pressing your feet up and down. As the elliptical trainer has gained popularity, it seems to have stolen a large part of the pedal-stepping audience, so most gyms have a token pedal stair-climber or two. On the other hand, the rolling staircase model seems to have come back into favor, possibly because it involves a heckuva workout. It's actually more intense than real stair climbing because it only goes up — and up and up.

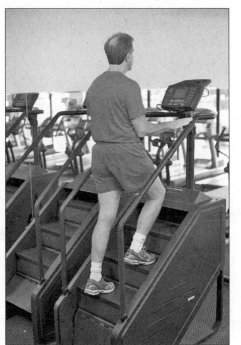

Figure 8-4:
The rolling staircase is a good calorie burner and butt toner.

Rolling staircases have been around a lot longer than steppers. At the turn of the century, federal prisoners were forced to climb on them to provide electrical power to the prison facility. When modern rolling staircases first came out, there were a few kinks to work out, like the fact that they had a habit of collapsing when in use. Liz had a client who came in for a workout on her wedding day. The stairs folded underneath her and she slid to the ground, breaking an arm and a leg in the process. We're happy to report that this defect has long since been fixed, and rolling staircases are as safe as any other piece of equipment in the gym, as long as you use them correctly. Plus, they offer a killer workout.

Who will like it

Women in particular love stair-climbers because these machines do a good job of toning the butt and thighs. People who want to get in shape for skiing, climbing, hiking, running, and, of course, stair-climbing races also love stair-climbers. The rolling staircase burns a ton of calories and is a good alternative workout for walkers and runners looking for a day off the road or mill.

This is a good time to clear up the myth that stair-climbing builds big, bulky muscles in your legs. The truth is that virtually any type of activity will increase the size of your muscles if you work very slowly against a lot of tension. And if you have a genetic predisposition toward building muscular thighs, you're pretty much going to fight against that no matter what you do. But for most people, this isn't an issue. The fact is, stair-climbing is a terrific way to burn calories, tone your legs, and help you climb real stairs more efficiently.

Why the stair-climber may not be your thing

Beginners may get frustrated because stair-climbing is no vacation in Maui. If you're a complete novice, you may not last 5 minutes, even on the lowest level. In this case, use other machines, such as the treadmill or stationary bike, until you build up some stamina and strength. Also, stair-climbing, especially the steppers, can be tough to get the hang of; novices sometimes find themselves sinking to the floor before they're able to get into the rhythm. Finally, stair-climbing bothers some people's knees. To minimize this problem, do exercises that strengthen your thighs, both front and back, because those are the muscles that hold your knees together.

Stair-climber user tips

Proper form is butchered on the stair-climber more than on any other single piece of machinery, especially the stair-stepper kind, but even people who use the rolling staircases aren't immune. We've seen people clutch the railings so tightly their knuckles turn white — or hug the console like it's a long-lost relative. Some less-informed exercisers think it's really cool to be able to climb at the machine's highest level, regardless of their form. It's not. When you clutch the rails (or lean forward), you transfer your weight from your legs to your arms or the machine, which drastically reduces the number of calories you burn and may cause wrist pain.

Fortunately, many stair-climber manufacturers have rectified this problem by designing handles that point straight up. This makes cheating more difficult. Still, we see people hanging on these newer handles. Here's how to use stair-climbers the right way:

- ✔ **Rest your hands — or better yet, your fingertips — lightly on the bar in front of you or on the side rails.** Don't grip the rails any tighter than you'd grip a paper cup. And never reverse your wrists so that your fingertips are pointing toward the floor and your elbows are turned up to the ceiling. You really should be able to use the stair-climber without holding on to the railing at all, but using the railing for balance (within reason) is okay. If you must hang on to keep up with the machine, you're going too fast.

- ✔ **Stand upright with a slight forward lean at the hips.** Don't overcorrect your form by standing upright like a Marine at inspection. A slight — and we mean slight — forward lean helps keep your knees from locking and protects your lower back from overarching.

- ✔ **Keep your entire foot on the pedal or the stair.** This helps your rear end and thighs get a full workout and prevents you from overburdening your calf muscles. On the rolling staircase, it also prevents you from stumbling.

- ✔ **On the rolling staircase, pick up your entire foot and place it back down again on the next step.** If you get lazy feet, you'll be rewarded with a stumbling motion that's a lot like when you get lazy feet on a real staircase. Whichever type of machine you use, dedicate at least part of your brain to concentrating on using correct form.

Rowing Machine

The rower isn't the most popular piece in the gym, but it should be, because it offers such a fantastic workout. Every gym typically has one tucked in a corner somewhere. Seek it out and at least give it the courtesy of one workout. Good rowers consist of a flywheel, a fan, and a cable with a handle attached to one end (see Figure 8-5). You pull the handle toward you as you slide the seat backward. The fan creates air resistance, which makes the movement feel pretty close to skimming across the water.

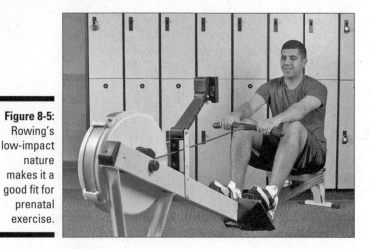

Who will like it

Anyone looking for a great total-body workout will love rowing. If you're trying to get in shape for a rowing or paddling sport, this is the way to go. Contrary to popular belief, rowing isn't bad for your back. If you row correctly, you initiate the movement from your legs and buttocks, which eliminates excess stress on your back muscles.

Why the rower may not be your thing

Some people get bored with rowing in a matter of seconds. Others are intimidated because rowing is not as natural as walking, running, or biking. We know one guy who smacked the handle into his forehead over and over again until some kind soul in the gym showed him the proper form.

Rowing-machine user tips

Experienced rowers make rowing look easy, but when you actually sit down at the machine, you may find that it takes a fair amount of coordination. Here are some tips to fine-tune the motion:

- ✔ **Think legs, legs, legs.** Concentrate on initiating the movement with your buttocks rather than your lower back. Don't fully straighten your knees. Even when you're completely extended, your knees should be a little soft.

✔ **Don't round your back.** Hunching over is the way to give yourself back pain. Don't lean all the way back at the end of the stroke, either. You're in proper position when your upper body is leaning backward about 45 degrees.

✔ **Pull the handle in a smooth, continuous stroke.** Don't stop at the most stretched-out and bent positions.

Can you trust the cardio calorie counters?

Most people do get a psychological boost from knowing how many calories they just burned from a cardio workout. There's just one problem: The information may not be accurate.

For the most part, the formulas used to calculate calories burned are derived from tests done on healthy young males — and in some cases, elite athletes working near their maximum effort. This does not always translate accurately for the rest of us. For instance, one study found that fitness equipment readouts may overestimate calorie count for obese women by as much as 80 calories for 30 minutes of moderate-intensity walking.

Other research has found that calorie predictions are skewed even further if you lean your body weight against the handrails, grip tightly, or otherwise position your body on a machine in a way that makes the exercise less strenuous. Some studies have shown that calculations can be off by as much as 50 percent.

Sometimes it's not the formulas or your technique that skew the calorie count; it's the deceptive marketing strategy of the machine's manufacturer. A researcher for one cardio-equipment manufacturer admitted to us that his company intentionally boosts the calorie information by as much as 30 percent so that people may, subconsciously, prefer their machines over other brands.

The most accurate machines tend to be the treadmill and the stationary bike because the contraptions have been so well-studied. In recent years, stair-climbers have adjusted calorie estimates drastically downward to better reflect reality.

The bottom line: Realize that the calorie figures are simply estimates. Use the calorie information to motivate you, but don't be a slave to it, and don't rely on the numbers to validate your efforts.

Chapter 9

Exercising Outdoors

· ·

· ·

*F*resh air: What a concept! With all the super-high-tech indoor exercise contraptions available these days, it's easy to forget you can get an effective workout in the great outdoors, often for no cost other than a pair of athletic shoes. You may even burn more calories per minute in the fresh air because outdoor activities sometimes involve more muscles than their indoor counterparts. For example, when you park yourself on a stationary bicycle, your upper-body muscles basically get a free ride — you can easily flip the pages of a magazine as you pedal away. But when you take your bike out for a spin, your chest, arm, abdominal, and back muscles are all called up for active duty, and you expend extra energy battling the wind.

In this chapter, we cover some of the most popular and invigorating outdoor fitness activities. We discuss what gear you need and how much it costs, and we offer training strategies and safety tips for rookies and klutzes alike.

Keep in mind that in addition to trying the activities covered here, such as walking and swimming, you also can have a blast in adult sports leagues, playing soccer, softball, basketball, rugby, and other sports that definitely aren't just for kids. Contact your local parks and recreation department to find out about leagues.

Walking

Can you really get fit by walking? Absolutely — as long as you walk long enough, hard enough, and often enough. (If you're asking, "How long?", "How hard?", and "How often?" check out Chapter 7.) One study found that among people who are successful in maintaining long-term weight loss, nearly 80 percent walk as their main physical activity.

The beauty of walking is that it's simply a matter of putting one foot in front of the other. Sure, walking burns fewer calories per minute than jogging, but most people last longer on a walk than on a run, so you can make up for the deficit. Plus, compared to runners, walkers enjoy a relatively low injury rate.

However, we're not going to sugarcoat this: Some exercisers find walking to be a big, fat bore. Some people combat boredom by heading for the nearest nature trail. The change of scenery (not to mention the change of terrain, sounds, and smells) can be very uplifting.

Essential walking gear

Although the rest of the animal kingdom does fine without the benefit of special equipment, human feet don't have adequate padding to meet the demands of walking in the modern world. You need a good pair of walking shoes to avoid foot, ankle, knee, hip, and lower-back problems. Expect to spend at least $50 for good walking shoes, which should hold up for 1,000 to 1,500 miles. (Running shoes usually have to be tossed after 400 to 500 miles.) Replace your shoes when the tread begins to wear thin or when the sides start to cave inward or outward.

Walking shoes may sound like a marketing conspiracy hatched by shoe-industry executives. After all, it's only walking — won't any pair of sneakers suffice? Actually, the concept of a walking shoe is a valid one. Walking shoes need to be more flexible than running shoes because you bend your feet more when you walk, and you push off from your toes with more oomph. Also, because your heels bear most of your weight when you walk, you need a firm, stable *heel counter,* the part of the shoe that wraps around your heel to keep your foot in place.

If you plan to hike or walk over rugged terrain, look for a walking shoe with treaded soles and added heel and ankle support. If you're focusing on speed walking or high mileage, go for a little more cushioning in the *midsole,* the area between the tread and the inside of the shoe. If you ultimately plan on graduating to running, you're probably better off buying a running shoe.

Walking with good form

Okay, we lied to you: There actually is more to walking than simply putting one foot in front of the other. The biggest mistake walkers make is bending forward, a sure way to develop problems in your lower back, neck, and hips. Your posture should be naturally tall. You needn't force yourself to be ramrod straight, but neither should you slouch, overarch your back, or lean too far forward from your hips. Relax your shoulders, widen your chest, and pull your abdominals gently inward. Keep your head and chin up with your shoulders over your hips and focus straight ahead.

Meanwhile, keep your hands relaxed and cupped gently, and swing your arms so that they brush past your body. On the upswing, your hand should be level with your breastbone; on the downswing, your hand should brush against your hip. Keep your hips loose and relaxed. Your feet should land firmly, heel first. Roll through your heel to your arch, then to the ball of your foot, and then to your toes. Push off from your toes and the ball of your foot.

Run through a mental head-to-toe checklist every so often to see how you're doing. To find out more about fitness walking (yep, there's plenty more to tell), read Liz's book *Fitness Walking For Dummies* (Wiley).

Walking tips for rookies

Although walking is the most basic of all fitness activities, novice fitness walkers can still benefit from the following pointers:

- ✔ **Increase your workout time gradually.** Most people can start off with five 10- to 20-minute walking sessions a week; after about a month, they can increase each workout by 2 or 3 minutes per week per session until walking 30 to 45 minutes is comfortable. Five days a week may sound like a lot, but an almost-daily walk makes it easier to get in the habit. Plus, for weight control, you probably need to walk at least an hour a day, five or six days a week.

- ✔ **Walk as fast as you comfortably can.** If you walk very fast — at a 12-minute-mile to 15-minute-mile pace — you burn more calories than when you walk at a 20-minute-mile pace. You may not be able to move at such supersonic speeds in the beginning, but as you get fit, you can mix in some fast-paced intervals. (For details about interval training, see Chapter 7.)

- ✔ **If you're walking on the shoulder of a road, walk against traffic so you can watch cars approach.**

- ✔ **Add some hills.** Walking over hilly terrain shapes your butt and thighs and burns extra calories — about 30 percent more calories than walking on flat terrain, depending, of course, on the grade of the hills.

- ✔ **Sneak in a walk whenever you can.** Leave your car at home and hoof it to the train station. Take a 15-minute walk during your lunch break. Traverse the airport on foot rather than on that automatic walking belt. It all adds up.

Running

Like walking, running is a workout that you can take with you anywhere. You don't need a rack on your car or a suitcase full of equipment; you just open the door and go. Plus, as any pathological runner will tell you, nothing is quite as satisfying as getting a good run under your belt. You work up a great sweat, you burn lots of calories, and your muscles and your brain feel pleasantly invigorated after you finish.

But beware: Many runners develop frequent, chronic injuries. Many people have joints that simply will not tolerate all that pounding. If you're not built to run, don't argue with your body. You can get in great condition in other ways. And if you're a beginner, it's probably safest if you start off alternating periods of walking with periods of running. For example, if you can walk for 30 minutes at a reasonably brisk pace and you're raring to go faster, start out by alternating 1 minute of running with 3 minutes of walking and gradually decrease the walk intervals as you increase the run intervals.

Essential running gear

Although you can spend hundreds of dollars on spiffy tights, fancy water bottles, MP3 holders, and running jackets that do everything but sing and dance, the only equipment that's truly essential for running is a good pair of shoes (although women will want a supportive jogging bra, too). Be prepared to spend at least $60 to $70 (and as much as $200) a pair, but know that a hefty price tag doesn't always correspond to the best shoe.

The shoe that's best for you depends on your weight, the shape of your foot, your running style, and any special problems you may have, such as weak ankles or bad knees. Try on several models at the store, and take each one for a test drive around the mall, or at least run a couple laps around the store.

Your running shoes should be fairly flexible, especially across the ball of the foot. Hold the shoe at both ends and bend it; it should break right at the ball of the foot. You want cushioning but not so much that you can't feel your foot hitting the ground. Look for a stable *heel counter* (the part of the shoe that wraps around your heel to keep your foot in place). If your foot slides around a lot, that can mean trouble down the road.

We recommend you take a week or two to run without indulging in running gear besides shoes and a sports bra. Then, if you're hooked, you may want to splurge on a few items that will truly make a difference, such as one of the watches or monitors described in Chapter 26 or a super-moisture-wicking top.

What's the deal with barefoot running?

A growing number of runners are shedding their chunky trainers in favor of shoes in a more minimalist category known as *barefoot runners* or *minimalist footwear*. Some of these shoes look like trimmed-down versions of regular running shoes. Others, like the Vibram FiveFingers, are quite odd, featuring separate compartments for each toe. (Trying to get all of your appendages separated and into the right compartment was a lengthy process that reminded Liz of helping her 4-year-old put on gloves.) According to proponents of this running-shoe breed, minimalists prompt you to shorten your stride to a more natural length and land closer to the ball of your foot than you do while wearing a typical running shoe; in theory, your feet and ankles become the flexible shock absorbers they were born to be, and you'll have fewer injuries than when you wear heavier, shock-absorbing versions of running shoes. Some preliminary research seems to support this claim, though only a very few studies have been done.

After testing several brands, we think minimalist footwear is great for speed work and running moderate distances, and they are plenty comfy. But we honestly have no idea how they'd respond by the 25-mile mark of a marathon. Heavier, inexperienced, and injury-prone runners may want to steer clear of this trend. Some runners report feeling sore after the first few runs, which makes sense when you consider that in a way, you're retraining your feet and ankles to fend for themselves.

Running with good form

Runners have a habit of looking directly at the ground, almost as if they can't bear to see what's coming next. Keeping your head down throws your upper-body posture off-kilter and can lead to upper-back and neck pain. Lift your head, keep your shoulders over your hips, and focus your eyes straight ahead.

Relax your shoulders, keep your chest lifted, and pull your abdominal muscles in tightly. Don't overarch your back and stick your butt out; that's one of the main reasons runners get back and hip pain.

Keep your arms close to your body, and swing them forward and back rather than across your body. Don't clench your fists. Pretend you're holding a butterfly in each hand; you don't want your butterflies to escape, but you don't want to crush them, either.

Lift your front knee and extend your back leg. Don't shuffle along like you're wearing cement boots. Land heel first and roll through the entire length of your foot. Push off from the balls of your feet instead of running flat-footed and pounding off your heels. Otherwise, your feet and legs are going to cry uncle long before your cardiovascular system does.

If you experience pain in your ankles, knees, or lower back, stop running for a while. Try switching to a lower-impact activity such as walking, cycling, or swimming, or stay off your feet altogether. If you don't, you could end up having to sit on the sidelines for months.

Running tips for rookies

These tips help you get fit and avoid injury while running:

- ✔ **Start by alternating periods of walking with periods of running.** For example, try 2 minutes of walking and 1 minute of running. Gradually decrease your walking intervals until you can run continuously for 20 minutes. Of course, sticking with a walk-run routine is fine; you're less likely to injure yourself that way.

- ✔ **Vary your pace.** Different paces work your heart, lungs, and legs in different ways. Experiment with the techniques described in Chapter 7.

- ✔ **Always run against traffic when running on the shoulder of a road.** This allows you to see oncoming cars and dive for the side of the road if necessary. Consider carrying a lightweight cellphone for emergencies, and always let someone know where you're running.

- ✔ **Don't increase your mileage by more than 10 percent a week.** If you run 5 miles a week and want to increase, aim to do 5½ miles the following week. Jumping from 5 miles to 6 miles doesn't sound like a big deal, but studies show that if you increase your mileage more than 10 percent per week, you set yourself up for injury.

Bicycling

Talk to a group of cyclists and, chances are, you're talking to a group of ex-runners. Cycling is perfect for people who can't take the relentless pounding of running or find the slow pace a real drag. Cycling is the best way to cover a lot of ground quickly. Even a novice can easily build up to a 20-mile ride. Cycling is also a great way to burn calories and spare the environment while you commute to work or get around town doing errands.

On the other hand, cycling can be a hassle. You can't just grab your shoes and head out the door. You need a trustworthy bike that is in good working order and set to your specifications. You also need to pump up your tires, make sure your seat bag has tools and a spare tube in case of a flat, and put on your helmet, gloves, and glasses. And even with all your protective gear, you can never be too cautious. Cycling is a low-impact sport — unless you happen to impact the ground, a car, a tree, a rut, or another cyclist.

Essential cycling gear

If you haven't owned a bike since grammar school, prepare yourself for sticker shock. *Mountain bikes,* the fat-tire bikes with upright handlebars, are somewhat less expensive than comparable *road bikes,* the kind with the skinny tires and curved handlebars. *Hybrid bikes* are — surprise! — a hybrid of the two. With an upright riding position, somewhat hefty frame, and tires of moderate width, hybrids are more comfortable than road bikes, lighter than mountain bikes, and stout enough to withstand potholes and other commuting hazards.

In all three categories, you won't find many decent bikes under $300; many cost more than $2,000. Don't take out a second mortgage to buy a fancy bike, but if you have any inkling that you may like this sport, don't skimp, either. You'll just end up buying a more expensive bike later.

What distinguishes a $300 bike from a $2,000 steed? Generally, the more expensive the bike, the stronger and lighter its frame. A heavy bike can slow you down, but unless you plan to enter the Tour de France, don't get hung up on a matter of ounces. Cheaper bikes are made from different grades of steel; as you climb the price ladder, you find materials such as aluminum, carbon fiber, and titanium. The price of a bike also depends on the quality of the *components* — the mechanics that enable your bike to move, shift, and brake.

Cheaper bikes come with *toe clips* (pedal straps) that enable you to pull up on the pedal as well as push down. But you can pull up even more efficiently with *clipless pedals,* which lock into cleats affixed to the bottom of your cycling shoes. These pedal systems are like ski bindings: You're locked in, but your feet pop out easily if you fall. To clip out, you simply twist your foot to the side.

Beginners usually have an accident or two with clipless pedals because they haven't developed the instinct to twist sideways. Suzanne once tipped over with both feet clicked into her pedals. We'll spare you the details of her injury, but let's just say that she ended up at the gynecologist.

Find a bike dealer you trust, and know that bike prices are negotiable. Ask the salesperson to throw in a few free extras, such as a bike computer to measure your speed and distance or a seat bag to carry food and tools.

Don't even think about pedaling down your driveway without a helmet snug atop your noggin. Cycling gloves make your ride more comfortable and protect your hands when you crash. Glasses are important to protect your eyes from the dust, dirt, and gravel.

Buy a pair of padded cycling shorts and a brightly colored cycling jersey so that you can easily be seen. Unlike cotton T-shirts, jerseys wick away sweat so that you won't freeze on a downhill after you worked up a big sweat climbing up. Plus, jerseys have pockets in the back deep enough to hold half a grocery store's worth of snacks. Always carry a water bottle or wear a *hydration pack,* a clever backpack-like water pouch that we describe in Chapter 26. Finally, carry gear to change a flat tire, and learn how to use it. There's no cycling equivalent of the auto club to come save you. Many bike shops offer free demonstrations on changing a flat and basic bike maintenance.

Cycling with good form

To protect your knees from injury, position your seat correctly (ask your salesperson for advice) and pedal at an easy cadence. *Cadence* refers to the number of revolutions per minute that you pedal. Inexperienced cyclists tend to use higher gears, which forces them to turn the pedals in slow motion; their legs tire prematurely, their knees ache, and they cheat themselves out of a good workout. Set your bike's gearing so you're pedaling comfortably. The faster cadence is easier on your knees.

Road cycling can wreak havoc on your lower back because you're in a crouched position for so long. Relax your upper body and keep your arms loose. Grasp your handlebars with the same tension that you'd hold a child's hand when you cross the street. Pedal in smooth circles rather than simply mashing the pedals downward. Imagine that you have a bed of nails in your shoes, and you have to pedal without stomping on the nails.

Cycling tips for rookies

You can learn a lot about cycling — and get faster in a jiff — by riding with a club or friends who have more experience. Here are some pointers to start your cycling career:

  ✔ **Remember that you are a vehicle and are required to follow the rules of the road.** Ride with traffic, not against it.

✔ **Stop at all signs and lights, and use those hand signals you learned in driver's ed.** Don't trust a single car, ever. Assume that the driver doesn't see you, even if he happens to be staring you in the face.

✔ **When you go off-road, start on wide fire roads rather than narrow "single-track" trails that require technical skills.** And don't think that you're immune to injury because there are no cars. More crashes happen on mountain trails than on the road because there are more obstacles and riders get careless and cocky.

✔ **Head into a turn at a slow enough pace that you maintain control, and never let your eyes wander from the road or trail.** Never squeeze the brakes — particularly the front brake — with a lot of pressure. You'll go flying over the handlebars, a maneuver known as an *endo,* and go right into a *face plant,* a maneuver that we think is self-explanatory.

In-Line Skating

Back in 1980, Rollerblade introduced a new kind of skate: Instead of two wheels at the toe and two wheels at the heel, the four wheels were positioned in a single-file line. This was the biggest innovation in skating since a 16th-century Dutchman patterned the first pair of roller skates after ice skates. In-line skating — often called *Rollerblading* — isn't as popular as it was during the early 1990s heyday, but it's still the skate of choice for more than 17 million people.

Skating is fun because it isn't as linear as running, walking, and cycling. You can curve, turn, glide, sprint, and spin. Skating is also a terrific tush toner because you push your legs out to the side, which works several seldom-used hip and glute muscles. Skating is a good calorie burner, too.

But in-line skating also can be dangerous. About 270,000 skaters per year wind up at the doctor or emergency room with injuries. Liz got a firsthand look at one of these injuries not long ago. While running over the 59th Street Bridge in New York City, Liz spotted a woman walking in bare feet and sobbing. The woman's entire left side was so bloody that she appeared to have been mauled by a tiger. It turns out the woman had attempted to skate over sharp metal teeth on the road — teeth designed to provide traction for cars during icy conditions in winter.

Most skaters use more common sense than that, but injuries are still common because the sport requires so much balance and concentration. Plus, stopping on in-line skates is darn tough. (See "Skating tips for rookies," later in this chapter, for stopping tips.)

Essential skating gear

Skating equipment isn't cheap — a good pair of skates costs between $70 and $500. (We suggest you rent several times before you buy.) Try on several pairs at the store and wear each for at least 10 minutes, until your feet start to get hot. Tilt your feet to the inside and the outside, putting plenty of pressure on your feet to make sure nothing hurts. Otherwise, you're asking for blisters. The boots should feel snug in the toe and heel. If your heel is loose, you won't have enough control when you skate.

In-line skates have more on conventional roller skates than just wheel placement. The wheels are faster, smoother, and more durable. Most skates have a plastic shell and foam-lined bootie, so they breathe more easily and conform to your feet much better than leather skates. You typically can get a more comfortable fit with skates that buckle rather than lace. Be sure to wear synthetic socks; cotton fibers retain moisture, which can irritate your feet.

A helmet is as essential for skating as it is for biking. A cycling helmet will suffice, but you can buy special in-line helmets with more protection at the rear of the head. Also crucial: wrist guards, knee guards, and elbow guards. Purchase safety equipment before you buy your skates so you won't be tempted to take a quick spin before suiting up.

Skating the right way

Keep your hands in front of your body at all times with your elbows in, your forearms straight ahead, and your palms down, as if you're placing your hands on a table. If you move your hands off center, your body is likely to follow. Keep your arms as still as possible — don't pump them back and forth.

Travel in a modified squat position, bending at the knees as if you're about to sit down. Keep your weight on your back wheel and push off straight with your heel. Pull your abdominal muscles inward and don't round your back. If you start to lose your balance, crouch lower — don't stand up straighter. If you veer off the pavement and onto mud or grass, run on your skates instead of stopping cold.

Skating tips for rookies

To find out whether skating is the sport for you, take a few lessons. (You can find an instructor through a skate shop, or call the International In-Line Skating Association for a referral.)

In the meantime, here are some suggestions to get started:

- ✔ **Practice first.** Head to a parking lot to practice skating, turning, and stopping. Stick to bike paths until you're quite comfortable skating, and when you do head for the open road, always skate with — not against — traffic. *Remember:* You're responsible for abiding by the same rules as motorists.

- ✔ **Don't expect brakes to bring you to a complete halt.** The best a novice can hope to do is slow down. To do this, simultaneously lean forward from your waist, tilt the braking skate up, and exert pressure on the heel pad while maintaining your balance. Skip hills until you master stopping, and always skate slowly enough that you feel as though you could stop at any time.

- ✔ **Don't skate on the side of a busy road, where a cyclist might ride.** Stick to bike trails, sidewalks, and other smooth, well-maintained, no-traffic areas.

- ✔ **Don't skate while holding anything in your hand, even a can of soda.** When you fall, your reflex is to save what you're holding, not to protect your body.

Exercising in Water

Exercising in the water is truly zero-impact. Although you can strain your shoulders if you overdo swimming, there's absolutely no pounding on your joints, and the only thing you're in danger of crashing into is the wall of the pool. You can get a great aerobic workout that uses your whole body. Plus, water has a gentle, soothing effect on the body, so any exercise you do in the water is helpful for those with arthritis or other joint diseases.

Swimming and other forms of water exercise are great for people who want to keep exercising when they're injured and for people who are pregnant or overweight. That extra body fat helps you glide along near the surface of the water, so you don't expend energy trying to keep yourself from sinking like a stone.

Lap swimming has the reputation of being drudgery — after all, the scenery doesn't change a whole lot from one end of the pool to the other. The trick is to use an array of gadgets that elevate swim workouts from forced labor to bona fide fun. You can even buy an underwater MP3 player with pretty decent sound or a special waterproof case to hold your standard MP3 player.

Essential water exercise gear

Obviously, a body of water is helpful — preferably one manned by a lifeguard. And in most instances, you must wear a swimsuit. By the way, we said *swimsuit,* not bathing suit. You don't want a suit that looks good while you're sunbathing but creeps up your butt when you get in the water.

If you exercise in a chlorinated pool, goggles are a must to prevent eye irritation and to help you see better in the water. Buy goggles from a store that lets you try them on. You should feel some suction around your eyes, but not so much that you feel like your eyeballs are going to pop out. You also need a cap so that your hair doesn't get plastered on your face or turn to straw from the chemicals.

As for the fun water gadgets: Many pools let you borrow equipment, but you can buy a whole set for less than $75. We especially like rubber swimming fins, which give you a lot more speed and power when you swim and water jog and give your legs a better workout.

You can use fins when you kick with a *kickboard,* a foam board that helps you stay afloat. But don't use fins so much that they become a crutch. As you get in better shape, you may want to switch from long swim fins to short fins, which make you work a lot harder. Don't swim with scuba fins; they're too big and too stiff.

Exercising with plastic paddles on your hands gives your upper body an extra challenge. Some paddles are flat and rectangular; others are shaped more like your hand, with a comfortable contour in the palm area. With both styles, you place your hand on top of the paddles and slip your fingers through a thick rubber band that secures your hand to the paddles. Paddles can help you perfect your swim stroke technique and increase the intensity of your workout, but use them sparingly; overuse can lead to shoulder injuries. When you swim with paddles, put a *pull-buoy* (a contoured foam wedge) between your thighs. This keeps your legs buoyant so that you can concentrate on using your arms rather than kicking.

Swimming with good form

If you swim for water exercise, you'll probably spend the bulk of your workouts doing the front crawl, also called *freestyle.* It's generally faster than the other strokes, so you can cover more distance. Don't cut your strokes short; reach out as far as you can, have your hand enter thumb-first so it slices the water like a knife, and pull all the way through the water so your hand brushes your thigh. Use an S-shaped sculling movement, where your hand moves out, then in, then out again across your body/thigh and out of the water. Elongate your stroke so that you take fewer than 25 strokes in a 25-yard pool. The fewer strokes, the better. Top swimmers get so much power from each stroke that they take just 11 to 14 strokes per length of a 25-yard pool.

Kick up and down from your hips, not your knees. Don't kick too deeply or allow your feet to break the water's surface. Proper kicking causes the water to "boil" rather than splash.

Breathe through your mouth every two strokes, or every three strokes if you want to alternate the side that you breathe on. You need as much oxygen as you can get. Beginners sometimes make the mistake of taking six or eight strokes before breathing, which wears them out quickly. To breathe, roll your entire body to the side until your mouth and nose come out of the water — imagine that your entire body is on a skewer and must rotate together. Don't lift your head out of the water to breathe — you'll spend a lot of energy doing that, and it'll slow you down in the water.

Swimming tips for rookies

Even if you're the queen of your kickboxing class or a champion at cycling uphill, you may still tire quickly in the pool at first. More than almost any other cardio activity, swimming relies on technique. The following tips can help you get the most out of your swimming workouts.

- ✔ **Take a few lessons if you haven't swum in a while.** Beginners waste a lot of energy flailing and splashing around rather than moving forward.

- ✔ **Break your workout into intervals.** For example, don't just get into the pool, swim 20 laps, and get out. Instead, do 4 easy laps for a warm-up. Then do 8 sets of 2 laps at a faster pace, resting 20 seconds between sets. Then cool down with 2 easy laps, and maybe a few extra laps with a kickboard. Mix up your strokes, too. The four basic strokes — freestyle, backstroke, breaststroke, and butterfly — use your muscles in different ways.

- ✔ **Try out a Masters swim club.** In this context, "master" means age 18 and over — not expert. You needn't be a fishlike swimmer to join one of these clubs, which are located at university and community pools nationwide and are geared toward adult swimmers of all levels. A coach gives you a different workout every time you swim and monitors your progress. Best of all, you have buddies to work out with. Don't worry about being slow; the coach will group you in a lane with other people your speed. If you have a competitive spirit, you can compete in Masters meets, where you swim against others who are roughly your speed.

✔ **If you find swimming a big yawn but enjoy being in the water, try water running or water aerobics.** Water running is a pretty tough workout because the water provides resistance from all directions as you move your legs. It's an excellent option for injured runners because, even though it's nonimpact and easy on your joints, water running helps maintain cardio conditioning. Don't assume that water aerobics are for little old ladies in flowered caps. With the right instructor and exercise program, you can get a challenging water-workout. Water running can be even tougher.

Getting your cardio in the snow

In some parts of the country, winter is so blustery that when you see someone walking, running, or cycling outdoors in the dead of January, you can only shake your head and say, "What, does that girl have brain freeze?" In these places, your best outdoor cardio options involve snow. We're talking about cross-country skiing and snowshoeing, activities that allow you to enjoy the elements rather than battle them.

Cross-country skiing burns mega calories and comes in two forms: classic and skate. On classic skis, you glide — or, more likely, shuffle — back and forth on long, skinny skis, primarily on groomed tracks. Skate skis are somewhat shorter and wider; you travel at a much faster clip, pushing your skis outward on wide, groomed trails, in a motion that resembles in-line skating. Classic skiing feels like a more natural motion and, for a novice, is far less demanding, both physically and mentally, than skate skiing, a.k.a. "skating." A beginner can go out for a casual classic ski and have a fine time with minimal or no instruction. A first-time skater attempting to wing it, even one fit enough to win triathlons, may well collapse from a combination of exhaustion and frustration. Skate skiing is ultimately a blast and in many areas has overtaken classic skiing in popularity, but the learning curve is darned steep.

Contrast this to snowshoeing, also an excellent calorie burner but one that requires no skill and minimal fitness and carries a lower risk of injury than any other snow sport. The term *snowshoeing* may conjure up images of bearded Scandinavian trappers slogging across the tundra, their boots strapped to giant wooden tennis racquets, but today's snowshoes are compact, with frames made of lightweight aluminum. High-tech fabric stretches across the frame, preventing you from sinking into the snow.

Downhill skiing and snowboarding are also popular cold-weather workout options. Sure, you get a free ride up the mountain, but you more than make up for it on the way down. Just ask your hips, thighs, and buttocks after a long day on the hill. Beyond that, downhill skiing and snowboarding are terrific activities for working on balance, coordination, and agility. Because these activities can be particularly hard on your body, we recommend taking a "get in shape for ski season" class at the gym or spending four to six weeks strength training prior to your first day on the slopes.

Though these activities tend to be expensive, many mountains offer excellent beginner packages that come with lift tickets, rental equipment, and a half or full day of lessons. Many also offer couples and family packages, including some free meals. Shop around online and see what you can find.

Part III
Building Muscle and Strengthening Bone

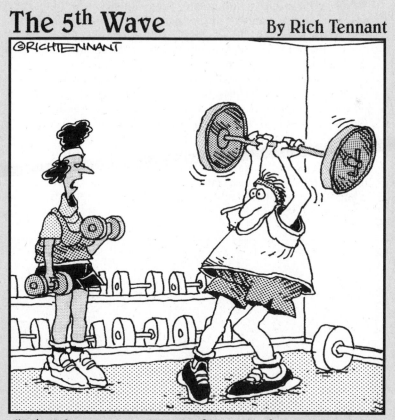

The 5th Wave   By Rich Tennant

"That's really great form—for someone taking his underwear off over his head."

In this part . . .

We give you the know-how to tone and strengthen your muscles and bolster bone density, whether you work out at home or at the gym. Chapter 10 gives you five great reasons to lift weights and answers important questions, such as, "Will weight lifting make me look like a professional wrestler?" In Chapter 11, we cover your major muscle groups so that you know your lats from your pecs from your delts. In Chapter 12, we explain the differences among barbells, dumbbells, and kettlebells (sorry, no mention of sleigh bells) and help you choose the best equipment for you. Chapter 13 helps you get started on a strength-training program. We discuss how much weight to lift, how many exercises to do, and how to use good form so you don't get injured. We also demonstrate a complete weight-training workout that you can perform either at a health club or at home.

Chapter 10

Why You've Gotta Lift Weights

Maybe you've never considered yourself the weight-lifting type. Maybe you suspect that the size of one's muscles is inversely proportional to the size of one's brain. Maybe when you see a hulking guy on the street, you think, "He may be able to bench-press my minivan, but I can read a menu in French."

The truth is that weight lifting is an incredibly smart thing to do. It's not just a form of narcissism, and it's not just for bodybuilders. Heck, these days, even 80-year-olds are pumping iron. In this chapter, we explain why you should, too. We also dispel popular weight-training myths and tell you what kind of results you can reasonably expect. If you think lifting weight seems too boring, too dangerous, too troublesome, or too likely to transform you into Hulk Hogan, we hope this chapter changes your mind.

First, a quick note: Throughout this book, we use the terms *weight lifting,* *weight training,* and *strength training* interchangeably, even though you don't necessarily need weight to build strength. *Resistance training* means the same thing, but we use that bit of verbiage sparingly.

Considering Five Important Reasons to Pick Up a Dumbbell

People who start lifting weights often tell you how much more fit, powerful, and energetic they feel . . . but enough about feelings. There's plenty of good, solid evidence that strength training does all that and more. We bet that at least one of the following reasons will get you to hoist some iron.

Staying strong for everyday life

If you don't use your muscles, they get smaller. This gradual slide toward wimpiness can begin as early as your mid-20s.

People who don't exercise lose 30 to 40 percent of their strength by age 65. By age 74, more than one-fourth of American men and two-thirds of American women can't lift an object heavier than 10 pounds, such as a small dog or a loaded garbage bag. These changes aren't the normal consequences of aging. They're a result of neglect — of experiencing life from a recliner and the front seat of an RV.

Fortunately, strength is one of the easiest physical abilities to retain as you get older; certainly, you can do a lot more to halt strength loss than you can to prevent wrinkling skin, fading eyesight, or increasing affection for network television. One study, which included men up to age 96, found that by lifting weight, most seniors can at least double — if not triple — their muscle power.

So if you rarely lift anything heavier than a cellphone, it's time to build enough brawn to get along in the real world. Increased strength is what you need to unscrew the top off a stubborn jar of pickles, hoist your kid onto the mechanical horsy, and close a suitcase that's too full. Even if you have the stamina to sprint the full length of an airport to catch your plane, it's not going to do you much good if you can't lug along that overstuffed luggage.

Keeping your bones healthy

Strong muscles and strong bones go hand in hand. The more weight you can lift, the more stress you can put on your bones; this stress is what stimulates them.

Most people start out with strong, dense bones — imagine them as poles of steel. But around age 35, most people — men included — begin to lose about ½ to 1 percent of their bone each year. For women, bone loss accelerates after menopause — 1 to 2 percent a year for the first five years and then about 1 percent annually until age 70. Then the loss slows back to ½ percent a year. In the five to seven years following menopause, women can lose up to 20 percent of their bone mass.

Ten million Americans are estimated to have *osteoporosis,* a disease of severe bone loss, and almost 34 million more are estimated to have low bone mass, placing them at increased risk for osteoporosis. When bones become extremely weak — picture them like chalk, porous and fragile — it doesn't even take a fall to break them. Someone with osteoporosis doesn't fall and break a hip; she breaks a hip and falls. An action as low-impact as a sneeze can cause a bone fracture in a person with osteoporosis.

Space cases: Losing bone density

The first astronauts to spend time in space experienced significant bone-density loss. In space, not only does no one hear you scream, but you're weightless — there's no load placed on your muscles and bones.

Because the low gravity of space has a muscle- and bone-wasting effect, astronauts consider serious strength training an essential part of their regimen. They can't lift chunks of iron while in orbit — dumbbells are subject to the same laws of gravity as any other type of weight — so astronauts use a series of very heavy rubber bands and springs, many of which are anchored in place. Liz visited the NASA training center in Houston a few years ago and had a lot of fun trying out the equipment and talking to the astronauts' trainers as well as several astronauts.

Osteoporosis causes more than 2 million fractures a year, mostly of the back, hip, and wrist; by 2025, the toll is expected to be 3 million broken bones, according to the National Osteoporosis Foundation. About half of those who break their hips never regain full walking ability, and many of these fractures lead to fatal complications. Women account for about 80 percent of osteoporosis cases, but following a hip fracture, the one-year mortality rate is nearly twice as high for men as it is for women.

However, if you do everything right, you can decelerate this bone loss significantly — by about 50 percent. If you've already lost a lot of bone, you may even be able to build some of it back.

Strength training alone can't stop bone loss, but it can play a big role. Also important are calcium, vitamin D, and aerobic exercise such as walking and jogging. (Swimming and cycling don't work as well because your body weight is supported, either by the water or the bike; when you have to support your own self, your bones respond by building themselves up.)

Preventing injuries

When your muscles are strong, you're less injury-prone. You're less likely to step off a curb and twist your ankle. Plus, as we explain in Chapter 15, you have a better sense of balance and surefootedness, so you're less apt to take a tumble during a weekend game of touch football. Research shows that one out of every three people over age 65 falls at least once a year. Almost 10 percent of older people who fall are hospitalized for an injury, and about half of those cases involve broken bones.

Looking better

Now let's talk about pure, unadulterated vanity. Aerobic exercise burns lots of calories, but weight lifting firms, lifts, builds, and shapes your muscles. A marathon runner may be able to go the distance, but he won't turn any heads on the beach if he has a concave chest and string-bean arms. (He may also be a faster runner if he pumped up a bit.)

The fibers that make up muscle lose shape when they're inactive. As one researcher told us, "If you take a chunk of muscle from an active person and look at it under a microscope, the fibers hold together well. If the person is inactive, the fibers look like gelatin." Squishy muscles, as you can imagine, don't do much for your appearance. For example, if your abdominal muscle fibers get soft, they don't do as good a job holding in your internal organs, and your belly looks poochier.

We want to be clear here: There's no such thing as *spot reducing* — that is, selectively zapping fat off a particular part of your body. But you can pick certain areas, such as your butt or your arms, and reshape them through weight training. And if you have wide hips or a thick middle, you can bring your body more into proportion by doing exercises that broaden your shoulders and back.

Weight training also makes you look better by improving your posture. With strong abdominal and lower-back muscles, you stand up straighter and look more svelte, even if you haven't lost an ounce.

Speeding up your metabolism

Metabolism is one of those buzzwords that never fades from the news. At gyms, health-food stores, and juice bars, you can buy pills, powders, and "thermogenic herbs" touted to rev up your metabolism (and thereby help you burn extra calories without trying). All these claims are bogus. The best way to increase your metabolism is to build muscle, which you can accomplish by lifting weights.

How does this work? First, a couple of definitions: Your *metabolism* refers to the number of calories you're burning at any given moment, whether you're watching the weather forecast or riding a bike. But when most people use the term, they're referring to your resting metabolism, the number of calories your body needs to maintain its vital functions. Your brain, heart, kidneys, and other organs are cranking away 24 hours a day, and your muscle fibers are constantly undergoing repair. All these processes require energy in the form of calories simply to keep you alive.

But here's the key: Your resting metabolic rate depends primarily on your amount of *fat-free mass* — everything in your body that's not fat, including muscle, bones, blood, organs, and tissue. The more fat-free mass you have, the more energy your body expends in order to keep going. Therefore, you want to build as much muscle as possible. You can't do anything to increase the size of your brain, but you certainly can make yourself more muscular, and lifting weights is the primary way to do just that.

Keep in mind, however, that packing on a few more pounds of muscle isn't going to turn your body into a calorie-burning inferno. For every 1 pound of muscle you gain, your body may burn an extra 10 to 15 calories per day. That's not a lot, especially if you compensate by eating one extra Hershey's Kiss (24 calories) per day. However, in the long run, even a small metabolic boost can be significant. If you burn an extra 25 calories per day, you can burn 9,125 calories in a year — enough to lose nearly 3 pounds, or at least prevent a 3-pound weight gain. Every little bit helps.

If that's not impressive, consider the flip side: If you don't lift weights, your metabolism will slow down every year, as your muscles slowly shrivel up. After age 40, metabolism typically slows by about 5 percent a decade. And with a more sluggish metabolic rate, you'll gain weight even if you eat the same amount of food. How's that for incentive to hit the weight room?

One final point: The metabolism-boosting benefits of weight lifting are particularly important if you're cutting calories to lose weight. Dieting alone tends to cause a loss in muscle as well as fat; if you lift weights while cutting back on your calorie intake, you can preserve muscle — and maintain your metabolism — while losing fat.

Building Muscle: Myths and Reality

There sure are a lot of misconceptions about weight training. Many people have no idea what changes to expect when they begin lifting weights, so they ask some not-so-dumb questions, like the ones that follow.

Looking at questions of strength

Discussions about strength training inevitably turn to questions of, well, strength. The following sections tease out the truth about increasing your muscle power.

How long does it take to get stronger?

You may be able to lift more weight after just one weight-lifting workout. This isn't because you've built up more muscle; it's mainly because your weight-training skills have improved. The first time you try the bench press, you waste a lot of energy trying to balance the bar, keep it steady, and move it in a straight line. But after you get the hang of the process — typically after one weight-lifting session — you're able to put all your energy into lifting the weight.

Another reason you develop strength after just a few weeks of working out is that, in a sense, your muscles have memory. Your nerves, the pathways that link your brain and muscles, learn how to carry information more quickly — much like the speed-dial feature on your telephone. So after learning an exercise, your brain tells your muscles, "You know what this is. Go for it."

During the first six to eight weeks that you lift weight, most of the strength you gain is due to skill and muscle memory. After that time, your muscles begin to grow. In other words, the *sizes* of your muscle fibers increase — you don't actually grow more muscle cells. Realize that some muscles gain strength faster than others. In general, large muscles, like your chest and back muscles, grow faster than smaller ones, like your arm and shoulder muscles. Most people can increase their strength between 7 and 40 percent after about ten weeks of training each muscle group twice a week.

Do some people have greater strength potential than others?

How much muscle power you develop depends on many things, including your age, sex, and body type (and, of course, your diligence). Every body type has a different capacity for building strength and muscle. For instance, men typically have the capacity for greater overall strength than women do because their bodies have a higher proportion of muscle and more of the strength hormone testosterone.

All the training in the world won't change your body type. If you start out short and narrow, weight training won't miraculously make you tall and broad. Weight training may, however, make you a fitter, more muscular version of short and narrow.

Seniors generally can't develop as much strength as young people, but it's not clear whether this is because of the normal aging process or years of inactivity. Look at Jack LaLanne, who worked out all his life. For his 80th birthday, he towed a rowboat across a river with his teeth.

Wondering about body shape

For many people, the allure of weight training is the promise of a buff or toned body to trot out on the beach. For others, the fear of turning into a muscle-bound hulk has them skipping the weights altogether. This section explains how you can really expect your figure to change.

How long will it take before my body looks better?

Most people start to see changes to their body after only a few weeks of weight lifting. Results depend on your body type, your starting point, and the amount of time and effort you devote to lifting weights. In general, those who have the farthest to go make the most dramatic changes.

Everyone notices the biggest improvements in the muscles that they use the least. The *triceps* (the muscles at the rear of your upper arm; see Chapter 11) are a classic example: You don't use them much in everyday life, so when you start targeting them with weight they become firmer fairly fast. The same goes for shoulders. Most people don't tend to carry much fat on their shoulders, so shoulders shape and tone relatively quickly.

Will weight lifting make me look like a professional wrestler?

Developing huge muscles is difficult for people with certain body types, and it usually comes only with a high-calorie diet mixed with intensive, consistent training. If you're lean and wiry to begin with, you'll probably add definition but not much size. The people most likely to build up their frames are those who have a muscular body type even before they start lifting.

About 99 percent of women — and a significant percentage of men — can't develop huge muscles without spending hours a day in the gym lifting some serious poundage. Even then, most women don't have the testosterone to add major bulk to their frames unless they take steroids — in which case, they may also end up with acne, a beard, liver cancer, uterus shrinkage, and a voice like Darth Vader's. Just the look you're going for, right?

Lifting may actually make you smaller. Because muscle is a very compact, dense tissue, it takes up less room than fat. At first, you may not lose any weight. You may even gain a few pounds, because muscle weighs more per square inch than fat, but your clothes may fit better. As we explain in Chapter 2, that number on your bathroom scale gives you incomplete information about how much fat you're carrying.

Working out the measurements of G.I. Joe

Apparently, an increasing number of men are harboring unrealistic expectations about their potential to get huge; when this gets really out of hand it becomes a full-blown mental disorder known as *muscle dysmorphia*. A few years ago, a Harvard psychiatrist came up with an interesting theory to explain why: outlandishly muscular toys. Over the last 30 years, G.I. Joe action figures have inflated into hulks with physiques that even top bodybuilders can't attain. The professor measured the waist, chest, and biceps of the action figures and then adjusted the numbers for a 6-foot man. In 1964,

G.I. Joe had 12.2-inch biceps; ten years later his "guns" had grown to 15.2 inches. By 1998, G.I. Joe's biceps measured a whopping 26.8 inches — nearly 7 inches larger than home-run record-holder Mark McGwire's.

For decades, Barbie — with her impossibly small waist and huge chest — has created unrealistic expectations for women and girls (if Barbie were full size, her measurements would be 32-17-28, typical of a woman suffering from anorexia); now, it seems that G.I. Joe is doing the same sort of damage in boys and men.

What if I want to get muscle definition like a soap star or action hero?

Lifting weight diligently will help shape your body, but you'll never see muscle definition if you have a thick layer of fat covering your muscles. *Muscle definition* means that you have so little body fat that you can see the outline of your muscles.

You begin to see a hint of definition when your body fat dips into the 20 percent to 22 percent range. At around 18 percent, muscle definition is really apparent. Below 15 percent, you develop an appearance that body-builders reverentially refer to as *ripped*. (We tell you all about body fat in Chapter 2.) We're not recommending that you try to get down this low, because it can be dangerously unhealthy; we do, however, want you to be aware that the buff, ripped look doesn't happen for most people with weight training alone. Also, keep in mind that you can still look firm, fit, and sexy even if you aren't ripped to shreds.

Asking about fat versus muscle

The following questions deal with weight lifting, muscles, and fat.

If I stop lifting weights, will my muscle turn to fat?

Will muscle turn to fat? Only if silver can be transformed into gold. Fat and muscle are two distinctly different substances. When you look at them under the microscope, fat looks like chicken wire, and muscle looks like frayed electrical wiring. If you stop lifting weights, your muscles simply *atrophy,* a fancy word for shrink. The main reason people may gain fat when they stop lifting weights is that they keep their calorie intake the same but are no longer burning as many calories throughout the day. Those extra calories are stored energy or fat.

Should I lose weight before I start lifting weights?

Actually, no. Start weight training right away. Weight training can speed up your metabolism and give you more muscle tone, better posture, and better body proportions. In addition, lifting weight can enhance your aerobic efforts. With stronger muscles, you have more staying power on the elliptical, and you're less apt to have a setback due to injury from your cardio workouts. For example, you may be working out like gangbusters when, suddenly, you feel a little twinge in your knee. You lay off for a couple days, which turns into a couple years. You may be able to prevent this whole incident by strengthening your knees. Plus, adding weight training to your new exercise program gives you more variety and helps keep you motivated.

Chapter 11

Your Muscles: Love 'Em or Lose 'Em

In This Chapter

▶ Discovering the formal names — and the slang — of your muscles

▶ Exploring what different muscles can do for you

▶ Finding out our favorite exercises for each muscle

There are 650 muscles in your body. We are happy to report that you don't need to memorize all of them. Consider, for example, the *extensor hallucis longus,* which extends your big toe. We don't want you to remember that one. In fact, we didn't even know that one — we had to look it up in our anatomy book. If you have any desire to find out more about that muscle, shut this book and apply to medical school.

In this chapter, we tell you about the 20 or so muscles that any conscientious exerciser should know. This chapter simply discusses the major muscles of the body; it doesn't show you a weight-lifting technique for that muscle group. However, we do list our favorite toning and strengthening exercises for each muscle group, and exercises are described in Chapter 13. To find out about other exercises that we don't list here, consult a trainer or our book *Weight Training For Dummies* (published by Wiley).

Seeing the Big Picture

What's the point of knowing major muscle groups? For one thing, you won't need an interpreter when a trainer, podcast instructor, or fellow gym member says, "Let's do lats and pecs today." Before you know it, you may be saying stuff like that, too. And you'll sound really impressive — like wine aficionados who say, "This chardonnay has a superior bouquet."

More important, knowing about all your major muscle groups helps you get a more complete workout. You'll know not to leave any muscle group out, and you'll understand, for example, why you should do several different shoulder exercises, rather than just one.

In addition, you'll take care to perform your exercises properly. For example, if you know where your biceps are, you'll realize exactly where you should feel the tension — and you can adjust your form if you don't feel the stress in the right spot. With many weight-training exercises, it's easy to emphasize the wrong muscle if you don't understand the purpose of the move. If you simply hop on a machine and pull some lever without knowing which muscle to focus on, you may be cheating yourself out of a good workout. See Figures 11-1 and 11-2 for a full view of your muscles.

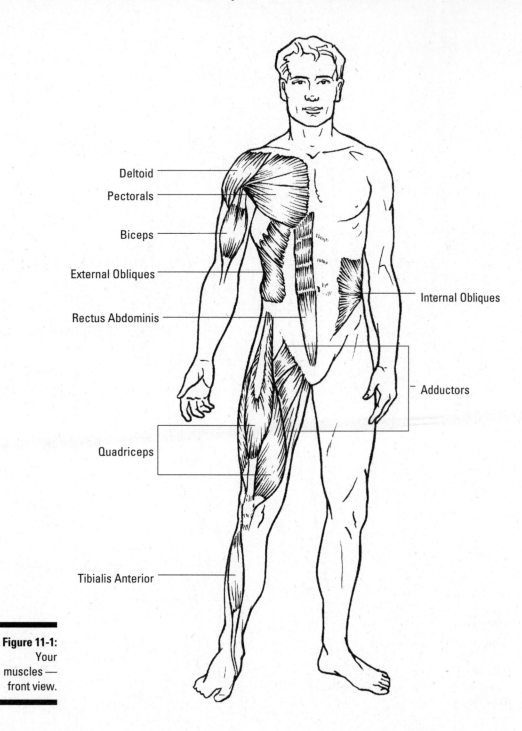

Deltoid

Pectorals

Biceps

External Obliques

Rectus Abdominis

Internal Obliques

Adductors

Quadriceps

Tibialis Anterior

Figure 11-1:
Your
muscles —
front view.

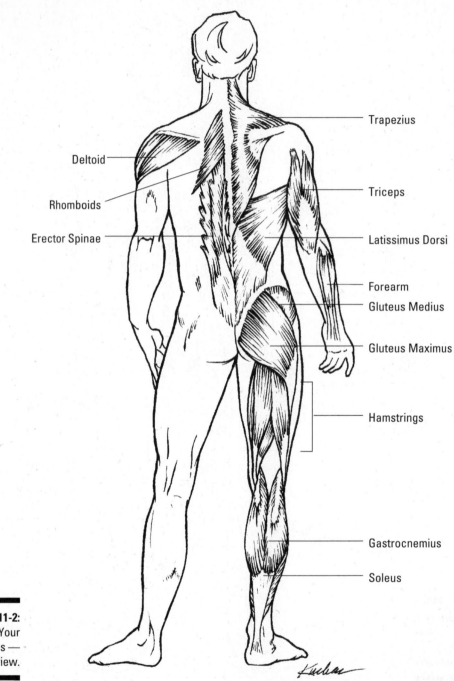

Trapezius

Deltoid

Rhomboids

Triceps

Erector Spinae

Latissimus Dorsi

Forearm

Gluteus Medius

Gluteus Maximus

Hamstrings

Gastrocnemius

Soleus

Figure 11-2:
Your
muscles —
back view.

Looking Over Your Shoulders

Strong shoulders are the key to building a strong upper body. Just about every exercise you can do for your chest and back involves your shoulders, too. If your shoulders are weak, you really limit the amount of weight you can use in the rest of your upper-body repertoire. In the following sections, we outline your shoulder muscles.

Deltoids

Given name: Deltoids; **Street name:** Delts

Whereabouts: Your *delts* wrap completely around the tops of your arms (see Figure 11-3). Cup your hand over your shoulder, and you get the idea. Now swing your arm around in a circle, raise it up above your head, and then swing it forward and backward. You can see what a versatile muscle your shoulder is. The front portion of the shoulder muscle is referred to as the *anterior delt,* the side is called the *medial delt,* and the back is called the rear or *posterior delt.* Go ahead, toss those terms around and amaze your friends.

Job description: Your delts help your arms move in a wide range of directions.

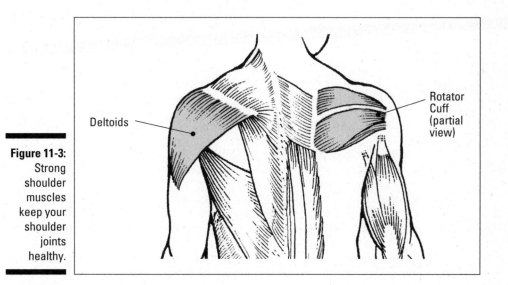

Figure 11-3:
Strong shoulder muscles keep your shoulder joints healthy.

The training payoff: You'll never have to wear shoulder pads if, heaven forbid, they ever come back in style. Also, strengthening your shoulders can help you avoid injuries such as shoulder dislocations or muscle tears. Shoulder joints are delicate and prone to injury; keeping your shoulder muscles strong and working them from every angle possible will keep your shoulder joints in good working order for years to come.

Strong shoulders also help you maintain good posture. With all the time you spend on the computer each day, balanced shoulder work to ensure that you can still sit and stand upright is essential.

Special tips: Be sure to target the front, middle, and back of your shoulders, as well as the delts as a whole, so make it a point to master several dumbbell exercises. We tend to like free weights better than machines for strengthening the shoulders. However, with the advent of swivel-resistance machines (described in Chapter 12), machines are doing a better job of mimicking free-weight movements. That said, figuring out how to use these machines can be challenging. As funny as it sounds, you may feel more comfortable starting with free-weight shoulder exercises and then graduating to free-motion-style machines.

Traditional shoulder machines, which move the weight along a fixed pathway, are still common and can be useful, but they also tend to be difficult to adjust and uncomfortable to use. Also, traditional machines are limiting. For example, no specific machine mimics the front shoulder raise.

Our favorite exercises: Shoulder press, lateral raise, front raise, and back delt fly.

Rotator cuff

Given name: Rotator cuff; **Street name:** Rotators

Whereabouts: Together, the four small muscles beneath your shoulder (refer to Figure 11-3) are called your *rotator cuff*.

Job description: Your rotator-cuff muscles hold your arm in its socket. You use these muscles to rotate the shoulder joint, such as when throwing or swimming. Baseball pitchers are frequently sidelined with rotator-cuff injuries.

The training payoff: By making a special effort to strengthen these commonly injured muscles, you're far less likely to tear or strain them. If you have weak rotators, you can damage them simply by carrying a briefcase or reaching across the table for turkey meatloaf — throwing a 90 mph fastball is not a prerequisite for injury (see Chapter 5 for info on injuries).

Special tips: In addition to doing rotator-cuff exercises, work your shoulders in a variety of directions. Your rotators are put into action whenever your deltoids are working; if your delts are weak and you do a heavy upper-body lift, you may do some serious rotator damage.

If you have chronic shoulder pain, check with your orthopedist to see whether you've injured your rotator cuff. Sometimes rotator tears can be corrected with exercise; other times, they require surgery.

Our favorite exercises: Internal and external rotation, performed with an exercise band, dumbbell, or weight plate or on a cable crossover machine.

Getting Your Back

We know a man in his early thirties who is a pretty good athlete but is constantly sidelined with lower back pain. As young as he is, he's often seen walking around the office bent over like a painful imitation of Groucho Marx. Could he benefit from doing some lower back strength training? Once he straightens up, we'll give him a lecture. The next sections cover the *erector spinae* (lower back) and other back muscles.

Trapezius

Given name: Trapezius; **Street name:** Traps

Whereabouts: Your *trapezius* is a fairly large, kite-shaped muscle that spans up into your neck, across your shoulders, and down to the center of your back (see Figure 11-4).

Job description: Your trapezius enables you to shrug your shoulders, like when someone asks your opinion on cap-and-trade versus a carbon tax. This muscle is also involved when you lift your arm, such as when hailing a cab.

The training payoff: A toned trapezius adds shape to your shoulders and upper back. Strengthening this muscle may also alleviate the neck and shoulder pain you may get if you carry your stress in your neck and shoulders.

Special tips: Give your trapezius extra attention if you often carry a backpack or laptop bag over your shoulder.

Our favorite exercises: Shrug or shoulder roll with a barbell, two dumbbells, or — if your neck is extremely weak and tight — no weight at all.

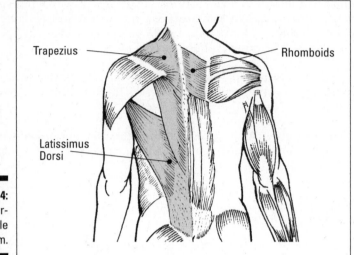

Figure 11-4:
The upper-
back muscle
team.

Latissimus dorsi

Given name: Latissimus dorsi; **Street name:** Lats (*Note:* Don't make the mistake of saying "laterals," as some less-informed exercisers do.)

Whereabouts: Feel the widest part of your back just behind your armpit — you've just found your *latissimus dorsi,* your largest back muscle. This muscle runs the entire length of your back, from below your shoulders down to your lower back (refer to Figure 11-4).

Job description: Your lats enable you to pull, like when you open a door against the wind or drag your Great Dane into the vet's office.

The training payoff: Well-toned lats make your hips and waist appear smaller by adding shape and width to your upper body. If you play sports — especially a racquet sport, golf, or hockey — strengthening your lats will enable you to power the ball or puck quite a bit farther. Runners, walkers, and cyclists also should focus on their lats to help counteract that tendency toward rounded shoulders, which are the result of weak rhomboids (see the following section) and other muscles of the upper and middle back, as well as the result of tight anterior and middle delts (discussed in the earlier "Deltoids" section) and pecs (see the later section "Checking Out Your Chest [Pectorals]").

Special tips: When you do lat exercises, think of your arms simply as a link between your back and the bar or dumbbell. Focus on working your back, not your arms.

Our favorite exercises: Lat pull-down machine, dumbbell row, dumbbell pullover, T-bar row, seated cable row, chin-up, and pull-up.

Rhomboids

Given name: Rhomboids; **Street name:** None — almost no one talks about them. (However, we did once hear them referred to as the "rheumatoids," a term we thought was better suited for an octogenarian garage band.)

Whereabouts: Your *rhomboids* are a small, rectangular group of muscles at the center of your back, hidden beneath your lower trapezius (refer to Figure 11-4).

Job description: Your rhomboids pull your shoulder blades together so you maintain good posture.

The training payoff: With strong rhomboids, you're less likely to hunch your shoulders forward.

Special tips: Focus on your rhomboids to avoid poor posture and potential injury.

Our favorite exercises: A low row machine, dumbbell back delt fly, and chin-up.

Erector spinae

Given name: Erector spinae; **Street name:** Lower back

Whereabouts: Your *erector spinae* run the entire length of your spine, but it's the lower third of this muscle group that you strengthen when you perform the exercises we mention in this section. The rest of this muscle group gets worked when you do upper-back exercises. Figure 11-5 shows where your erector spinae are located.

Job description: Your lower-back muscles are responsible for straightening your spine — for example, when you stand up after tying your shoes. They also work in tandem with your abdominals to keep your spine stable when you move the rest of your body, like when you're sitting in your car and you reach around for something in the back seat.

The training payoff: We consider the erector spinae part of your *core,* a term that refers to all the muscles that wrap around your lower spine and support your body.

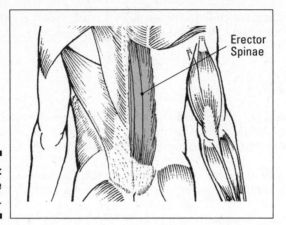

Erector
Spinae

Figure 11-5:
A look at the
lower back.

Though the front core muscles — the abs — get all the attention, strengthening the lower back muscles is just as important for avoiding pain and injury. All the core muscles work in harmony. One weak link throws the whole core out of sync, leaving you vulnerable to injury. Strong lower-back muscles are also very important for posture.

Special tips: The lower back is an injury-prone area. If you have constant lower-back pain, ask your doctor to recommend exercises for your specific problem. Also, be sure to stretch your thigh and hip muscles to help support your lower back.

Our favorite exercises: Pelvic tilt and back extension on the floor or on a hyperextension bench; we also like Pilates and yoga for strengthening all core muscles.

Checking Out Your Chest (Pectorals)

The fibers of your chest muscles spread out like a fan, connecting to your arms, ribs, collar bone (clavical), and breastbone (sternum). For this reason, your chest muscles respond well when you work them from a variety of angles. For example, you can do chest exercises while lying flat on your back on a bench, reclining at various angles, sitting upright, standing, or lying facedown (like when you do push-ups). Ask a trainer to show you several chest exercises so you can vary your workouts.

Given name: Pectorals; **Street name:** Pecs

Whereabouts: Place your hand on your chest as if you're pledging allegiance to the flag. You've found your *pecs*. See Figure 11-6.

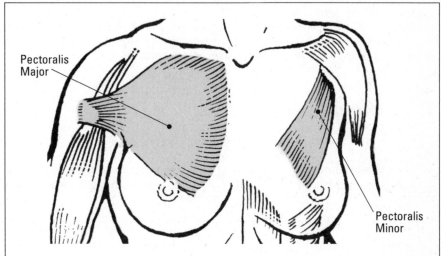

Figure 11-6: You work your pectorals when you do chest exercises.

Job description: Thanks to your pecs you can push — a shopping cart, a lawn mower, or your child's sled down the hill. You also use your pecs to wrap your arms around something, like when you give your mom a bear hug.

The training payoff: You need strong chest muscles for sports like tennis, golf, and football. In women, flabby pecs often translate into bra overhang. It may look like your bra doesn't fit (which can be the case), but just as often the culprit is the relaxed and flaccid muscle that resides underneath the breasts spreading outward. With strong pecs, you look great in tight T-shirts.

Special tips: For women — it's important to understand that your pecs are not your breasts; in fact, they reside directly underneath your breast tissue. However, toning your pecs can lift your breasts and make them appear firmer.

For men — don't become obsessed with bench-pressing to the point of excluding all other exercises. Men with overdeveloped chest muscles and wimpy legs resemble hard-boiled eggs on toothpicks. Besides, doing too much chest work sets you up for shoulder injuries.

Our favorite exercises: Bench-press, chest press machine, dumbbell fly, push-up, and incline dumbbell press.

Taking Up Arms

Take a survey of today's TV stars, celebutantes, and music artists, and you can see that firm arm muscles are in style. Even department-store mannequins now have toned arms. Be sure to give your front and rear arm muscles equal time; if one of these muscle groups is disproportionately stronger than the other, you're at greater risk for elbow injuries.

Biceps

Given name: Biceps; **Street name:** Bi(s) or guns

Whereabouts: Your *biceps* are the two muscles at the front of your upper arm (see Figure 11-7) — the ones that pop up when you flex like a bodybuilder.

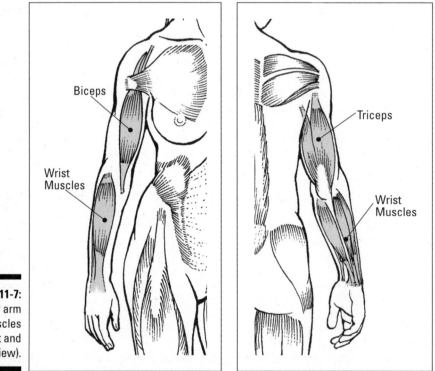

Figure 11-7: Your arm muscles (front and rear view).

Job description: Your biceps are responsible for bending your elbow. When you pick up this book or when you turn the pages, you use your biceps.

The training payoff: With strong biceps, lifting a stack of newspapers or carrying an armload of wood is easier. Your biceps also help out your back muscles when you pull a really stubborn weed out of your garden. Plus, strong biceps make you look buff.

Special tips: Many people have sloppy posture when they do biceps exercises — they rock their bodies back and forth to hoist the weight up. Not only is this posture dangerous for your lower back, but it also makes life too easy for your biceps. Pay special attention to form on bicep exercises, and don't use more weight than you can handle.

Our favorite exercises: Dumbbell biceps curl, concentration curl, barbell biceps curl, and tubing biceps curls.

Triceps

Given name: Triceps; **Street name:** Tri(s)

Whereabouts: Your *triceps* are located at the back of your upper arm (refer to Figure 11-7).

Job description: Your triceps do the opposite of what your biceps do; that is, your triceps straighten your elbow. Your triceps help out your chest muscles when you push something, like when you push your armoire into just the right spot in your bedroom after years of tripping over the leg on your way in the door.

The training payoff: Triceps exercises help firm up *bingo arms.* That's when the backs of your arms flap loosely away from the bones — a condition common among people whose main form of physical activity is playing bingo.

Special tips: The triceps make up two-thirds of your upper-arm size, so if you want a nice pair of arms, work these muscles. Working your triceps is especially important if you often hold a briefcase or handbag while your arm is straight. If your triceps are weak — and that's common because these muscles don't get much work in daily life — you may be prone to elbow pain.

Our favorite exercises: Triceps kickback, bench dip, triceps press-down, and triceps-extension machine or dumbbells/barbells.

Forearm muscles

Given name: Wrist extensors and flexors; **Street name:** Wrist or forearm muscles

Whereabouts: These muscles run from the bottom of your elbow to your wrist (refer to Figure 11-7).

Job description: Your *forearm muscles* bend and move your wrists. They're also a link between your upper body and any barbell, lever, or dumbbell you move. If you don't have the wrist strength to grip a barbell, you're certainly not going to be able to bench-press, even if your chest muscles are strong.

The training payoff: Powerful wrist muscles give you a stronger grip for weight lifting. Wrist strength also can help prevent tennis elbow (see Chapter 5) and *carpal tunnel syndrome* — a painful irritation of wrist nerves resulting from repetitive motions such as typing or certain assembly-line tasks, like tightening a bolt with a wrench.

Special tips: To ensure that you develop adequate wrist strength, wrap your hand firmly around the barbells or dumbbells you use.

Our favorite exercises: Dumbbell wrist curl and reverse wrist curl; we also like to do these with a bar or on a cable machine.

Getting a Core Understanding of the Abdominals

Developing a toned, flat abdomen has long been a national obsession. Most fitness magazines don't let a month go by without an article titled "Midriff Madness!" or "Flatten Your Tummy in 3 Minutes a Day!" But don't delude yourself: All the abdominal exercises in the world won't make your tummy pancake flat; in order to whittle your middle, you need to lose the extra body fat stored on top of your abdominal muscles. Still, ab training is a must, both for good posture and for the prevention of lower-back pain.

Actually, it's somewhat outdated to refer to working your middle as *ab training*. Those in the know refer to it as *core training* to reflect the idea that all the muscles that wrap around your spine work in conjunction with each other to support and stabilize your body as you move, or to protect your body while a single part of you is moving. For instance, when you toss the keys to your teenager, your core muscles tighten as you follow through with your arm so your spine doesn't do too much of the work — and so you don't fall over at the thought of your 16-year-old behind the wheel.

Rectus abdominis and company

Given name: Rectus abdominis; **Street name:** Abs (***Note:*** Don't refer to your abdominals as your stomach, which is the organ responsible for digesting food.)

Whereabouts: Your *rectus abdominis* is a flat sheet of muscle that runs from just under your chest down to a few inches south of your belly button (the top of your pelvis). See Figure 11-8.

This is one long, continuous muscle; you don't have "upper abs" and "lower abs," as many people mistakenly think. Although you can do exercises that emphasize the upper or lower portions of your rectus, all abdominal exercises do involve the entire muscle.

The muscle just below the rectus abdominis is the *transverses abdominis,* the deep stabilizer of the trunk. It's responsible for protecting the trunk and spine; think of it as the body's internal weight-lifting belt.

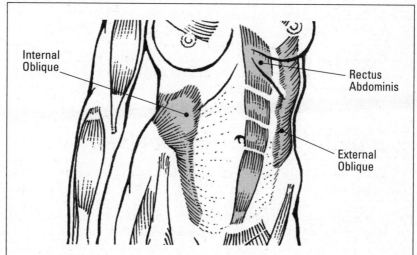

Figure 11-8: Your main abdominal muscles.

Job description: Your rectus allows you to flex your spine and pull your torso or chest toward your hips, and it works with your lower-back muscles to keep your torso stable while you move the rest of your body. For example, when you're shoveling dirt in your garden, your arms are moving, but you have to brace your body to get enough leverage and to protect your lower back.

The training payoff: Appearances aside, strong abs improve your posture by making it easier to stand up straight. Plus, they're important for guarding against lower-back pain.

Of course, the obvious reason to train your abdominals is to firm up your midsection. If your abs are really toned and you don't have much excess fat around your middle, you can see six distinct sections of the muscle. This is known as *washboard abs* or the *six pack*. But having such a firm midriff is not worth fixating on — for most people, washboard abs are not a realistic proposition. Even people with relatively low body fat tend to store at least some fat around the middle.

Special tips: Those full sit-ups you did back in high school gym class won't do the job — plus they're hard on your back, especially if you lock your feet under a couch. Although many gyms have abdominal machines, we prefer floor exercises, Pilates, yoga, and moves performed with a physioball or BOSU (devices we describe in Chapter 12).

We especially like doing abdominal exercises while leaning on a physioball. To prevent yourself from sliding off the ball, you have to keep adjusting your body position; this forces you to work your abs more completely, hitting deeper muscle fibers that don't get much of a workout while doing conventional crunches.

As for those ab-strengthening gadgets advertised on TV infomercials, you're better off spending your money on a Chia Cat Grass Planter.

Our favorite exercises: We love exercises that emphasize the rectus and transverses but integrate the entire core; these include the plank and crunches done on a physioball.

Internal and external obliques

Given name: Internal and external obliques; **Street name:** Obliques or the waist

Whereabouts: Your *internal and external obliques* run diagonally down the sides of your rectus abdominis (refer to Figure 11-8).

Job description: Your obliques enable you to twist from the waist or do a side bend.

The training payoff: Strong obliques are essential for preventing lower-back pain. They work with your rectus abdominis and lower-back muscles to support your spine.

Special tips: Placing a pole across your shoulders and twisting from side to side can wreak havoc on your lower back, especially if you do this movement a zillion times.

Our favorite exercises: We love the bicycle crunch and side plank.

Bringing Up the Butt and Hips

If your rear end and hips are larger than you'd like them to be, don't be afraid to strengthen these muscles with weights. With the right workout program, these muscles can look firmer and more shapely, not bigger and bulkier. Also, strengthening your butt and hip muscles can help prevent hip and lower-back injuries. If your job requires you to sit on your rear end all day, doing exercises that target these muscles is a good idea.

Gluteus maximus

Given name: Gluteus maximus; **Street name:** Glutes, buns, or butt

Whereabouts: This muscle is the largest muscle in your body — as if you need anyone to tell you that. Your two *glutes* (left and right cheeks) span the entire width of your derriere (see Figure 11-9).

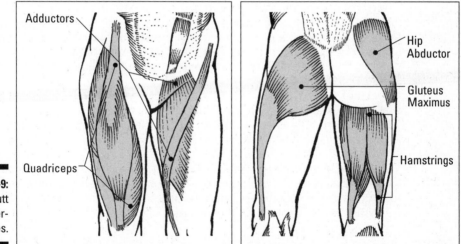

Figure 11-9:
Your butt and upper-leg muscles.

Job description: Your glutes extend your hips and help you jump, climb stairs and hills, and straighten your leg behind you. You also use your gluteus maximus when you stand up from a sitting position.

The training payoff: Training your glutes can lift your butt, make it rounder, and give it more shape. You also need your glutes to get off the couch so you can go work out.

Special tips: Some glute exercises, such as the squat and the lunge, can be hard on your knees, so pay extra attention to your form. When you bend your knees, your kneecaps should move in the direction that your toes are facing, and they shouldn't shoot out past your toes.

Our favorite exercises: Lunges, single-leg squat lunge, and leg-press machine.

Hip abductors

Given name: Hip abductors; **Street name:** Outer thighs or outer hip

Whereabouts: The meatiest part of the side of your hips (refer to Figure 11-9).

Job description: Your *abductors* help you slide your leg out to the side, like when you go skating or step aside so someone can get past you. These muscles also help your gluteus maximus (or butt) rotate your hips outward.

The training payoff: Working your abductors can firm up your outer thighs and prevent hip injuries. Athletes, seniors, and anyone who wants to prevent having a hip replacement should pay special attention to strengthening their hip muscles. You need strong abductors for running, jumping, pedaling, kicking, and skating — just about any movement that involves your lower body. Strong abductors also are important for maintaining a natural walking stride. If your hip abductors are weak, you tend to shuffle along.

Special tips: Some exercise programs advise you to do hundreds of leg lifts to tone this area, but following this advice won't get you anywhere. Work your outer thighs as you would any other muscle group — by doing 8 to 15 moderately challenging repetitions.

Our favorite exercises: Wide sides, sometimes called *sumo squats,* also known as *squats where you step out to the side and then step back in again;* we don't love the abductor/adductor machines because they aren't terribly effective for toning that saddlebag area.

Leg adductors

Given name: Leg adductors; **Street name:** Inner thighs

Whereabouts: Your *adductors* are several muscles that run from inside your hip to various points along your inner thigh (refer to Figure 11-9). You don't need to know each by name.

Job description: Your adductors help you move one leg in front of the other, especially moving your leg to the midline of your body.

The training payoff: When you sit astride a horse or motorcycle, your inner hips squeeze inward to keep you from sliding off. You also use your inner-thigh muscles for skating, soccer, and swimming the breaststroke.

Special tips: Forget the ThighMaster and the other "thigh toner" gadgets you see advertised on TV. You can work your inner-thigh muscles more effectively by adding exercise bands to floor exercises or by using machines in the gym specially designed to focus on these muscles.

Don't become fixated on toning your inner thighs; the *New England Journal of Medicine* reported about a woman who had overused a thigh-toning gadget to the point that all the tendons of her inner thighs became inflamed. Ouch.

Our favorite exercises: As for hip abductors (see the preceding section), wide-stance squats do a good job; also effective: doing a sumo squat and then standing up and sweeping your leg through the center, as if you're kicking a soccer ball.

Looking at Your Legs

Keep in mind that if all goes well, your legs will be carrying you from here to there for the rest of your life. So treat them with respect. By strengthening your leg muscles, you can head off many common knee and ankle injuries. And by staying healthy, of course, you can stay active. You can work out more and develop lean, toned legs that power you up a hill and look good in shorts.

Quadriceps

Given name: Quadriceps; **Street name:** Quads

Whereabouts: Your *quadriceps* are the four muscles at the front of each thigh (refer to Figure 11-9).

Job description: Your quadriceps straighten your knee and flex your hip.

The training payoff: You need strong quads for walking, running, climbing, skiing, skating, hopping, skipping, and jumping. Keeping your quads strong can help prevent knee problems. (If you already have knee pain, check with your doctor to find out which exercises are best for you.)

Special tips: Don't worry if you feel an intense burning sensation when you do leg extensions. This is one of the few exercises that completely isolates the quads, which causes them to tire quickly.

Our favorite exercises: Single-leg squat, lunge, leg press, and single-leg raise.

Hamstrings

Given name: Hamstrings; **Street name:** Hams

Whereabouts: Your *hamstrings* are the three muscles at the back of your thigh (refer to Figure 11-9).

Job description: Your hamstrings work in opposition to your quadriceps; in other words, your hamstrings bend the knee and extend the hip (as in walking backwards). They also help out your glutes when you move from a sitting to a standing position (see the "Gluteus maximus" section earlier in this chapter).

The training payoff: Hamstring injuries are pretty common (if not properly strengthened and flexible) because hamstrings tend to be weak compared to quads. Weekend warriors are especially prone to hamstring pulls, usually when they sprint or jump suddenly, like when they leap for a fly ball during a game of pick-up softball. Suzanne even had a friend who pulled a hamstring muscle while bowling, just as he released the ball.

Special tips: Because your hamstrings are susceptible to pulls, make sure they're adequately warmed up before you perform strengthening or stretching exercises, and always stretch them after a workout. For tips on warming up, see Chapter 6.

Our favorite exercises: Lying hip raises, seated leg curl machines, modified straight-leg deadlifts.

Gastrocnemius and soleus

Given names: Gastrocnemius and soleus; **Street name:** Calves

Whereabouts: Your *gastrocnemius,* also called your gastroc, is the large diamond-shaped muscle that gives shape to the back of your lower legs. (To see precisely what the gastroc looks like, pedal behind any top-notch cyclist.) The *soleus* resides underneath the gastroc (see Figure 11-10).

Job description: Your calf muscles allow you to stand on your tiptoes and spring off the ground whenever you jump for joy.

The training payoff: Strong and shapely calves don't just look good; they also give you staying power when you take those long, romantic walks or wait in a three-hour line for concert tickets. Plus, you need strong calves for dancing, jumping, running, and hopping.

Special tips: With calf exercises, some people find it more effective to use slightly lighter weights and do a few more repetitions — say, up to 25 — than with most other muscle groups. The muscle tissue in your calves is made specifically for endurance (walking and standing), so it takes more repetitions to reach the deepest fibers.

Our favorite exercises: Standing calf raise, seated calf raise.

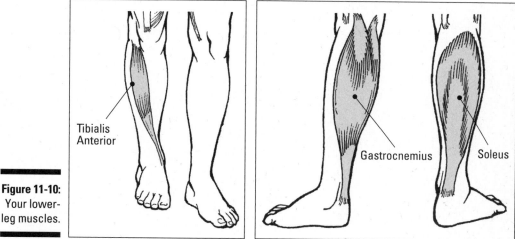

Figure 11-10: Your lower-leg muscles.

Tibialis anterior

Given name: Tibialis anterior; **Street name:** Shins

Whereabouts: The *tibialis anterior* is the largest of several muscles that run from the top of your foot up the lower leg to the outside of the shin bone, near the knee (refer to Figure 11-10).

Job description: Your shin muscles enable you to pull your toes toward your shin, as when you pick up your foot when walking or running.

The training payoff: *Shin splints* — throbbing pain at the front of your ankles caused by any sort of irritation or inflammation in the shins — are fairly common among walkers, runners, dancers, and aerobicizers who overdo it (see Chapter 5). You're especially prone to this injury if your shin muscles are weak compared to your calf muscles.

Special tips: If you do get shin splints, stay off your feet for a few days until the pain subsides. Icing and stretching can help speed recovery. For tips on icing, see Chapter 5.

Our favorite exercises: You're not likely to find a special machine at the gym to work your shins, so you can simply sit down in a chair or on a bench and tap your toes 20 times in succession.

Chapter 12

Demystifying Strength Equipment

· ·

In This Chapter

▶ Figuring out weight machines

▶ Using dumbbells and barbells

▶ Strengthening with cable pulleys and kettlebells

▶ Toning with tubes, bands, and balls

▶ Using your body as weight equipment

· ·

Some weight-lifting contraptions look like the convergence of a gynecological examination table, a minimalist sculpture, and an all-terrain vehicle. It's only natural to stare at them and think: Where do I sit? What do I push? Has anyone ever been flattened by one of these things?

As far as we know, no one has ever had any midair collisions on the Ab Flyer or time-traveled to somewhere dangerous with 6 Second Abs. Strength equipment is not as complicated as it appears. Still, you need to know what the heck you're looking at and how to use each device safely. In this chapter, we cover the vast array of strength-training equipment that you can use at home or at health clubs, including the latest developments in machines, free weights, and other strength tools. We explain the pros and cons of each type of device and help you choose the best equipment for your goals. For advice on buying strength equipment for your home, see Chapter 19.

Using Weight Machines

If you can unfold a lawn chair, you're more than qualified to operate a weight machine. It all comes down to two relatively simple acts: You adjust your seat and then you either push or pull a bar or a set of handles. These handles are connected to a cable, chain, or lever, which, in turn, is attached to a stack of rectangular weight plates. Each plate in the stack weighs between 5 and 20 pounds, depending on the make and model, and has a hole drilled in the center. If you want to lift 30 pounds, you stick a metal peg, called a *pin,* into the hole on the plate marked "30." When you pull the machine's handles, the cable picks up 30 pounds.

You may also come across machines that don't have a weight stack. Instead, you adjust the poundage by sliding donut-shaped weight plates onto a thick peg. Jargon-heads call these *plate-loaded machines.* The weight plates are the same ones used for loading up barbells. (See the "Cutting Loose with Free Weights" section later in this chapter for details about weight plates.) One popular brand of plate-loaded machines is Hammer. Many plate-loaded machines are designed so that each arm or leg works independently of the other, a feature we like because it forces your weaker side to work hard. Some non-plate-loaded machines like FreeMotion and certain lines of Cybex are designed to have a lot of wiggle in the movement, so they feel more like using free weights than standard machines.

Try every machine in your gym at least once. Different brands generally differ in the size and shape of the pulleys; the angles of the bars, seats, and weight stacks; and the type of seat and handle adjustments. You may like the Nautilus leg machines but prefer the FreeMotion Dual Cable Cross for the upper body. Even if the machines are all the same brand, you may feel more comfortable using, say, the vertical chest press rather than the horizontal one.

The weight machines designed for home use — called *multi-gyms* — generally aren't as sophisticated as health-club machines, but in many cases, your muscles won't know the difference.

What's new in weight machines

In recent years, companies such as FreeMotion and Matrix have led the way in machine innovation. Compared to traditional machines, which follow a rigid movement path when you push and pull, FreeMotion machines force you to work harder. Compared to traditional machines, which follow a rigid path of movement when you push and pull, these machines require the use of additional, deeper muscles to keep you from wobbling as you do the movement. As a result the exercises are more *functional* — that's fitness code for more translatable into everyday movement patterns. Also, the give and take makes these types of machines more comfortable than some of the traditional machines. Virtually every major weight equipment manufacturer has its own version of FreeMotion-type machines, which we call *swivel-resistance equipment.*

Swivel-resistance machines are a bit harder to get the hang of at first, so seek out guidance from a trainer at your gym. If you're intimidated by even the thought of walking into a club, you may want to start with traditional machines and later graduate to swivel-resistance machines.

While swivel-resistance machines represent somewhat of a return to the basics of weight training, another trend points in the high-tech direction: computerized weight machines. Here are some features:

- **Computerized resistance:** Instead of putting a pin in a hole or loading a plate onto a bar, you press a button indicating how much weight you want to lift in pounds or kilograms.

- **Videos:** These machines feature videos demonstrating proper technique.

- **Workout data:** Some machines store your personal information, such as your body weight and how many reps you did the last workout; either you punch in your personal code or carry around a chip or fob that you wave at the machine.

   You may even be able to download the information to a computer so that you can slice and dice your workout in any number of ways. For example, you may graph your progress on the lat pulldown based on how much you've increased the weight in the last six weeks or chart the increase in total number of sets and reps that you average per workout.

If you're a data lover, you'll embrace this trend. Our experience is that exercisers are often ambivalent about computerized weight equipment. Although the video displays are intended to make things simpler for novices, they often add an unnecessary layer of intimidation onto what may already be a daunting situation. Veterans may find all the bells and whistles cumbersome. Personally, we favor some tradition: When we use computerized machines, we miss the clanging and banging of a weight stack.

The advantages of traditional weight machines

Machines are ideal for beginners because weight machines are quite safe. If you can't muster the strength to finish an exercise, you don't have to worry about dropping a bar on your chest.

Most traditional machines require little coordination; they basically hold your body in position and guide you through the motion. Consider the shoulder-press machine: You simply sit in a chair and push the handles up — all your effort goes into lifting those handles. But if you're shoulder pressing with a swivel-resistance machine or barbell (defined in the "Cutting Loose with Free Weights" section later in this chapter), you not only have to push the bar up but also have to keep it balanced and steady. Initially, your arms may wobble back and forth. Even after you get the hang of it, the exercise always requires a certain amount of balance and coordination.

Another plus for traditional machines: They're helpful for isolating a particular muscle group. *Isolating* is just gymspeak for zeroing in on one muscle (actually, using a single joint in a motion) rather than getting several muscles or joints into the act. This is useful if you're trying to correct a specific weakness. For example, if your hamstrings (rear thigh muscles) are wimpy, you can use a machine that holds your whole body still while you bend your legs to target these muscles. With free weights, you generally can't strengthen your hamstrings without working your front thigh and butt muscles, too.

Finally, machines — at least those with weight stacks — let you get in a faster workout with less stopping and starting to adjust the weights. Instead of sliding weight plates on and off or removing free weights from the rack, you simply place a pin in a hole and adjust the seat. This makes it easy to work out with a partner who is using much heavier or lighter weights.

If your gym has 10 or 12 machines grouped in a circle, square, or similar shape, you can move from one right to the other, exercising your whole body in less than 20 minutes. Typically, machines that work your larger muscle groups (chest, back, butt, and thighs) come before machines that work your shoulders and arms.

The drawbacks of traditional weight machines

The following sections cover some of the limitations of traditional weight machines.

Interest

Machine circuits can get pretty boring — for you and your muscles. You need to stimulate your muscles with at least occasional changes in your workout. Typically, a gym has only two or three machines for each muscle group; however, with free weights, you can strengthen each muscle with dozens of exercises.

You may want to stick to machines initially but plan to mix in some free weights or swivel-resistance machines after a month or two of working out two or three days a week.

Fit

Every weight machine won't fit every body. Most machines are designed for people of average height, so if you're shorter than 5'4" or taller than 6'2", you may not be able to adjust the seat to fit your body. (Figuring out which machines don't fit may take you a while, however. Unlike amusement parks, gyms don't post height-requirement signs.) Manufacturers have tried to get around the height problems by offering a variety of pads to sit on or stick behind you, but they don't work for everyone.

Some brands of machines tend to fit specific populations better than others. For instance, Technogym and Icarian are a bit larger than average, so smaller women have a hard time using many of their machines. If a machine feels uncomfortable to you — even if you're of average height — try another machine that targets the same muscle group or head for the free-weight area.

Muscle isolations

Another drawback of machines is that many of them isolate each muscle group. We know we said this was an advantage, but it can be a flaw. Because you rarely isolate your muscles in everyday life — even doing something as simple as opening a door requires multiple muscles working in harmony — it doesn't always make sense to train them that way in the gym. The trend in weight training these days is toward *functional* workouts — that is, using gym exercises for the purpose of making real-life activities easier. Often, this goal conflicts with isolation training.

We think a mix of functional and isolation training is just fine for beginners. As you become more expert or clearer about your goals, you will probably gravitate toward more functional training. However, bodybuilders are a good example of experienced weight lifters who do a lot of isolation training specifically to make their bodies look a certain way. But even they do some functional training, too.

Portability

One final reason to venture beyond machines: You can't take 'em with you. If you're on vacation and your hotel gym has nothing more than a pile of dumbbells, you need to know what to do with them. Don't give yourself another excuse to blow off a workout.

Special tips for using weight machines

Don't let weight machines scare you. Use the following tips to look like an old pro next time you go to the gym:

- ✔ **Make the adjustments.** Don't just hop on a machine and start pumping away. If the last guy who used it was a foot taller than you are, you may find yourself suspended in midair in the middle of the exercise.

  To adjust a machine, you usually have to adjust a lever, shift the seat up or down, and then readjust the lever. Adjusting the seat is a hassle at first, but if you don't do it, you set yourself up for an injury and an uncomfortable series of repetitions. Also, you cheat yourself out of a good workout.

For instance, if you don't adjust the biceps-curl machine correctly, you may compensate by using your back muscles, thereby defeating the purpose of the exercise.

Let a trainer show you how to adjust each machine to fit your body. In general, line up the joint that you're trying to move (your knees, for example) with the joint of the machine that's moving. You shouldn't have to strain in any way to do the movement. If you begin to feel any discomfort, particularly in your joints, stop the exercise and readjust the seat or position, as needed.

✔ **Check the weight stack before you lift.** Never begin the exercise without checking where the pin has been inserted or the dial has been set. If someone has *racked* the machine (put the pin all the way on the bottom or dialed up the highest amount of weight so the entire weight stack is captured), either your eyes are going to pop out of your head or you're going to be mighty embarrassed when you can't budge it.

When you first learn to use a machine, write down the weight and seat adjustment ("leg extension: 30 lbs., second setting") on a card or in a workout log. Carry these notes with you and update them regularly.

✔ **Remember the name of each machine.** You should not refer to the lat pull-down as "that one where you pull down that bar thingy." Knowing what to call each contraption reminds you what the heck you're doing — you'll remember that you're working your lats *(latissimus dorsi),* assuming you remember what those are. (If you don't, see Chapter 11.) Most machines have some sort of name plaque or label. If you don't see one, ask the trainer on duty what the machine is called. Some now have computers that talk to you and remind you how to use them.

✔ **Stay in control.** If the weight stack bangs and clangs like a junior-high marching band, you're probably lifting too fast. Many machine manufacturers recommend taking two slow counts to lift the weight stack up and four slow counts to lower the weight stack down. You may feel more comfortable speeding it up to a two-two count.

✔ **Don't stick any body part near a weight stack that is being lifted or lowered.** Liz saw a woman place her hand on a weight stack as she pulled out the pin. Sixty pounds of weight came crashing down on the woman's palm. She was rushed to the hospital, where her hand was repaired with eight stitches. Liz also saw a woman with long hair lean over to pull out a pin before lowering the weight stack; the last 4 inches of her hair got pressed between the weights. Fortunately, Liz and other staff members were able to rectify the situation without giving the woman a new hairstyle.

✔ **Change the weight in the smallest increment possible.** Most machines have plates hanging on the frame or built into the weight stack that weigh one-quarter or one-half as much as a full plate. Instead of increasing your weight by an entire plate, you can place this thin rectangle on top of the stack, slide a doughnut over, or dial in a small increase. Cybex, for example, has come up with an ingenious way to increase weight by one-third of a plate, a system used on some of its machines. Each machine has an abacus-like apparatus linked to the stack of 20-pound weight plates. To increase the weight, you slide a weighted disk toward the stack, increasing the weight by 5 pounds. There are three disks per abacus, allowing you to go from 10 pounds to 15 pounds to 20 before moving on to a new plate.

Cutting Loose with Free Weights

Free weights are nothing to be afraid of. They're simply bars with weight plates on each end, and they're perfectly suitable for people who don't envision a Mr. Olympia title in their future. The long bars are called *barbells,* and the short bars are called *dumbbells* (see Figure 12-1). It takes two hands to hoist a barbell. You can lift a dumbbell with one hand, although you may do some exercises using two hands on a single dumbbell.

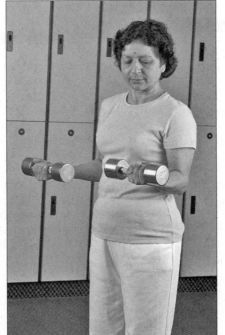

Figure 12-1:
You can use dumb-bells for hundreds of exercises.

Building muscle on the cheap

Weight is weight, and sometimes in a pinch, household items can be mighty effective for building strength. For instance, you've probably heard that soup cans are mmm-mmm good for dumbbell substitutes, and this is true. However, cooking-oil or cleaning-oil bottles filled with sand, pebbles, or water can be a better alternative. Many of these bottles are designed with an indent in the center, making them easier to grip. You also can fill plastic shopping bags with fruit, books, cans or whatever and hold the bags by the handles for exercises such as squats and lunges. Just be careful about using bags for overhead movements; you don't want a swinging bag full of pears to clunk you in the head. You may fill a backpack and wear it to add resistance to lunges, squats, or even push-ups.

Just make sure the weight is as even as possible for both sides of your body. Don't do squats with your hardcover *Harry Potter* collection in one bag and packages of lasagna noodles in the other. If you're curious, weigh the items on your bathroom scale so that you have an idea of how much you're lifting or whether you've chosen an item that's suitably heavier than the last.

At most gyms, you find a wide array of dumbbells, lined up from lightest, usually 2 pounds, to heaviest, as much as 200 pounds. At larger gyms, you also find a selection of bars with plates welded to each end, starting with 20 pounds and increasing in 10-pound increments.

Virtually every gym has bars without weight plates on each end. The *long bar* (also called an *Olympic bar*) alone usually weighs 45 pounds. To increase the poundage, you slide *weight plates* — round plates with a hole through the center — onto each end. You then secure the plates with clips called *collars,* which are a safety requirement in many facilities. An assortment of these weight plates, typically from 2½ pounds to 45 pounds, sits on a rack near the bars. If you want to lift 75 pounds, you add a 10-pound plate and a 5-pound plate to each side of the 45-pound bar. After you finish, be sure to remove these plates and put them back in their proper place. Otherwise, you risk unfriendly stares from the staff and the guy or gal who uses the bar after you.

Some plates, such as those made by Iron Grip, are easier to carry than the traditional ones because they have handles built in. Imagine the difference between carrying a suitcase with a handle and without. We suspect they prevent back problems caused by improperly lifting standard weight plates. The handles also keep the plates from slipping and dropping to the floor.

The advantages of free weights

Free weights are much more versatile than machines. Whereas a weight machine is designed for one particular motion, a single pair of dumbbells can be used to perform literally hundreds of exercises. For instance, you can push dumbbells overhead to work your shoulders, press them backward to tone your triceps, or hold one in each hand while you squat to strengthen your thighs and butt muscles. You can change the feel and emphasis of an exercise by simply altering the way you grip the bar.

Another important benefit of free weights is that they work your muscles in a way that closely mimics real-life movements. Machines tend to isolate a particular muscle so the rest of your muscles don't get any action. But free-weight training requires several muscles to move, balance, and steady a weight as you lift and lower it. Free-weight exercises allow you to strengthen muscles that wouldn't get much work if you were doing isolation exercises with machines. Some people find they gain strength when they do the majority of their exercises with free weights.

The drawbacks of free weights

For some novices, free-weight exercises are hard to get the hang of. You need more instruction than you do with machines — there are a lot more mistakes to make and injuries to avoid.

Anyone using free weights needs to be very careful, even with light weights. Debbie Bacon of Phoenix, Arizona, learned this lesson the hard way. While waiting for her husband to come home late one night, Debbie decided exercising might help her stay awake. She was doing shoulder exercises with 7-pound dumbbells when she got so tired that she lost control of the weights and they crashed together. Unfortunately, her right index and ring fingers got in the way. The incident involved a fractured fingertip and a piece of acrylic nail that got lodged where it shouldn't have been. But we'll spare you the gory details. Suffice it to say that free weights require your full attention.

Also, free-weight exercises require more balance than machine moves. If you're short on time, a free-weight workout probably will take you longer than a machine workout. Instead of simply putting a pin in a weight stack, you may have to slide weight plates on and off a bar. But if a gym has various free weights available without having to change plates, this may not be the case.

Special tips for using free weights

Here are a few tips to make free-weight training safe and fun:

✔ **If you're using very heavy weights, enlist a spotter.** Don't hesitate to ask for assistance if you think you may have trouble completing a set. A spotter — someone who watches as you lift weights to ensure your safety, shown in Figure 12-2 — is particularly helpful when you graduate to a heavier weight. You can enlist help from a health-club staff member or ask anyone nearby who doesn't look too busy. (This is a good way to make friends at the gym, too.)

Fill your spotter in on your game plan. Mention how many reps you think you can do and on which rep you think you'd like to call in the cavalry. For details on acting as a spotter, see the sidebar "Giving a spot."

✔ **Be careful when you lift a weight from a rack and when you put it back.** Never pick up a weight off the floor without bending your knees and tightening your abs.

✔ **Never drop the weights carelessly when you've completed a set.** The loud clang is sure to annoy your fellow lifters, and the weights may roll away and land on someone's toes — or bounce and crash into a mirror. Don't laugh; we've seen it happen more than once.

✔ **Use two hands when lifting plates.** This is the same command we bark at our children when they're helping us empty the dishwasher. Remember that plates are weight, too, and you can just as easily hurt yourself placing a weight on a bar as you can performing an exercise. Don't attempt to lift a weight plate onto a bar if it's too heavy for you.

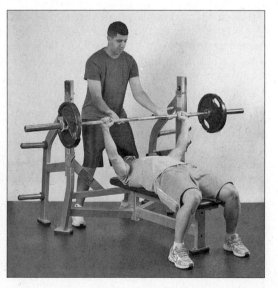

Figure 12-2:
Always use a spotter when lifting a heavy weight.

Giving a spot

If you spend enough time in the gym, sooner or later someone is going to ask you, "Hey, mind giving me a spot?" He's not asking you to buy him a puppy; he would like assistance with his next set. You should be flattered at the request, but be aware that spotting is an awesome responsibility. It falls on your shoulders to prevent the weight from, well, falling on the guy's shoulders.

Here's how to handle the job of spotting a fellow weight lifter:

✔ **Pay attention at all times.** Don't get into a heated discussion about the Second Amendment. You need to be ready, on a split-second's notice, to lift the bar off your spottee's chest if his arms give out. Politely tune out the rest of the world until your spottee completes his set.

✔ **Ask your spottee where he'd like you to place your hands.** There are several schools of thought on this subject. You can rest a fingertip or two on the bar at all times so you can give instantaneous help when your spottee calls for it — usually during the last repetition or two. Some people, including us, find that position annoying, because it diminishes the feelings of glory you experience when you complete a set by yourself. We prefer the ready-willing-and-able spotting technique. That is, have your hands poised a couple inches from the bar; touch the bar only when your spottee begins to struggle. Some spotters also place their hands on the joint or limb doing the movement, as close to the bar as possible (for example, on the wrists).

✔ **If you don't think you can handle spotting someone, say so.** In order to spot someone bench-pressing 100 pounds, you don't need to be able to bench 100 pounds yourself — you're just there to help out. However, this is no time for heroics. If you have trouble lifting the 5-pounders off the rack, you're not a candidate for this job.

✔ **Use proper posture.** This means not rounding your spine, keeping a good center of gravity, and making sure you're in a stable position. This is the strongest position to help someone complete their lift without destroying your back.

✔ **Don't over-spot.** You're there to help the guy, not do the work for him. When you're spotting someone on the bench press, don't lean directly over the bar, grip it with both hands, and pull it up and down. With a little experience, you'll be able to provide just the right amount of additional effort that the person needs to complete the exercise. (If you're the one being spotted, you may want to say something like, "Don't help me until I really need it." You can also scream, "I got it! I got it!" if it looks like your spotter is going to prematurely swoop in to help.)

✔ **Always offer encouraging words.** Say things like, "It's all yours! You got it! You got it! All you!" This gives your spottee inspiration to squeeze out that last repetition. Plus, it makes everyone else in the gym glance over in admiration.

✔ **No matter which end of the spot you're on, pleasant breath is a must.** Remember, you'll be breathing forcefully right into someone's face. You don't want to find a bottle of Scope waiting for you in your locker.

Using benches with free weights

A bench can help you get a better workout. Some benches are flat, and some are upright, like narrow chairs with high, padded backs. Others are adjustable so you can slide them to an incline or decline position.

Here are some tips for using benches:

✔ **Experiment with the angle of the bench, especially for chest exercises.** Inclining the bench a few degrees allows you to work the muscle fibers of your upper chest. (But attempting chest exercises at too high an angle can put your shoulder joint in jeopardy.) Declining the bench emphasizes your lower chest. You can use a slightly different angle each workout if you want.

✔ **Use a bench for support.** When you're doing overhead lifts or bicep curls, adjust the seat so it's upright, and sit snugly against it. This position protects your back and makes the exercise more effective. You won't be able to rock your body back and forth to build momentum to hoist the dumbbell. You have to rely solely on the muscle power of your biceps. However, you'll still have to stop yourself from arching the small of your back off the bench when the weight gets heavy.

✔ **Use weight-lifting benches for one activity only: lifting weights.** Don't use a bench to change a light bulb at home, and don't use it at the gym to take a nap. Never use a weight bench as a step bench. (You can, however, use your step bench as a weight bench as long as you're not lifting dumbbells heavier than, say, 30 pounds.)

✔ **Keep your feet flat on the floor or flat on the bench, whichever is more comfortable.** You can keep your feet up in the air if you want to work your core muscles more thoroughly.

Note that you don't need an actual bench to perform "bench" exercises. You can use a *physioball,* a thicker, sturdier version of a beach ball that we describe in Chapter 15. Performing strength moves while sitting or lying on a ball forces your core muscles to work extra hard to keep you from rolling off. A step bench, used in step aerobics, can double as a weight bench. So can a BOSU, a half-ball described in Chapter 15.

Pulling Your Weight with Cable Pulleys

At most gyms, you see a box full of ropes, straps, handles, short bars, long bars, V-shaped bars, and bars shaped like a handlebar mustache. This paraphernalia looks like a pile of junk excavated from someone's garage. But in fact, these are the attachments you can clip onto a cable machine to do a wide variety of exercises. The *cable machine* consists of a cable and a round pulley attached to a metal frame. There are one-tower and two-tower versions. With a two-tower cable pulley, you can stand between the towers and work both sides of your body.

Note: Swivel-resistance machines are more formalized versions of cable machines and work on a similar principle as the traditional cable machines that we're talking about here. (For more on swivel-resistance machines, see the earlier section "What's new in weight machines.")

The advantages and disadvantages of cable pulleys

Cable pulleys are a cross between machines and free weights. On the one hand, the cable is hooked up to a stack of weights, so nothing can come crashing down. On the other hand, the motion isn't guided — you're free to pull the bar down the way you want to, and you're free to make lots of mistakes. Like free weights, cable machines require a certain amount of control and instruction.

Also like free weights, cable pulleys allow you to perform a wide variety of exercises. For instance, to strengthen your back, you can pull down a bar clipped to a high pulley — one that's attached all the way at the top (see Figure 12-3). To strengthen your biceps, you can pull up on a low pulley — attached near the bottom of the frame, typically a few inches from the floor. To strengthen your chest, you can grab a high pulley on each side of the frame and pull both handles toward your chest, as if you're going to wrap your arms around someone.

Special tips for using cable pulleys

Don't be afraid to play around with the different types of adjustments. Attaching a new bar is easier than it looks, and you may find that, when working your triceps, a V-shaped bar feels more comfortable than a straight bar. When you do make the switcheroo, you may need to adjust the amount of weight you're using. Even if you're doing the very same exercise, you may use more weight pulling down the V-shaped bar than you would pulling down the straight bar.

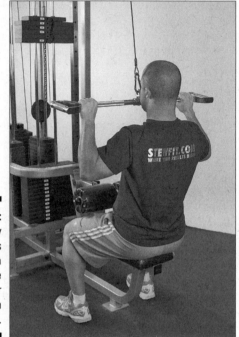

Figure 12-3:
Cable pulley machines are a versatile tool for strength training.

Getting into the Swing of Things with Kettlebells

A *kettlebell* is a cast-iron weight that looks like a bowling ball with a handle, or a bit like the kind of tea kettles that sit atop wood-burning stoves to keep the humidity down.

Kettlebells range in weight from about 1 pound up to 70 pounds, though most people don't venture much over 20 pounds.

To train with a kettlebell, you pick up the weight with both hands and swing it through a motion, using your entire body to control the weight so that you don't accidentally toss it, or yourself, through a plate-glass window. We tell you in Chapter 13 to lift weights slowly so that you don't create extra momentum in your movements, but kettlebells throw caution to the wind and ask you to put a lot of momentum into your lifting movements. When you swing the bell correctly, you appear to be tossing a bucket of water to put out a fire. See Figure 12-4.

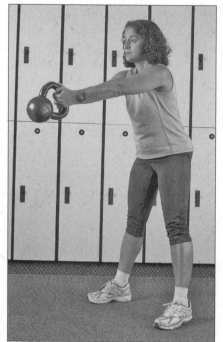

Figure 12-4:
Use good
control
when you
swing a
kettlebell.

The advantages of kettlebells

Though kettlebells are all the rage at trendy American training studios, they actually date back to Tsarist Russia. A 1913 article in the Russian magazine *Hercules* states, "Not a single sport develops our muscular strength and bodies as well as kettlebell athletics." That may be a bit of an exaggeration, but there is good reason that kettlebells are reportedly popular among the Russian Special Forces, the FBI Hostage Rescue Team, and the Secret Service Counter Assault Team: Kettlebells can be a great tool to help get you in phenomenal shape.

Because more muscle groups are involved in the swinging (and controlling the swing of) a kettlebell than during the lifting of dumbbells, some people consider a kettlebell workout more effective at building functional strength, as well as promoting balance, coordination, flexibility, and agility. Certainly, the workout yields great results for the core muscles, which bear the main responsibility for keeping the motion from getting too wild. The shape and handle of the kettlebells allow you to perform exercises that simply aren't possible in any other way.

The drawbacks of kettlebells

Kettlebell workouts are fun, but we do offer a caveat: There isn't much room for error. Without proper instruction, you can throw out your back, torque your hip, or succumb to some other pretty serious injury.

Special tips for using kettlebells

Learn proper kettlebell form by taking a class with an expert instructor before you strike out on your own or even try a DVD workout. If you practice impeccable form and don't overdo the weight, you can be one of those people who train for years with kettlebells and never get hurt.

Stretching Your Routine with Tubes and Bands

Exercise tubes are like the thick rubber tubes you can find in a medical-supply store — they just come in brighter colors. Some exercise tubes have handles or buckles attached to each end, or they come in a kit with attachable plastic bars and door attachments. You also can buy *exercise bands,* which are long, flat sheets of strong rubber.

The advantages of tubes and bands

You can exercise virtually every muscle group in your body with bands and tubes, although tubes work better for some exercises, and bands work better for others. You just have to experiment. For instance, here's how you can use bands to work both of your biceps at once: You stand on the center of the band and hold an end in each hand, with your elbows by your sides; see Figure 12-5a. Bend your arms without moving your shoulders and curl your hands up toward your shoulders as shown in Figure 12-5b. Lower your arms slowly so the band doesn't just snap back into place. (You can find a whole chapter full of band exercises in our book *Weight Training For Dummies,* published by Wiley.)

Bands and tubes take up zero space, and they're portable. They give you an instant strength workout, whether you're in a small studio apartment, in a hotel room, or on a camping trip in the Mojave Desert.

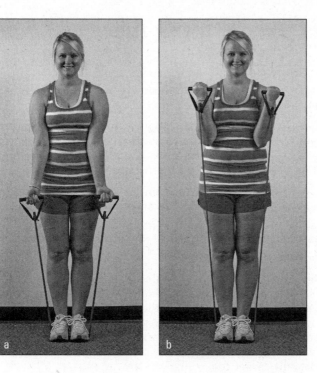

Figure 12-5:
You can use
exercise
tubes to
strengthen
virtually
every
muscle in
your body.

Bands and tubes are easy to adjust, too; to make an exercise tougher, just use a shorter or thicker band or step farther away to stretch the band farther and increase the level of resistance.

They're also cheap: You can purchase a couple of bands for around $10. Even if you go hog wild, you'd have trouble spending more than $100 on a set of bands, a travel bag, and a DVD explaining how to use the bands.

The drawbacks of tubes and bands

If a band or tube slips, you can get snapped in the face or groin. Ouch. Also, reproducing the same amount of work from one workout to the next is difficult. You know when you're lifting a 20-pound dumbbell or a 50-pound weight stack, but bands and tubes have no comparable measuring system. They simply come in different resistances: usually light, medium, heavy, and extra-heavy. (There's no universal code for color. One company's yellow band may be the easiest resistance, whereas another company's yellow band may be the most difficult. Look for band thickness.) Also, know that there's a limit to how much strength you can gain with bands.

Special tips for using tubes and bands

When you're using bands and tubes, keep the following tips in mind:

- ✔ **Lift and lower the band or tube slowly.** If you move carefully, you'll feel your muscles working in both directions.

- ✔ **Don't wrap the band or tube so tightly around your palms or feet that you cut off the circulation to your hands or feet.** Instead, wrap it loosely several times so that it forms loops, the way you wind a dog's leash around your hand. Never tie it tightly around your wrist or ankle, either.

- ✔ **When you wrap a band or tube under your feet, make sure that it's secure.** You don't want a band to slip out from under you.

- ✔ **Use bands or tubes that are specifically designed for exercising.** Inspect them frequently for holes and tears, and replace them when they're worn.

- ✔ **Experiment with different varieties.** Bands and tubes come in many shapes, sizes, and colors and with myriad doodads to add or clip onto them. Some tubes have hard handles, others have fabric handles, and some have none. Brands featuring three bands braided together provide a unique sense of resistance. They're readily available on dozens of Web sites, virtually any sporting goods store, and now even at places like Walmart and Target.

Training with Weighted Balls

Medicine balls are among the oldest forms of strength training in existence. Reports of Persians tossing weighted balls back and forth to rehabilitate from injury date back more than 3,000 years. Ancient Greek Olympians used weighted balls for training and rehabilitation. A bit more recently, balls became popular with *plyometrics,* a type of exercise that involves quick, explosive movements to develop speed, agility, and coordination along with strength.

Medicine balls come in different varieties and typically weigh 1 to 25 pounds. The most popular balls look like the kickball your gym teacher used to torture you with in junior high, except they're a lot heavier. Others look like multi-colored basketballs with a shoelace built in to keep the ball in a very tight shape. Some have handles or straps.

The advantages of medicine balls

Medicine balls are useful in much the same way as kettlebells: The momentum generated by tossing and catching them forces you to work some of the deep support muscles that don't see much action during straight-up weight training.

Medicine balls needn't be tossed around, however. You can use them as you would any conventional type of resistance. For example, when you perform a lunge, you can hold the ball to your chest to add resistance; the ball adds an element of balance to the move as well. See Figure 12-6.

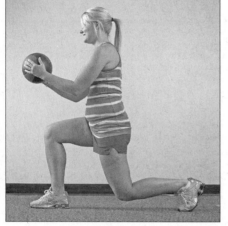

Figure 12-6:
The medicine ball is a good way to add resistance to exercises like the lunge.

We like medicine balls for certain exercises. Take that lunge again: One of our favorite versions is tossing the ball to a partner as you lunge out and then catching it as you stand up. The ball takes a very basic exercise and turns it into a full-body workout.

The drawbacks of medicine balls

Medicine balls aren't as easy to use as dumbbells because you can't grasp them fully, and they may seem cumbersome at first. If you're not careful, they can slip out of your hands during use. Also, you need to buy several different sizes to ensure you have the proper resistance for a range of exercises, from squats to walking lunges to core training.

Special tips for using medicine balls

Keep the following tips in mind when using medicine balls:

✔ **Practice good form.** Many medicine-ball exercises involve catching, throwing, and tossing, all movements that have great capacity to get you in shape, along with the capacity to cause injury if you twist too abruptly or whack yourself with the ball.

✔ **Control your movements.** Even when you're using medicine balls during plyometric exercises, which are quick and explosive, always stay in command of your body.

✔ **Don't overdo it.** Medicine-ball work can be intense, so a little goes a long way. Work these exercises into your routine gradually.

Rounding out a workout with other gadgets

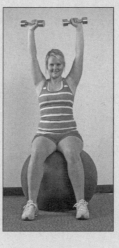 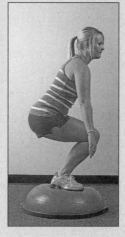

Don't confuse medicine balls with physioballs, also known as *stability balls* or *exercise balls.* A physioball, shown on the left, looks more like a beach ball, except it's sturdier and larger. In weight training, physioballs are mostly useful as a bench or as a method of challenging your balance. However, physioballs can be thrown around like medicine balls and used to offer resistance to exercises. Because they're comparatively lighter, the challenge comes more in handling the size rather than extra weight.

A BOSU, shown on the right, is a variation on a physioball. Essentially, it's half a physioball that has been mounted to a plastic platform. You can stand on a BOSU — either on the ball side or platform — as you do your squats or biceps curls. This is another way of adding core stability challenge to a movement without adding resistance.

There are plenty of other gadgets that can be used in weight training, from weighted gloves to the Pilates *magic circle,* a round metal ring that you squeeze with your arms or thighs. The options are too numerous to mention and are constantly changing. We recommend trying any gadgets that seem useful and appealing, but don't feel that you need to spend all your cash on weight-training tools. You can get a great workout sticking to the basics.

Relying on Your Body as Strength Equipment

You can't get any more basic than lifting your own self! Yes, your very own body can function as strength equipment. You can lift it, lower it, curl it, twist it, and bend it in all sorts of ways that are designed to increase your strength. We're talking leg lifts, push-ups, pull-ups, and the like. When you move your body weight, you're fighting gravity — and that can be a considerable fight.

The advantages of using your body weight

You don't require any storage space and you certainly can take yourself anywhere. Plus, push-ups and pull-ups are impressive, and they call upon just about every muscle in your upper body. If you're really serious about building upper-body strength, add push-ups and pull-up-type exercises to your strength-training routine.

Also, using your own body weight can be a way to start out doing an exercise that eventually will require some type of resistance. For example, when you first try a squat (see Chapter 13), simply bending and straightening with your body will be plenty of resistance, thank you very much. After a while, you'll have to make the exercise more challenging by using free weights, bands, a machine, or a ball.

The drawbacks of using your body weight

Ever try a pull-up? They're darned hard. Most people can't do pull-ups until they've spent at least a few months lifting weights. And then, eventually, they have the opposite problem: The pull-ups become too easy. To continue making progress, you may need to invest in equipment or join a gym. (But trust us: It's likely to be a long time before you need to do pull-ups while wearing a weight belt with a hubcap-sized weight plate dangling from it.)

Special tips for using your body weight

Keep the following tips in mind when using your body weight:

- ✓ **Your body is resistance.** Do keep this in mind. As with any other form of resistance, you can overdo it if you're not careful. Start out slowly, and progress with care. If you haven't worked out in a while, using just the weight of your body can leave you very sore indeed.

- ✓ **Change up your exercise.** As we've said, you don't necessarily need to add more resistance to a body-weight exercise to make it more challenging. Other ways to push yourself include adding a few more reps, upping the number of sets, slowing down your reps, or changing your body position.

Chapter 13

Designing a Strength-Training Program

*I*f you walk into a gym and observe the members lifting weights, you notice something striking: Every lifter is doing something different. Some are pumping their dumbbells slowly; others are swinging large casks of metal like they're trying to toss them over a wall. Some pull down a bar 6 times and move on to the next machine; others pull down that bar 15 times, rest, and then do it again — and again. The fact is, you could lift weights for the next 50 years and never do the same workout twice.

To a novice, the endless possibilities may seem daunting. Worry not: All the exercises are really variations on the same set of classic moves, and the routines follow a basic set of principles. In this chapter, we explain how to create a sound, sensible workout so that you make the best use of your time and energy. We don't want you flailing around your gym or basement wondering which exercises to do, how to perform them properly, how much weight to lift, and so on.

The exercises we show in this chapter include variations done with both free weights and machines. After you master these, you may want to try some of the more advanced exercises we demonstrate in *Weight Training For Dummies* (Wiley). In the meantime, we recommend consulting a qualified trainer at least once before you embark on a strength-training program. (See Chapter 20 for tips on finding a competent trainer.)

The Building Blocks of a Strength-Training Workout

This section covers the basic principles of a good strength-training program — how much to lift, how quickly and how many times to raise and lower each weight, and so on.

Note: Before designing a strength-training program, you need to know two key terms: rep and set. *Rep* is short for *repetition* — one complete motion of an exercise. Suppose you're doing a leg lift. When you lift your leg and then lower it back down, you've completed one rep. A *set* is a group of consecutive repetitions. For example, you can say, "I did two sets of ten reps on the chest press." This means that you did ten consecutive chest presses, rested, and then did another ten chest presses.

Choosing your weight

Here, we discuss how heavy your weights should be and how to know when you're ready for more.

How much weight should I lift?

To increase strength and help build strong bones, you need to lift an amount that stresses your muscles and bones. So although we can't tell you a specific amount to lift, we can tell you that it has to be enough so that you feel challenged. No matter how many repetitions you do, always use a heavy enough weight so that the last rep is a struggle but not such an effort that you compromise good form. After about six weeks of strength training, you may want to go to *muscular failure* (that is, your last repetition is so difficult that you can't squeeze out one more).

Be sure to adjust the amount of weight you use for each exercise. In general, use more weight to work larger muscles like your thighs, chest, and upper back, and use less weight to exercise your shoulders, arms, and abdominals. But even when doing different exercises for the same muscle group, you're likely to need a variety of weights. For example, you typically can handle more weight on the flat chest-press machine than you can on the incline chest-press machine. This is because the incline machine involves more of the shoulder, a muscle group that's much smaller than the chest and isn't able to press as much weight.

Using a training log, online tracker, or notepad, write down how much weight you lift for each exercise so that next time around, you don't have to waste time experimenting all over again. (Some fitness facilities have machines that allow you to record and store your info right there or on a chip or card you carry with you.) But don't lock yourself into lifting a certain amount of weight every time. Everyone feels stronger on some days than on others. Just because you can do a triceps push down with 15 pounds on Monday doesn't mean you'll be able to do it on Wednesday. Listen to your body. It'll tell you what it can and can't handle.

How do I know when I'm ready to lift more weight?

As your muscles gain strength, you need to gradually increase the load on them by increasing the amount of weight you lift. Graduating to a heavier weight is one of the most rewarding aspects of lifting weights. If you track your progress in a log, you'll have a record of just how far you've come.

It won't take long to outgrow the weights you use during your first workout. When you can easily do the maximum number of reps you're aiming for, increase the weight by the smallest increment possible and drop down to fewer reps. You know you're lifting too much weight if you can't complete your repetitions with good form and if you feel the need to grunt. Or you fall off the bench!

Not all muscles improve at the same rate. After a month of weight training, you may jump up 20 pounds on a chest exercise but only 5 pounds on a shoulder exercise. But you also probably started out using a smaller weight on shoulders to begin with. Because the chest is a much larger muscle than the shoulder, it has greater strength potential. The relative amount of weight you increase may be the same for both muscle groups.

Planning your workout

The following sections address the questions of how many reps, how many sets, and how often you should lift.

How many reps should I do?

The number of reps you should do depends on where you are in your training (new, experienced, coming back from a long layoff) and your goals:

- ✔ To become as strong and as big as your body type will allow, do 3 to 8 reps per set with a very heavy weight.

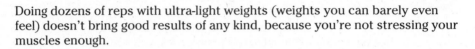

✔ To tone your muscles and develop the type of strength you need for everyday life — moving furniture or shoveling snow — aim for one set of 10 to 12 repetitions.

Doing dozens of reps with ultra-light weights (weights you can barely even feel) doesn't bring good results of any kind, because you're not stressing your muscles enough.

If you have a few different goals in mind, you can mix and match the number of reps you do per workout. If you want to get bigger and stronger and also improve the endurance of those muscles, you can do a heavy workout one day and a lighter workout the next time out. Or you can train in cycles: Do several weeks of heavy training (heavier weights and fewer reps) followed by several weeks of light training. Keep track of how you feel; your body may respond better to one type of training than another.

How many sets should I do for each muscle group?

There's no simple answer. Several studies show that doing one set per muscle builds just as much strength as doing three sets per muscle, at least for the first three or four months of training. So here's our advice: If you're a novice or if you're starting again after a layoff, begin with one set of 10 to 12 repetitions, and make sure your last rep feels challenging. You should feel like you have control of the weight but if you did one more rep, you may not be able to make it all the way. Most people can increase their initial weights after two to four weeks of training; at that point, consider adding a second or even third set for each muscle group. However, if your goal is simply to build enough strength for good health, one challenging set may be sufficient. Just make sure you perform a balanced workout, giving each muscle group equal time. Performing, say, three sets of a chest exercise but only one set of a back exercise can lead to injury.

How often do I need to lift weights?

Start by lifting two or three days per week for several weeks, completing one set of 10 to 12 reps and then increasing in either sets or weight based on your exercise goals. If your aim is maximum strength, targeting each muscle three times a week may not give your muscles enough chance to rest. In that case, cut back to two workouts per muscle group per week.

If you really get into weight training, consider doing a *split routine,* in which you exercise some of your muscles during one workout and then come back a day or two later to exercise the others. You still work each muscle at least twice a week, but because you don't train every muscle during every workout, you can devote more energy to the muscles you're focusing on that day — and each of your muscles still gets enough rest.

Splitting your routine is a good idea if you're serious about building muscle and if you have free time in small chunks. You may be fresher and more motivated if you walk into the gym knowing that, today, you have to work only your chest, triceps, and shoulders. You probably work these muscles harder than if you try to fit all your muscle groups into one workout.

Here are the two most popular ways of splitting a routine:

> ✔ **Push/pull:** Work your *pulling muscles* (your back muscles and biceps) on one day, and during the next session, work your *pushing muscles* (your chest and triceps). You can fit in your leg, shoulder, and abdominal exercises whenever you want. Following is an example of a push/pull routine.

Day	*Muscles Worked*
Monday	Push (chest, triceps, shoulders, lower-body exercises)
Tuesday	Pull (back, biceps, abdominals)
Wednesday	REST
Thursday	Push (chest, triceps, shoulders, lower-body exercises)
Friday	REST
Saturday	Pull (back, biceps, abdominals)
Sunday	REST

> ✔ **Upper body/lower body:** Work your upper body one day and your lower body the next. You fit in your abs two to four times a week whenever it's convenient. (See Chapter 11 for definitions of various muscles.)

Day	*Muscles Worked*
Monday	Upper body (back, chest, shoulders, triceps, biceps)
Tuesday	Lower body (glutes, quadriceps, hamstrings, calves, abdominals)
Wednesday	REST
Thursday	Upper body (back, chest, shoulders, triceps, biceps)
Friday	REST
Saturday	Lower body (glutes, quadriceps, hamstrings, calves, abdominals)
Sunday	REST

Whatever workout schedule you design, make sure each muscle group gets at least one full day of rest between sessions. You can lift two days back to back, but you don't want to lift with your upper body, for example, two days in a row. Lifting weight literally creates tiny little tears in your muscles. They need those 48 hours to recover and rebuild. (You can do cardio on consecutive days because it's much easier on your muscles than weight training.) If you don't rest in this way, you may wind up sore and more prone to overuse injuries. (Keep in mind that perpetual soreness can be a sign of overtraining.) Besides, overworking a muscle may weaken it, defeating your purpose for training.

Considering time and speed

In the next sections, we discuss how long you should take to raise and lower a weight (faster isn't always better!), and we give you tips on resting between sets.

How fast should I do my reps?

Take a full 2 seconds to lift a weight and 2 to 4 seconds to lower it. If you lift more quickly than that, you may hear a lot of clanging and banging (of the weights). Plus you'll end up relying on momentum rather than muscle power. Going slow and steady yields better results because more of your muscle gets into the act.

How long should I rest between sets?

The amount of rest you take in between sets is another variable that you can toy around with. If you're a beginner, rest about 90 seconds between sets to give your muscles adequate time to recover. As you get in better shape, you need less rest — only about 30 seconds — before your muscles feel ready for another set. If you follow a chest exercise with, say, a thigh exercise, you typically need less rest than if you do consecutive exercises for the same muscle group, such as two chest exercises in a row.

After the first few weeks of training, you can fine-tune the amount of rest you take between sets according to your goals. If you're using really heavy weights and doing fewer reps in order to bulk up, you can take up to 5 minutes between sets so that your muscles can pump out their greatest effort each time. Of course, 5 minutes is a long time to sit around at the gym; Suzanne recently saw a guy studying Chinese characters during his lengthy rest periods. That seemed like a good use of time.

If you're short on time or you like a fast-paced workout, try *circuit training:* You move quickly from exercise to exercise with little or no rest at all. Circuit training does a decent job of building strength, and it can be a good substitute for an aerobic workout, especially if you start and end with a fairly long aerobic warm-up and cool-down. However, it doesn't give you quite the same benefits of either. That said, we love circuit training and often use it in our own workouts. You also see this type of strength training in clubs aimed at beginners, like Curves, because it's easy, fast-paced, and, believe it or not, fun to do. Just know that if you're serious about making real gains, you need to slow it down and do some focused strength training, too.

Setting up and changing your routine

Here, we address questions related to your workout routine — how to order the exercises and how to know when you're ready for change.

In what order should I do my exercises?

In general, exercise larger muscles before smaller ones. Work your back and chest before your shoulders and arms, and work your butt before your thighs and calves. Smaller muscles assist the larger muscles. If the smaller muscles are too tired to pitch in and do their job, they give out long before your big muscles get an adequate workout. For example, your biceps help out your upper back when you do a *lat pull-down,* an exercise where you pull a bar down to your chest. If you work your biceps first, they'll be too tired to do their job during the pull-down, and your back muscles won't get as good a workout.

As for which muscles to start with — chest, back, or legs — that's up to you. You may want to begin with all your chest exercises and then move on to your back. Or you can alternate chest and back moves. You can fit your core exercises in whenever you like, as long as you remember to do them. (See the "Considering your core" section for more on exercising your abdominals.)

How often should I change my routine?

Some people change some or all of their exercises every time they work out. There's no hard-and-fast rule on this subject, but we recommend that you try at least one new exercise every month. After you have a basic routine, such as the one we demonstrate in the last section of this chapter, expand your repertoire so you have more options to choose from. Varying your exercises keeps you more interested and can help you get better results. If you stick with the same routine month after month, year after year, your muscles adapt to those exercises; but by working your muscles from a variety of angles, you involve more muscle fibers and keep your muscles challenged.

Changing your exercises isn't the only way to keep you — and your muscles — stimulated. You also can play with other variables, such as how many sets and reps you perform and how much rest you take between sets.

Consider trying *periodization,* a method of organizing your workout program into several periods, each lasting about four weeks. Each phase has a different emphasis:

- ✔ The first month you may do a basic routine, using moderate weights and performing one set of 8 to 10 reps of each exercise.

- ✔ In the next period, you may go for more strength, lifting heavier weights, doing 6 to 8 repetitions and taking more rest between sets.

- ✔ In the third phase, you may focus on building stamina, doing 10 to 12 repetitions and taking less rest between sets.

Periodization is great if you're a beginner, because it helps you focus on one goal at a time.

Advanced weight-training techniques

We call the following techniques advanced, but novices can use them, too, after they have some experience and base fitness.

✔ **Super set:** You do two consecutive sets of different exercises, preferably ones that exercise opposite muscle groups (like quadriceps and hamstrings) without resting in between. For example, you can do one chest exercise immediately followed by a different chest exercise and then take a rest. The idea is to completely tire out the muscle — to work it so hard that you reach the deepest muscle fibers. You also can do a super set with exercises that target different muscle groups, like a chest exercise followed by a leg exercise. With this type of super set, you don't rest between exercises — the purpose is simply to save time.

✔ **Pyramids:** You do multiple sets of an exercise, increasing the weight for each set while decreasing the number of reps. You may do a light warm-up set for ten reps, then a heavier set for eight reps, then an even heavier set for six reps, and so on, until you reach a weight at which you can

do only one rep. You don't have to go all the way down to one rep for your workout to be considered a pyramid. The idea is to work up slowly and fatigue the muscle.

✔ **Negatives:** Someone helps you lift a weight, and then you're on your own for the lowering, or *negative,* phase of the lift. Your muscles generally can handle more weight when you lower a weight than when you lift it, so this technique gives you a chance to really tire out your muscles. ***Note:*** If you're a beginner, don't try negatives. They can cause significant muscle soreness.

✔ **Breakdowns (also called *drop sets* or *descending sets*):** You lift a heavy weight, and as soon as you exhaust the muscle — however many reps it takes — you pick up a lighter weight and squeeze out a few more reps. You may do ten reps of an exercise and then drop 5 pounds and try to eke out three or four more reps. The theory is that you use more of your muscles this way. You have to dig deeper because the muscle fibers you normally use are already pooped out.

Considering your core

Abs are everywhere these days, from infomercials featuring belly-blaster products to the covers of fitness magazines, promising ten steps toward washboard abs. To have great-looking abs — and who doesn't want that? — you need to develop the abdominal muscles through strength training. This section outlines which muscles to target and provides tips on how to do core exercises.

Which muscles should I work to get great abs?

Instead of limiting your focus to "abs," we suggest you think "core." This way, you don't limit your training to the long, flat sheet of muscle that runs down your middle (your rectus abdominis) but instead train your entire waistline in 3D, including the sides (obliques), the back (erector spinae), and the deepest ab muscles (transverse abdominals). We describe these muscles in depth in Chapter 11.

The reason core training is so important is that those muscles typically work together, whether in real life or in a workout; in trainer's jargon, this is called "functional training." You rarely find yourself in any situation that calls for bending forward from the waist quickly 20 times in a row (as you do with crunches), but you often find yourself using your core to brace your body as you bend down to pick up a package or to twist around to grab a grocery bag from the back seat of your car. So, to avoid injury and to get better results from your workout, you should start thinking — and working out — in core terms.

How can I get my midsection in shape?

Keep in mind that you can never achieve that rock-hard, six-pack look if you have a beer belly sitting on top of your middle. If you're overweight, core strength training will hone those middle muscles, but you won't see any definition until you lose body fat.

There are more theories about core training than there are about the Kennedy assassination. Here's our take on getting your midsection into shape:

- **Don't do core exercises every day.** Your core muscles, like all your other muscle groups, need a day of rest between workouts. Besides, they tend to get a workout no matter which muscles you're working. When you do push-ups, for example, you may be concentrating on toning your arms, shoulders, and chest, but your core is working extra hard to protect your back and maintain form.

- **Do up to three sets of 10 to 25 reps.** You sometimes do more reps of core exercises than of moves targeting other muscle groups because adding resistance to core exercises is difficult and because you use your core moves somewhat differently than many of your other muscles by alternating muscles. Whereas most muscles are moving, pushing, or pulling, the core muscles' main job is to brace your body or shift slightly and constantly to protect your spine and hold your body in position. However, if you're able to whip off 100 reps of a core move, you're doing the reps too quickly or with poor form, or the exercise is too easy for you.

As with any other exercise, you should be struggling on the last repetition. Doing 100 continuous reps of any ab exercise is inefficient and a waste of time. In fact, one of the core moves we show you later in this chapter, the plank, can give you an amazing workout in just one rep.

✔ **Stay away from ab machinery.** Instead, stick with exercises performed on the floor, such as the plank and back extension and moves performed with a physioball. We're not fond of most abdominal weight machines because they tend to overuse the lower-back or hip muscles and aren't very functional. Nor do we like those abdominal infomercial gadgets that you can strap over your knees, press on your stomach, or stick under your butt; they force you to pay money for something you don't need.

The only type of ab device we're not entirely opposed to are ab-roller contraptions. An ab roller can function like training wheels on a bike, guiding you through the correct path of motion until you're strong enough and skilled enough to perform it on your own. However, when you're past the remedial stage of core training, forgoing the ab roller and performing other core exercises under your own power is recommended.

Lifting Safely and Effectively

This section offers general rules for lifting weights safely. We include tips on warm-ups, breathing, posture, proper movement, and more.

Lifting weights the right way

The way some people lift weights, you'd think they were in labor or impersonating a mountain gorilla. Grunting, screaming, and rocking back and forth are not indications of proper weight-lifting technique.

We've seen people invent some pretty outrageous exercises. One guy bent over, picked up a very heavy dumbbell, lifted it straight over his head so that he almost fell backward, and then threw it to the ground so hard that it bounced and broke a mirror. He seemed quite pleased with himself.

Whether you're performing the exercises that we feature later in this chapter — or any other exercise you try — the following rules always apply:

✔ **Always warm up.** Before you lift a weight, do at least 5 minutes of slow, rhythmic movement to get your muscles warm and pliable. If you're doing lower body, you can pedal easily on a bike or do a slow trot. If you're going to do arm exercises and don't have access to any upper-body cardio machines, such as an elliptical trainer with arm handles or a rower, do a few minutes of arm swings.

✔ **Concentrate on your form.** Good form is always more important than lifting a lot of weight. Don't arch your back, strain your neck, or rock your body to generate momentum. Not only can these maneuvers cause injury, but they also make the exercises less effective.

✔ **Increase your weight by the smallest possible increment.** Jumping from a 5-pound weight to a 10-pounder doesn't sound like a big leap, but think about it: You're doubling the load on that muscle. If you're using a 5-pound weight, move up to a 6-, 7-, or 8-pounder.

✔ **Remember to breathe.** In general, exhale forcefully through your mouth as you lift the weight and inhale deeply through your nose as you lower it. Although proper breathing is important for speeding oxygen to your muscles, don't get hung up on the mechanics. Some people spend so much time trying to get the correct breathing pattern down that they lose track of what they're doing.

Just don't overdo the breathing, because overly forceful breathing can leave you feeling lightheaded. And don't hold your breath. You can bring about sharp increases in your blood pressure, and you can even faint from lack of air. (*Note:* Holding your breath is okay during extremely heavy lifts, because it protects your spine by bracing it with the pressure from the held breath. But unless you're aiming to lift world-record amounts of weight, don't hold your breath.)

✔ **Use a full range of motion.** In other words, pull or push as far as you're supposed to. (If you're not sure, a trainer can show you the correct range of motion for each exercise. See Chapter 20 for tips on finding a personal trainer.) Using the full range of motion enhances your flexibility.

You don't want to go past a natural range of motion, because this can cause injury to the joint. For example, lifting dumbbells out to the side above shoulder level puts too much stress on the shoulder. Sitting down too far when you squat can cause knee injuries.

✔ **Pay attention.** Remind yourself which muscle you're working, and focus on that muscle. It's easy to do lat pull-downs without challenging your lats. And it's easy to do abdominal crunches without really working your abs. (See Chapter 11 for a rundown of the major muscle groups.)

Suzanne recently watched a guy perform abdominal crunches with the sports section of the newspaper lying on his lap. He tried to steal a glance at the paper every time he curled his torso up. We suspect his abs aren't getting much in the way of results, although he is definitely up on the basketball scores.

✔ **Never work through an injury.** If you feel pain, review your technique and slow down the pace to make sure you're performing the move correctly. If you're using good form and you still hurt, skip the exercise for now. You may want to try it again after you've been exercising for a few weeks. Or you may need to try a different exercise that targets the same muscle.

Making sense of the instructions

You may notice that in exercise descriptions, people use a few phrases over and over again. Here's a brief explanation of these phrases, which you're likely to hear from trainers and group-exercise instructors:

- ✔ **"Pull your abdominals in."** This doesn't mean to suck in your gut or hold your breath. Simply pull your abs slightly inward, a movement also known as *tightening* or *contracting* your abs. You're gently pulling your belly button up and in toward your spine so you immediately feel taller and thinner. This position helps give your torso stability while you exercise, protecting your spine from injury and ensuring that you're actually using the muscle you're intending to work.

  Imagine that you're wearing a pair of jeans that's one size too small; when you pull your abs in, it's like tightening the jeans another two sizes down.

- ✔ **"Stand up tall."** You don't need to stand like a guard at Buckingham Palace, but do lift your chest and keep your head centered between your shoulders. No slumping allowed!

  Imagine you have a string attached to your breastbone and someone is standing above you, giving it a gentle tug upward.

- ✔ **"Tilt your chin toward your chest."** Tilt your chin just enough to fit your closed fist between your chest and chin. This position lines up the vertebrae of your neck with the rest of your spine. If you tilt your chin back or drop it toward your chest like you're sulking, you put excess pressure on your neck.

Following a Simple Total-Body Workout

In this section, we provide you with a *total-body workout* — a snazzy term referring to a routine that covers all major muscle groups in your body.

Do all the exercises in the order we list them, which is roughly largest to smallest muscle group. We're big believers in doing full-body workouts, even when your goals are very specific. This is a good way to build a balanced body and avoid injuries. You can perform this routine either at home or at the gym. All you need for this workout are dumbbells (four to eight pairs should suffice) and a weight bench (you can substitute a physioball or an aerobic step bench for a regular weight bench). In case you have access to health-club machines, we include a second exercise, which we call a *gym alternative,* for each muscle group. The machines at your gym may not be exactly the same as the ones we mention, so you may have to ask for help adapting them.

The workout will take you 15 to 20 minutes to complete, depending on how much rest you take between sets, how many reps you do, and how experienced you are. We don't give specific weight recommendations because there are such vast differences in what people are capable of lifting, but keep in mind the rules we lay out earlier about reps, form, and amount of weight to lift for each exercise.

We emphasize dumbbell exercises because you can easily perform them at home or at the gym. The particular dumbbell exercises that we show here are all suitable for beginners; they don't require the brawn of an NFL defensive end or the coordination of an Olympic gymnast. Also, many of these moves perform double or triple duty; for example, the squat works three lower-body muscles — your front thighs, rear thighs, and derriere — in a single exercise.

The machines we show here generally mimic the dumbbell moves, working your muscles with a similar movement and from similar angles. Virtually every health club has these machines, in addition to other contraptions that work your muscles in different ways, and we highly recommend exercising each muscle group from a variety of angles. After you become familiar with the basic exercises shown here — in about six to eight weeks — we suggest you consult a trainer, a DVD, a podcast, the Web, or other books to expand your repertoire.

Don't worry: Our directions are in plain English, not like those assemble-it-yourself furniture manuals. For each exercise, we tell you which muscles the move targets. Then, where appropriate, we identify potential joint injuries and remind you to pay special attention if you've ever injured the joint in question. We also note which exercises are functional and which are isolation moves. *Functional* is a buzzword that simply lets you know that the move works several muscle groups at once and thus is likely to translate to the way you use your body in everyday life and in sports and fitness activities.

We're starting to see some trainers go too far with the concept of functional movement. For example, one well-known trainer put out a series of DVDs mocking all isolation movements. He made some valid points but lost us when he began demonstrating moves like kneeling on top of a physioball while raising a bar with one hand and bouncing a basketball with the other. That didn't strike us as particularly functional. Perhaps it's helpful to the college and pro athletes this particular trainer works with, but for a beginner, this is overkill. You're far better off starting out with some isolation moves that teach you how to use your body and that build basic strength, so we include some isolation moves as well.

Squat

In addition to strengthening your butt muscles, the *Squat* also does a good job of working your quadriceps, hamstrings, and core. Think of all the times you need to get out of a chair or stand up — the Squat helps you do that with ease. If you have hip, knee, or lower-back problems, restrict the distance your knees travel during this exercise by bending only part of the way down. The Squat is one of the quintessential functional moves.

Getting set

Place your hands on your hips or hold dumbbells with your arms down at your sides. Stand with your feet as wide apart as your hips and place your weight slightly back on your heels. Pull your abdominals in and stand tall with square shoulders (see Figure 13-1a).

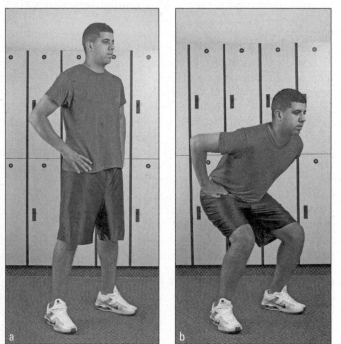

Figure 13-1:
The Squat strengthens your butt and thigh muscles.

The exercise

Sit back and down, as if you're sitting into a chair. Lower as far as you can without leaning your upper body more than a few inches forward as shown in Figure 13-1b. Don't lower any farther than the point at which you're parallel to the floor, and don't allow your knees to shoot out in front of your toes. As soon as you feel your upper body fold forward over your thighs, straighten your legs and stand back up. Don't lock your knees at the top of the movement.

Technique tips

Keep these tips in mind as you perform the Squat:

✓ Keep your head up and eyes focused on an object directly in front of you. Your body tends to follow your eyes, so if you're staring at the ground, you're more likely to fall forward. Imagine balancing a book on top of your head.

✓ When you stand back up, push through your heels rather than shifting your body weight forward. Don't let your heels (or toes) lift off the floor.

✓ Try not to arch your back as you stand up.

Gym alternative: Leg-press machine

The leg-press machine is an excellent Squat alternative for those who have chronic knee problems or who don't have good balance. Set the leg-press machine so that when you're lying on your back, your shoulders fit snugly under the shoulder pads and your knees are bent to an inch or so below parallel to the foot plate. Place your feet as wide as your hips with your feet pointing forward. Grasp the handles.

Pull your abdominals in and keep your head and shoulders on the back pad. Push upward until your legs are nearly straight, just short of locking. Then bend your knees, controlling the weight as you go down, until your thighs are parallel to the foot plate.

One-Legged Squat

The *One-Legged Squat* is one of the best functional exercises to work the butt, thighs, and core. It's especially effective because it adds an element of balance and coordination to the movement, much like what's often called for in real life. The exercise may look a lot like the basic Squat, but it feels completely different; you feel the muscles of the base leg, the one with the foot on the floor, working deeply and completely while the muscles of the other leg are constantly shifting to maintain balance (see Figure 13-2). That said, most beginners are up to the challenge.

Getting set

Place your hands in one of three positions: on your hips, elbows bent in front of you at chest level, or holding dumbbells with your arms down at your sides as shown in Figure 13-2a. Stand with your right foot on the floor directly under your hip and your left foot a few inches in front with your heel up and toe pressed firmly into the floor. Shift your weight slightly back on your right heel. Pull your abdominals in and stand tall with square shoulders.

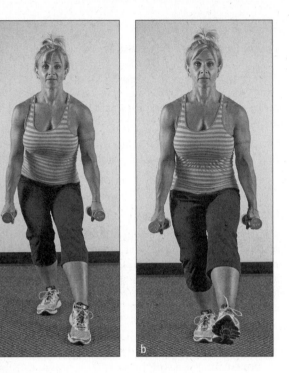

Figure 13-2:
The One-Legged Squat resembles the basic Squat but requires balance.

The exercise

Sit back and down into the base leg, as if you're sitting into a chair. Lower as far as you can without leaning your upper body more than a few inches forward or losing your balance. Don't lower any farther than the point at which you're parallel to the floor, and don't allow your knees to shoot out in front of your toes. After you feel your upper body fold forward over your thighs, straighten your legs and stand back up. Don't lock your knees at the top of the movement. Switch leg positions and repeat.

Here are a couple of ways to make this exercise easier or harder:

✔ If you haven't developed enough balance to do this exercise, place your hand lightly against a wall or lightly hold on to a sturdy object. The trick is to use support to keep you balanced but not rely on it too heavily; otherwise, you miss a lot of the benefit of this exercise.

✔ If you find that balancing during this move is ridiculously easy, try lifting your toe off the floor as you squat (refer to Figure 13-2b) or placing the toe behind your other leg as if you're in a curtsy. For even more of a challenge, do this move perched atop the dome side of a BOSU ball.

Technique tips

As you perform the One-Legged Squat, follow the basic Squat technique tips: Keep your head up and your eyes straight ahead. Instead of shifting your weight forward, push through your heels as you stand, and don't let the heels lift off the floor. Try not to arch your back.

Gym alternative: Leg-press machine

This is an excellent One-Leg Squat alternative for those with chronic knee problems or iffy balance. It's also a pure isolation move for each leg you're targeting, so you really feel those muscles working. Set the leg-press machine so that when you're lying on your back, your shoulders fit snugly under the shoulder pads and your right knee is bent to an inch or so below parallel to the foot plate. Lift your left foot off the plate or cross your left ankle over your right thigh. Grasp the handles.

Pull your abdominals in and keep your head and shoulders on the back pad. Push upward until your right leg is nearly straight, just short of locking. Then bend your knee, controlling the weight as you go down, until your thigh is parallel to the foot plate. Switch legs and repeat.

One-Arm Dumbbell Row

Exercising your upper back without machinery isn't easy, but this functional move is one that does a good job. The *One-Arm Dumbbell Row* also strengthens your core, biceps, and shoulders in a way that you use them to saw wood, pick things up off the floor, or lift up a piece of furniture. Be especially careful if you have lower-back problems.

Getting set

Stand to the right of your weight bench, holding a dumbbell in your right hand with your palm facing in. Place your left knee and your left hand on top of the bench for support. Let your right arm hang down and a bit forward. Pull your abdominals in and bend forward from the hips so that your back is naturally arched and roughly parallel to the floor and your right knee is slightly bent. Tilt your chin toward your chest so that your neck is in line with the rest of your spine (see Figure 13-3a).

The exercise

Bend your right arm until your elbow is pointing to the ceiling, your upper arm is parallel to the floor, and your hand comes to the outside of the rib cage as shown in Figure 13-3b. Lower the weight slowly back down.

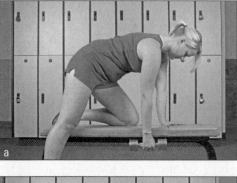

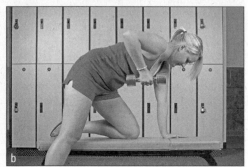

Figure 13-3:
The
One-Arm
Dumbbell
Row is a
great way
to work your
upper back.

Technique tips

Keep these tips in mind as you perform the One-Arm Dumbbell Row:

- ✔ Concentrate on pulling from your back muscles (right behind and below your shoulder). Don't just move your arm up and down. Although your arm is moving, this is a back exercise. Think of your arm as a hook that connects to the weight and is pulled by the back.

- ✔ Keep your abs pulled in tight throughout the motion.

- ✔ Don't let your back sag toward the floor or hunch up.

- ✔ Pull your shoulders back and down to set the shoulder blades.

Gym alternative: Seated row machine

Set your seat height so that when you grasp the handles, your arms are level with your shoulders. Sit tall in the seat, facing the weight stack with your chest against the pad.

Remaining tall, pull the handles toward you to lift the weight stack. When your hands are a few inches in front of your chest, slowly straighten your arms to lower the weight.

Dumbbell Chest Press

The *Dumbbell Chest Press* closely mimics the Bench Press — the all-time favorite exercise among serious weight lifters everywhere. This exercise works your chest muscles, along with your shoulders and triceps. You should lower and lift the dumbbells only a few inches to avoid overstraining these joints.

Getting set

Lie on the bench with a dumbbell in each hand and your feet flat on the floor (or place your feet up on the bench if it's more comfortable). Push the dumbbells up so that your arms are directly over your shoulders. Pull your abdominals in, and tilt your chin toward your chest (see Figure 13-4a).

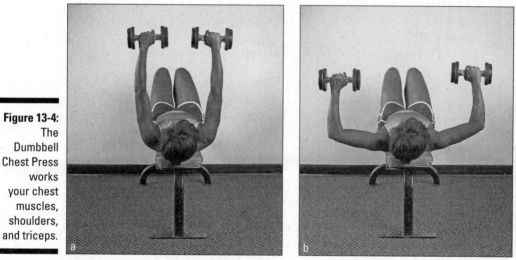

Figure 13-4: The Dumbbell Chest Press works your chest muscles, shoulders, and triceps.

The exercise

Lower the dumbbells down and a little to the side (see Figure 13-4b) until your elbows are slightly below your shoulders. Roll your shoulder blades back and down, like you're pinching them together and accentuating your chest. Push the weights back up, taking care not to lock your elbows or allow your shoulder blades to rise off the bench.

Technique tips

Keep in mind the following tips as you perform the Dumbbell Chest Press:

✔ Let your back keep a natural arch so that you have a slight gap between your lower back and the bench.

✔ Don't contort your body in an effort to lift the weight. Lift only as much weight as you can handle while maintaining good form.

✔ When pressing the dumbbells up, they don't need to touch each other.

Gym alternative: Vertical chest-press machine

Sit so that the center of your chest lines up with the center of the horizontal set of handlebars. Press down on the foot bar so that the handles move forward. Grip the horizontal handles and push them forward, straightening your arms. Lift your feet from the foot bar so that the weight of the stack transfers into your hands. Slowly bend your arms until your elbows are slightly behind your chest, and then push the handles forward until your arms are straight. After you complete the set, put your feet back on the foot bar and let go of the handles before you lower the weight stack all the way down.

Dumbbell Shoulder Press

The *Dumbbell Shoulder Press* targets your shoulders, placing some emphasis on your middle deltoid triceps and upper back. It's great to develop your shoulders for everyday use because you use them just about any time you push or pull with your upper body. Use caution if you have lower-back, neck, or elbow problems.

Getting set

Hold a dumbbell in each hand and sit on a bench with back support. Plant your feet firmly on the floor about hip-width apart. Bend your elbows and raise your upper arms to shoulder height so the dumbbells are at ear level. Pull your abdominals in so there is a slight gap between the small of your back and the bench. Place the back of your head against the pad (see Figure 13-5a).

The exercise

Push the dumbbells up and directly over your head (see Figure 13-5b); the ends of the dumbbells can touch lightly. Then lower the dumbbells back to ear level.

Technique tips

Keep these tips in mind as you perform the Dumbbell Shoulder Press:

✔ Keep your elbows rigid without locking them at the top of the movement.

✔ Press your back against the back support without flattening out the curve in your back, or sit forward and keep your core tight.

> ✔ Bring your arms and elbows down, keeping your elbow joints in line with your shoulders.
>
> ✔ Don't wiggle or squirm in an effort to press the weights up.

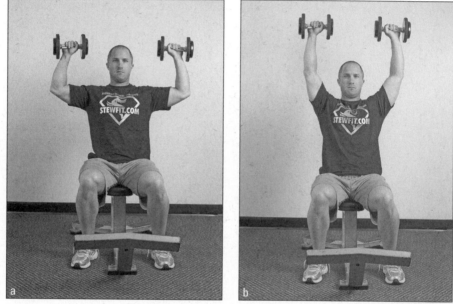

Figure 13-5:
The Dumbbell Shoulder Press works out your shoulders, triceps, and upper back.

Gym alternative: Shoulder-press machine

Set your seat height so that the shoulder-press machine's pulley is even with the middle of your shoulder. Hold on to each of the front handles. Pull your abdominals in tight, but allow a slight natural gap to remain between the small of your back and the back pad.

Press the handles up without locking your elbows. Lower your arms until your elbows are slightly lower than your shoulders.

Back Delt Fly

The *Back Delt Fly* is an excellent functional move for strengthening the back of your shoulders and upper back and for improving your posture. It opens up the chest and strengthens the back to help you stand up taller.

Getting set

Hold a dumbbell in each hand and sit on the edge of the bench. Lean forward from your hips so that your upper back is flat and above parallel to the floor. Let your arms hang down so that your palms are facing each other and the weights are behind your calves and directly under your knees. Tuck your chin toward your chest and pull your abdominals inward (see Figure 13-6a).

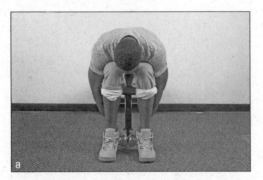

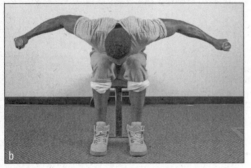

Figure 13-6:
The Back Delt Fly helps improve upper-body posture.

The exercise

Raise your arms up and out to the sides, bending your elbows a few inches as you go until your elbows are level with your shoulders; see Figure 13-6b. Squeeze your shoulder blades together as you lift. Slowly lower your arms back down.

Technique tips

Keep these tips in mind as you perform the Back Delt Fly:

- ✔ Use very light weights.

- ✔ Do not allow your body to pop up and down or let the weights swing. Always keep the movement under control.

- ✔ Keep your wrists straight.

To make this move more functional, try it while standing, leaning forward, or balanced on one foot. We also like this move done kneeling and working one arm at a time.

Gym alternative: Cable Back Delt Fly

Attach a horseshoe handle to the upper cable pulley and stand next to the tower so that your left side is nearest to it. Grasp the handle with your right hand and step about an arm's length away from the tower. Stand with your feet hip-width apart and bend forward from the hips. Pull your abs in toward your belly button. Rest your left hand on the tower or, if you feel secure in your balance, rest it on your left thigh. Lift your right arm up and to the side in an arc pattern; squeeze your shoulder blades together at the top of the movement and then slowly lower back to the start. Complete all reps and repeat with your left arm.

Dumbbell Biceps Curl

The *Dumbbell Biceps Curl* targets your biceps, the muscles you rely on to hold heavy objects and look buff in sleeveless shirts. Use caution if you have lower-back or elbow problems.

Getting set

Hold a dumbbell in each hand and stand with your feet as wide apart as your hips. Let your arms hang down at your sides with your palms forward. Pull your abdominals in, stand tall, and keep your knees slightly bent (see Figure 13-7a).

The exercise

Curl both arms upward until they're in front of your shoulders as shown in Figure 13-7b. Slowly lower the dumbbells back down.

Technique tips

Keep these tips in mind as you perform the Dumbbell Biceps Curl:

- Keep your knees slightly bent and your posture tall. Don't lean back or rock your body forward to help lift the weight.
- Keep your elbows as close to your body as you can without supporting your elbows on the sides of your stomach for leverage.
- Don't rest when you reach the top or bottom of the exercise; instead, keep a constant tension on the biceps.
- Lower the weight back to the starting position slowly and with control.

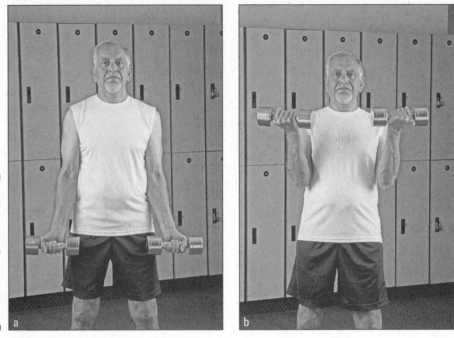

Figure 13-7: Keep your elbows close to your body while performing the Dumbbell Biceps Curl.

Gym alternative: Cable Curl

Place the pulley on the lowest setting and clip on a short straight bar. Stand facing the machine with your feet hip-width apart and grasp the bar in both hands so that your arms are in front of you, hands directly in front of your thighs.

Strengthening the wrists

One way to avoid a painful injury known as *tennis elbow* is to strengthen your wrists. One of the simplest weight-lifting exercises for your wrists is the *dumbbell wrist curl:*

1. **Form a 90-degree angle between your forearm and bicep; lay your forearm on a table or weight bench, palms facing up.**

2. **Placing a dumbbell in your open hand, close your fingers and hand around the dumbbell, and roll the dumbbell up until your wrist is flexed.**

3. **Return to your starting position and repeat for a set of eight to ten reps.**

Bend your elbows and pull the bar upward until your elbows are at shoulder level. Then slowly lower the bar back down. *Note:* Some gyms have free motion triceps machines where you can perform this same movement.

Triceps Kickback

The *Triceps Kickback* works your triceps, which assist the chest in just about every pushing movement. Use caution when doing this move if you have elbow or lower-back problems.

Getting set

Stand to the right of your weight bench, holding a dumbbell in your right hand with your palm facing in. Place your left lower leg and your left hand on top of the bench. Lean forward at the hips until your upper body is at a 45-degree angle to the floor. Bend your right elbow so your upper arm is parallel to the floor, your forearm is perpendicular to it, and your palm faces in. Keep your elbow close to your waist. Pull your abdominals in and bend your knees slightly (see Figure 13-8a).

The exercise

Keeping your upper arm still, straighten your arm behind you until your entire arm is parallel to the floor and one end of the dumbbell points toward the floor (see Figure 13-8b). Slowly bend your arm to lower the weight. After you complete the set, repeat the exercise with your left arm.

Technique tips

Keep these tips in mind as you perform the Triceps Kickback:

- ✔ Keep your abdominals pulled in and your knees relaxed, and don't allow your back to round.
- ✔ Don't lock your elbow at the top of the movement. Straighten your arm, but keep your elbow slightly bent.
- ✔ Don't allow your upper arm to move or your shoulder to drop below waist level.
- ✔ Keep your wrist straight.

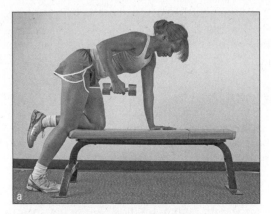

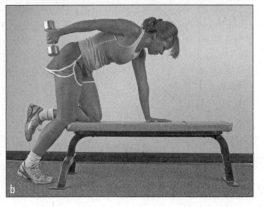

Figure 13-8:
Make sure your shoulder doesn't drop below waist level during the Triceps Kickback.

Gym alternative: Cable Triceps Extension

Set the cable machine on the highest pulley and clip a short straight bar on to it. Stand facing the machine with your feet hip-width apart. Hold the bar so that your hands are placed on top of the bar. Step a few inches away from the machine and bend your arms so that they're alongside your waist and your forearms are parallel to the floor.

Straighten your arms straight down to lift the weight stack, and then slowly bend your arms to lower the weight. *Note:* Some gyms have a free-motion-style machine that allows you to perform the same movement.

The Plank

The *Plank* is probably the best all-around functional exercise for the core because it integrates all the core muscles to hold your body into position. Because the positioning is fairly easy to grasp and there isn't a lot of movement involved, it's a good beginner exercise. The plan is also a good advanced exercise because you can make it more challenging simply by holding the position longer. Pay special attention to your form if you have lower-back or neck problems. We don't offer a machine alternative for this move because we don't think there is a suitable one. Instead, our alternative abdominal move uses a large plastic ball known as a *physioball*.

Getting set

Kneel on the floor on your hands and knees so that your palms are directly under your shoulders and your knees are directly under your hips. Bend your elbows and place the bottoms of your forearms on the floor; clasp your hands together as shown in Figure 13-9a. Next, pull your bellybutton in toward your spine and extend your legs out straight behind you so that you're now balanced on your forearms and the underside of your toes; see Figure 13-9b. Your legs can either be squeezed together or a small distance apart, whichever is most comfortable for you.

The exercise

Hold this position, taking care not to let your back sag or your butt lift above the rest of your body; in other words, your body, from the top of your head to your heels, should form one straight line. Stay in position for 10 slow counts, making sure to keep breathing. When you're done, bend your knees to the floor and sit back on your heels to give your lower back a stretch; see Figure 13-9c. Do 1 to 3 reps.

Make the exercise harder or easier by adjusting the length of time you hold the position. If this is too challenging, you can stay on your knees rather than lengthening your body and then gradually progress to a Full-Body Plank as you get stronger.

Technique tips

Keep these tips in mind as you perform the Plank.

- ✔ **Focus on maintaining a straight line.** Be aware of keeping your core strong and tight.
- ✔ **Don't hold your breath.** Continue deep inhales and exhales.

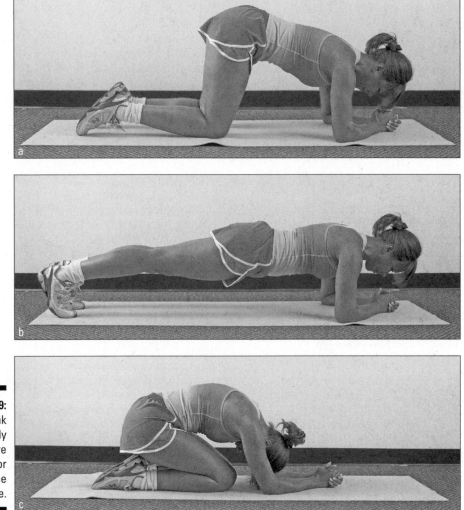

Figure 13-9:
The Plank is a highly effective exercise for working the core.

Gym alternative: Ball Plank

Kneel in front of a physioball and place your hands on top of the ball, shoulder-width apart with your arms straight but elbows relaxed. Stretch your legs out behind you so that you're balanced on your palms and the underside of your toes; your legs can either be squeezed together or a small distance apart, whichever is more comfortable. Maintain a straight line from the top of your head to your heels by pulling in your core muscles.

Hold the position for 5 counts. You may have difficulty keeping the ball from wobbling or rolling around; if so, you can start with the ball against the wall. Try to hold it still by maintaining good form and a strong core. If the ball keeps slipping out, that's okay. Eventually, you'll be able to keep the ball still. The ball adds an element of instability to the exercise, so the core gets a much deeper workout than during a basic plank.

Opposite Extension

The *Opposite Extension* both stretches and strengthens your lower back. It's the perfect complement to the Plank to develop a strong, balanced midsection. Use caution if you have a lower-back problem or experience lower-back pain while performing this exercise. If you do feel pain, try lifting only your legs and leaving your arms flat on the floor.

Getting set

Lie on your stomach, face down, with arms straight out in front of you, palms down, and legs straight out behind you. Pull your abs in, as if you're trying to create a small space between your stomach and the floor (see Figure 13-10).

Figure 13-10:
The Opposite Extension stretches and strengthens your lower back.

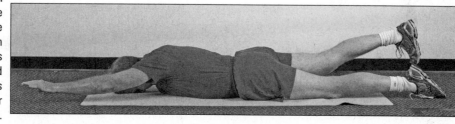

The exercise

Lift your left arm and right leg about 1 inch off the floor, and stretch out as much as you can. Hold this position for 5 slow counts and then lower your arm and leg back down. Repeat the same move with your right arm and left leg. Continue alternating sides until you complete the set.

Technique tips

Keep the following tips in mind as you perform the Opposite Extension:

✔ Exhale as you lift your arm and leg, and inhale as you lower them.

✔ Pretend that you're trying to touch something with your toes and fingertips that are just out of reach.

✔ Work for precision rather than height.

✔ Lift your arm and leg at the same time and to the same height.

Gym alternative: Ball Back Extension

Kneel on a physioball and place your hands behind your head. Lean forward and lengthen your body so your torso is resting against the ball and you're firmly balanced on your toes. Make sure your spine forms a straight line from your tailbone to your neck. Lift your chest upward a few inches, hold a moment, and then slowly lower back down.

Cross your arms over your chest, pull your abs in, and lower your upper body a few inches by bending forward at the hips. Raise back up, using your lower back, so your body is parallel to the floor.

Part IV
Limbering Up with Flexibility, Balance, and Mind-Body Exercise

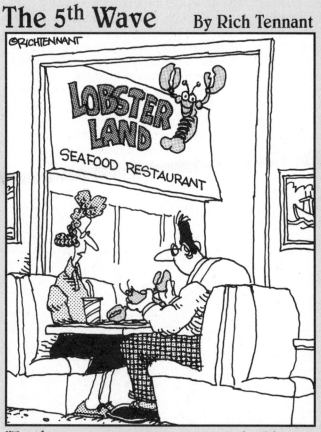

The 5th Wave   By Rich Tennant

LOBSTER LAND
SEAFOOD RESTAURANT

"Is there a way you can explain Pilates to me without using the carcass of your lobster?"

In this part . . .

In this part, we introduce you to the two most neglected yet equally important components of fitness: flexibility and balance. In Chapter 14, we make a darn good case for taking five minutes out of each day to stretch. We also cover the basic rules of stretching and present a head-to-toe stretching workout that doesn't require the flexibility of a Cirque du Soleil troupe member. Chapter 15 focuses on balance. We present four easy-to-follow balance tests, along with exercises to help you move more gracefully and prevent unnecessary falls. Chapter 16 is all about yoga, one of the best ways to improve flexibility while also strengthening your core muscles and de-stressing. We explain the different styles of yoga and show you a few basic poses. In Chapter 17, we explain what Pilates is and why it's worth adding to your fitness repertoire.

Chapter 14

Flexibility Training: Getting the Scoop on Stretching

*S*tretching may be the most misunderstood aspect of fitness. You see people at the park bending over to touch their toes and think: Hmm . . . should I be doing that? How many seconds should I hold a stretch like that? Should I do it before I exercise or afterward?

Truth is, even exercise scientists don't agree on all the ins and outs of stretching, also known as *flexibility training*. And even we admit that finding the motivation to stretch can be tough. After all, getting your fingertips to touch behind your back is not exactly a process that puts a blowtorch to fat.

In this chapter, we set the record straight on what stretching can and can't do for you. (**Hint:** It can do a lot.) Fortunately, you needn't be able to do full splits to reap the benefits of stretching, and you can fit a stellar flexibility program into a few minutes a day. Whether you find stretching a relaxing pastime or a chore on par with cleaning your oven, this chapter shows you how to make the most of flexibility training.

Understanding Why You Need to Stretch

Stretching is the key to maintaining your flexibility — in other words, how far and how easily you can move your joints. Here are some good reasons to make stretching part of your exercise routine:

✔ **Maintaining good posture:** Flexibility is one of the keys to good posture, helping you look better and avoid muscle pain. When your front neck muscles are short and tight, your head angles forward. When your shoulders and chest are tight, your shoulders round inward. When your lower back, rear thigh, and hip muscles are tight, the curve of your back becomes exaggerated.

✔ **Reducing back pain:** A regular stretching routine also can reduce pain and discomfort, particularly in your lower back. In fact, the pain often lessens when you begin doing simple stretches for your lower-back and rear-thigh muscles.

✔ **Correcting muscle imbalances and improving coordination:** Say that your front-thigh muscles are strong but your rear thighs are tight and weak. (This is a common scenario.) As a result, you end up relying on your front thighs more than you should. Chances are you don't even notice this, but it throws off your movement in subtle ways — you may have a short walking stride or bounce too high off the ground. Muscle imbalances can eventually lead to injuries such as pulled muscles. They also contribute to clumsiness, which in itself can lead to injury.

✔ **Keeping your range of motion later in life:** As you get older, your tendons (the tissues that connect muscle to bone) begin to shorten and tighten, restricting your flexibility. Scientists also suspect that collagen, one of the main materials in connective tissue, becomes denser with age, so your movements become less fluid. Studies show that by the time people are in their seventies, many people can move the majority of their joints only half as far as they could in their prime.

As you lose flexibility, you walk more stiffly and with a shorter stride and therefore have more difficulty stepping up to a curb or bending down to pick up trash. The danger is that you're at greater risk of falling, and this risk, combined with bone-density loss, can become a life-threatening situation. The good news: Stretching your rear-thigh, hip, and calf muscles can greatly reduce this risk, regardless of your age.

✔ **Performing better in sports:** Flexibility is a key performance factor for many sports. Clearly, gymnasts, dancers, and skateboarders need a great deal of flexibility to excel. Swimmers need good shoulder flexibility. Runners, walkers, and cyclists require some flexibility but less than athletes in other sports (in fact, some studies have shown that having too much flexibility in certain sports, such as running and cycling, actually increases chances of injury). The point is that there seems to be an optimal amount of flexibility, depending on which activities you tend to pursue, but even the least athletic among us require a basic amount of stretching. (For more info on stretching and injury prevention, see the sidebar "Can stretching prevent injury?")

Can stretching prevent injury?

Can stretching prevent injury? The jury is still deliberating this one, and the body of evidence is contradictory. On the one hand, research shows that an active warm-up routine combined with preworkout stretching can significantly reduce the risk of injury to the muscles and their connective tissue while you're exercising. This is probably because the warm-up/stretch combinations heat up and elongate the muscles. However, this combo does not seem to diminish overuse injuries or injuries that happen when you aren't exercising.

Other studies show that stretching without a warm-up does not reduce injury rates at all, probably because it may actually make the joints less stable and less able to react quickly to sudden movements. Research does show that a warm-up without stretching can help prevent injury, so when it comes to injury prevention, it's unclear how important stretching is. But this much is clear: Preworkout stretching alone, without a warm-up, is not a good idea.

A few studies suggest that over the long term, postworkout stretches can improve strength and endurance performance and lower the risk injury. Just don't expect stretching to make your muscle less sore. For example, stretching right after running a marathon will not make you feel less stiff or achy the next day. It may even slightly increase your chances of getting hurt.

Nevertheless, we continue to see runners swinging their legs up on the hood of a car to stretch their hamstrings before heading out for a run and walkers hanging their heels off the edge of a curb before they take a step. So ingrained is this preworkout stretch ritual that the message does not seem to be getting through to the average exerciser. Top athletes do seem to get it: When you watch any Olympic or professional competition, you see the athletes doing active warm-ups and using techniques known as PNF (proprioceptive neuromuscular facilitation) or Active Isolated stretching. Olympic swimmer Dara Torres actually hired two stretchers to travel with her in order to keep her muscles supple enough to continue swimming at the top of her game into her forties. Even yoga and Pilates, which are very flexibility-based disciplines, use active warm-up techniques before moving into static positions.

Whether stretching reduces injury remains unclear, but regardless of whether you stretch before working out, continue to keep in mind the numerous other great reasons to take up flexibility training.

Deciding When to Stretch

Contrary to popular opinion, stretching is not the first thing you should do when you walk into the gym or arrive at the park for a jog. Don't stretch your muscles until you've at least warmed up thoroughly (see Chapter 6 for warm-up basics).

Before a workout, warm up and *then* stretch, or leave your stretching until after you're done exercising. We think stretching at the end of your workout, after you've finished exercising but before you shower, may be the most convenient and beneficial time to stretch. A postworkout stretch is a great way to relax and ease back into the rest of your day.

Be sure to stretch after — not before — you cool down (see Chapter 6 for more on cool-downs). Putting your head below your heart right after a workout can cause fainting and nausea. Before you lie down to stretch, make sure that you aren't feeling breathless and that your heart rate has dipped below 100 beats per minute and dropped at least 20 beats from when you stopped exercising.

Exploring Stretching Techniques

There are several different schools of thought on how to stretch. Here are four of the most common:

- **Static stretching:** You move into a position and hold yourself in place for at least 15 seconds. The idea here is that you gradually stretch the muscle to the point of its limitation. This is the most common type of stretching, and most experts consider it very safe.

- **PNF stretching:** This technique has a name that, in our opinion, sets a new standard for fitness jargon: *proprioceptive neuromuscular facilitation*. PNF involves tightening a muscle as hard as you can right before you stretch it. The theory behind PNF is that the act of tightening, or squeezing, causes the muscle to become relaxed and more "receptive" to the stretch. So after you tighten your hamstring for a few seconds, you're able to stretch it a little bit farther than usual immediately after you release the tension. PNF stretching is best done with a partner, and some gyms offer 45-minute private training sessions entirely devoted to this type of stretching.

- **Active Isolated Stretching (AIS):** Using a rope, towel, belt, or band, you tighten the muscle opposite the muscle you're targeting for a stretch. Then you move the targeted muscle into a stretched position and hold it for about 2 seconds — that's right, 2 seconds — just long enough to elongate the muscle without triggering the rebound reflex. The *rebound reflex,* also known as the *stretch reflex,* is an automatic defense mechanism that causes muscles to tighten up and spring back to prevent tearing when they have been pulled too hard or too far or for too long.

  The theory behind AIS is that when you *contract,* or shorten, a muscle, the opposite muscle has no recourse but to relax and lengthen. You repeat the process 8 to 12 times in each position before moving on to the next stretch.

Let's roll! Doing a little massage

You may see people in the gym sitting or lying on a large foam tube, rolling it back and forth like they're rolling out cookie dough. In fact, they are doing a technique called *myofascial release,* a fancy name for self-massage. The theory is that the roller stretches muscles and tendons as it loosens up soft tissue and scar tissue and increases blood flow.

We like rollers. They seem particularly effective for loosening the sides of the hips in an area known as the *iliotibial* (IT) band, for treating shin-splint pain, and for stretching any unusually tight muscle. You simply place your weight on the roller and roll it back and forth under the offending muscle. Or you move into a stretch and roll the device underneath the muscle while you remain in the stretch position.

There's little research here, but as with massage, many people feel that using rollers makes their muscles feel better. And there is research to show that any type of massage can be effective for increasing circulation and breaking up *muscle adhesions,* areas where muscle fibers are bunched together as if they are taped or glued together.

If your gym doesn't have a foam roller, you can pick one up on the cheap. A small one will run you about $15. You can get a similar effect from placing handballs in strategic places. For example, lie on your back and place the ball on the inside of your shoulder blade or gently sit on one and roll it back and forth. We don't recommend using an actual rolling pin, though; it will be too hard and painful to use.

So which type of stretching works best? There isn't a consensus among fitness professionals or exercise scientists. Static stretching seems to be the safest and easiest to learn though not necessarily the most effective. However, some exercise experts theorize that conventional stretching techniques can damage muscles by pulling on them too hard and triggering the rebound reflex.

PNF and Active Isolated Stretching may well be the most effective, according to some studies, but these methods require more knowledge and skill and, in the case of PNF, the convenience of a partner.

 We recommend starting out with static stretching. As you gain some experience and your muscles begin to feel more well-oiled, doing some PNF or Active Isolated Stretching is probably a good idea. In the next sections, we give you a complete static routine and a sampler of PNF and AIS.

Still Life: Doing Static Stretching

If you consider stretching too boring, too painful, or too complicated, you'll like this section. We introduce some guidelines for static stretching and get you started with a thorough basic stretching routine.

Following a few rules of static stretching

Watch runners at the park or weight lifters at the gym. Chances are they have the wrong idea about stretching. Maybe they'll grab their heel for a split second to stretch their front thigh, or bend over for a moment to touch their toes. We've watched entire classes of boot-campers start off by flopping over and grabbing their ankles with their knees locked tight in place. It's enough to make us cringe, and that sort of "stretching" isn't going to make you more flexible. It may even injure you.

Here are the basic rules for a useful and safe flexibility workout:

✔ **Stretch as often as you can — daily, if possible.** Stretch after every workout, both cardiovascular and strength. If you stretch on days when you don't work out, warm up with a few minutes of easy movement like shoulder rolls, gentle waist twists, or light cardio activity. The American College of Sports Medicine (ACSM) recommends stretching at least three to five days a week, although we think that stretching five to seven days is ideal for most people. Stretching three times a week seems to improve the bendiness of joints much more than stretching once a week, but stretching even more often seems to provide at least some additional benefits.

✔ **Move into each stretching position slowly.** Never force yourself into a stretch by jerking or snapping into position. Blasting yourself into a stretch can sometimes be too much of a shock to a muscle and may cause an injury.

Never bounce. After you find the most comfortable stretch position, stay there or gradually deepen the stretch. Bouncing only tightens your muscle — it doesn't loosen it. Forceful bouncing increases the risk of tearing a muscle.

✔ **Notice how much tension you feel.** A stretch should rate anywhere on your pain meter from a feeling of mild tension to the edge of discomfort. It should never cause severe or sharp pain anywhere else in your body. Focus on the area you're stretching, and notice the stretch spread through these muscles.

✔ **As you hold each position, take at least five deep breaths.** Deep breathing promotes relaxation. The consensus seems to be that holding a static stretch for 15 to 30 seconds is ideal. We suggest that you get out a stopwatch and time your stretches until you get a sense of exactly how long 30 seconds really is.

✔ **Perform each stretch two to four times.** Here again, studies compiled by the ACSM find this regimen to be the most effective.

✔ **Stretch *all* your muscles.** Just because you stretch out your shoulders does not mean your hamstrings are any less tight. For stretching to be really effective, you have to take a full-body approach. Remember that old song "Dem Bones," which says "the thigh bone connected to the hip bone"? This is absolutely true of stretching. Any joint that is tight can throw off your posture or your stride or cause you discomfort.

Trying a simple static stretching routine

This section features a no-brainer stretching routine that won't pull your hamstrings like a rope in a tug of war. After you master these moves, the workout should take about five minutes.

Keep in mind that this is just a starting point. We think it's a great idea to learn additional stretches; you can choose from literally hundreds, as you find out if you take up yoga, Pilates, or martial arts. Varying your flexibility routine allows you to stretch your muscles at a number of angles. Plus, you'll be able to give the necessary extra attention to the muscles you use most in your particular workout. For example, if you're a tennis player or rower, you may want to do a few extra upper-body stretches.

Neck Stretch

This stretch is designed to loosen and relax the muscles in your neck. To do the Neck Stretch, stand or sit comfortably. Drop your left ear toward your left shoulder, and gently stretch your right arm down and a few inches out to the side (see Figure 14-1), using your opposite hand to assist the stretch by gently pressing on the side of your head. Repeat the stretch on your right side.

As you perform the Neck Stretch, be sure to keep your shoulders down and relaxed.

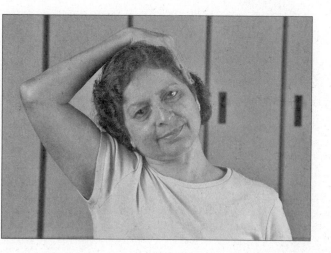

Figure 14-1:
The Neck Stretch loosens and relaxes the muscles in your neck.

Chest Expansion

This stretch targets your shoulders, chest, and arms and helps promote good posture. Sit or stand up tall and bring your arms behind you, clasping one hand inside the other (see Figure 14-2). Lift your chest and raise your arms slightly. You should feel a mild stretch spread across your chest.

Keep in mind the following tips as you perform the Chest Expansion:

- ✔ Resist arching your lower back as you pull your arms upward.
- ✔ Try to keep your shoulders relaxed and down.
- ✔ Don't force your arms up higher than is comfortable.

Back Expansion

This move stretches and loosens your shoulders, arms, and upper- and lower-back muscles. Here's how to do it: Standing tall with your knees slightly bent and feet hip-width apart, lift your arms in front of you to shoulder height. Clasp one hand in the other. Drop your head toward your chest, pull your abdominals inward, round your lower back, and tuck your hips forward so that you create a C shape with your torso. Stretch your arms forward so that you feel your shoulder blades moving apart and you create an "opposition" to your rounded back. You should feel a mild stretch slowly spread through your back and shoulders. (See Figure 14-3.)

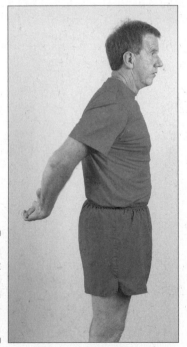

Figure 14-2:
The Chest Expansion promotes good posture.

Keep in mind the following tips as you perform the Back Expansion:

✔ Keep your abdominal muscles pulled inward to protect your lower back.

✔ Lean only as far forward as you feel comfortable and balanced.

✔ Keep your shoulders down and relaxed.

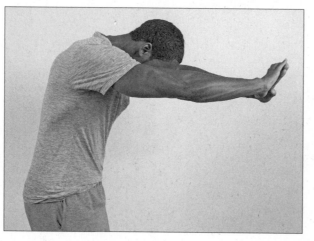

Figure 14-3:
The Back Expansion stretches your shoulders, arms, and back.

Standing Hamstring Stretch

This is a great stretch for your hamstrings (rear-thigh muscles) and your lower back. If you have lower-back problems, do the same exercise while lying on your back on the floor and extending your leg upward.

Stand tall with your left foot a few inches in front of your right foot and your left toes lifted. Bend your right knee slightly and pull your abdominals gently inward. Lean forward from your hips and press your buttocks backwards as if you're preparing to sit down, and rest both palms on top of your right thigh for balance and support (see Figure 14-4). Keep your shoulders down and relaxed; don't round your lower back. You should feel a mild pull gradually spread through the back of your leg. Repeat the stretch with your right leg forward.

Keep in mind the following tips as you perform the Standing Hamstring Stretch:

✔ Keep your back straight and your abs pulled inward to make the stretch more effective and to protect your lower back.

✔ Don't lean so far forward that you lose your balance or feel strain in your lower back.

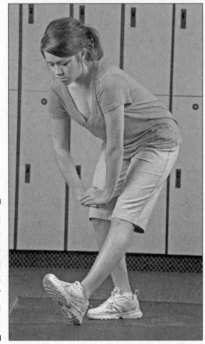

Figure 14-4:
The
Standing
Hamstring
Stretch
targets your
rear-thigh
muscles.

Standing Quad Stretch

This stretch focuses on the quadriceps (front-thigh muscles). Be extra gentle with this stretch if you're prone to knee or lower-back pain. If back pain is an issue for you, you can do a similar stretch while lying on your side, bending your top knee and bringing your heel toward your buttocks.

Stand tall with your feet hip-width apart, pull your abdominals in, and relax your shoulders. Bend your left leg, bringing your heel toward your butt, and grasp your left foot with your right hand (see Figure 14-5). You should feel a mild pull gradually spread through the front of your left leg. Then switch legs.

Keep these tips in mind as you perform the Standing Quad Stretch:

- ✔ Hold onto a chair or the wall if you have trouble balancing.
- ✔ Don't lock the knee of your base leg.
- ✔ If you're more comfortable, hold your foot with the hand on the same side.

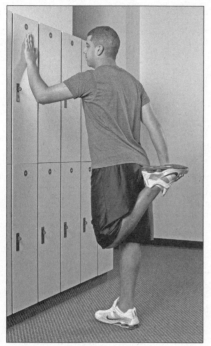

Figure 14-5:
The
Standing
Quad
Stretch
targets your
front-thigh
muscles.

Double Calf Stretch

This stretch offers some relief for the calf muscles, which tend to be tight and bunched up from daily activities such as walking and standing.

Stand with your feet together, toes facing forward, about 2 feet from a wall that you're facing. Pull your abdominals gently inward and don't round your lower back. With straight arms, press your palms into the wall and lean forward from your ankles, keeping your heels pressed as close to the floor as possible (see Figure 14-6). You should feel a mild stretch spread through your calf muscles.

Keep in mind the following tips as you perform the Double Calf Stretch:

- ✔ Keep both heels flat on the floor or as close to the floor as your flexibility allows.

- ✔ Keep your abs pulled in to prevent your lower back from sagging or arching.

- ✔ To increase the stretch, bend your elbows, leaning your chest toward the wall.

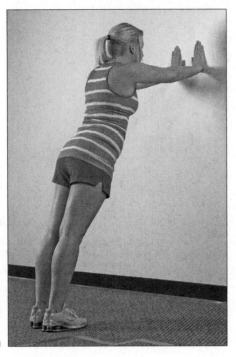

Figure 14-6:
The Double Calf Stretch helps relieve tightness in your calf muscles.

Hip Stretch

This stretch is great for your outer hips and lower back. You can do this stretch while sitting or standing, but we like performing it from a lying position because it's easier to control the tension.

Lie on your back with your knees bent and feet flat on the floor. Lift your left leg up and place your ankle across your right thigh, a few inches below your knee so that your left knee is pointing out to the side as much as your flexibility allows; see Figure 14-7a. While keeping both knees bent, lift your right foot until your right thigh is perpendicular to the floor, and thread your hands through the center of your legs so that you can clasp your right leg. Gently pull your right leg toward your chest. (See Figure 14-7b.)

You'll feel this stretch in your outer thigh and buttocks and perhaps in your lower back. If you're very tight in your arms or shoulders, you may feel it there, too.

Here are a couple of tips to keep in mind:

- ✔ To increase the stretch, keep your right hand on your thigh and, pulling it gently toward you, place your left palm gently on your left thigh just below your knee. Press your left knee outward and away from you.

> ✔ If any of this is just too hard, simply stay in the start position with your left ankle perched on your right thigh and gently pressing your left knee outward.

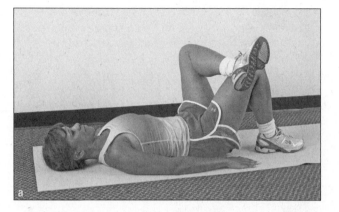

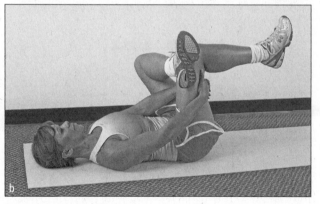

Figure 14-7:
The Hip Stretch increases hip and glute flexibility.

Butterfly Stretch

This exercise stretches your inner thighs, groin, hips, and lower back. Take extra care to lean forward from your hips rather than rounding your lower back. This exercise may also cause some knee discomfort.

To do the Butterfly Stretch, sit up tall with the soles of your feet pressed together and your knees relaxed to the sides as far as they'll comfortably go as shown in Figure 14-8a. Pull your abdominals gently inward and lean forward from your hips. Grasp your feet with your hands and carefully pull yourself a small way farther forward (see Figure 14-8b). You should feel the stretch spread throughout your inner thighs, the outermost part of your hips, and lower back.

Keep in mind these tips as you perform the Butterfly:

- ✔ Increase the stretch by carefully pressing your thighs toward the floor as you hold the position.
- ✔ Don't hunch your shoulders up toward your ears or round your back.
- ✔ To reduce stress on your knees, move your feet away from your body. To increase the stretch, move your feet toward your body.

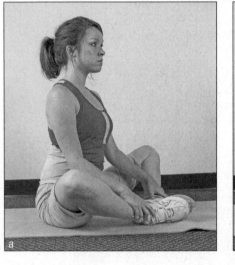
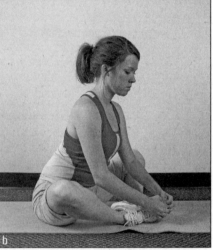

Figure 14-8:
The Butterfly Stretch targets your inner thighs, groin, hips, and lower back.

Trying Alternative Stretches

If you're curious about Active Isolated Stretching (AIS) or PNF — the alternative stretching techniques we describe earlier in this chapter — or if you're particularly inflexible, give the following stretches a try. You may find these more comfortable to do and perhaps even more effective.

Testing out Active Isolated stretches

Active Isolated Stretching (AIS) involves tightening opposing muscles before moving into a stretch. We particularly like AIS for people who don't exactly have the flexibility of a ballerina. When you're inflexible, holding a stretch for even ten seconds can seem like a lifetime. If static stretching is just too much to bear (many runners fall into this category), AIS may feel more tolerable.

The following sections introduce some Active Isolated stretches focusing on your legs — the front and back of your thighs and your calf muscles. You will need a rope, towel, or belt.

Active Isolated Hamstring Stretch

This move stretches your rear thigh muscles. To do this stretch, place a rope around your right foot and lie on your back, keeping your left leg straight (strive to place your left calf on the floor). Straighten your right leg, straighten your right knee, and use the rope to pull your right leg toward your chest (see Figure 14-9). Do your best to relax your head and neck toward the floor. Hold for 2 seconds, and then release, allowing your right leg to relax for a few seconds. Repeat for a total of 8 to 10 counts. If necessary, do an additional set of 8 to 10 repetitions.

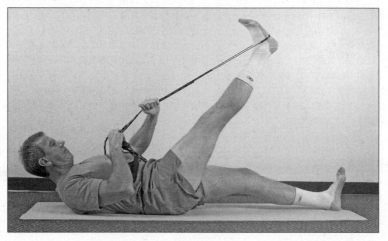

Figure 14-9:
The AIS
Hamstring
Stretch.

Active Isolated Quadriceps Stretch

You may not even know your quads (thigh muscles) are tight, but as soon as you do this stretch, you'll know. Although you may feel like a contortionist, work through this exercise to get a fantastic stretch in your quads.

With a rope wrapped around your right foot, lie on your left side. Bend your left leg and tuck your knee up to your chest. Then bend your right leg and pull your right foot toward your butt. Pull the rope tight and hold for two seconds (see Figure 14-10). Release, allowing your right leg to relax for a few seconds. Repeat for a total of 8 to 10 counts. If necessary, do an additional set of 8 to 10 repetitions.

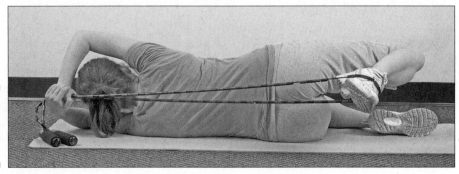

Figure 14-10:
The AIS Quadriceps Stretch.

Active Isolated Calf Stretch

This stretch keeps your calf muscles loose and supple. To do it, sit up and wrap the rope around your right foot; your left foot can be either bent or straight. Straighten your right knee and pull your right foot straight back toward your chest. Next, lean your upper body forward about 10 degrees, and hold for 2 seconds (see Figure 14-11). Leaning forward is critical. If you simply pull your foot toward your chest without the forward lean, you won't get much of a stretch. Release, allowing your right leg to relax for a few seconds. Repeat for a total of 8 to 10 counts. If necessary, do an additional set of 8 to 10 repetitions.

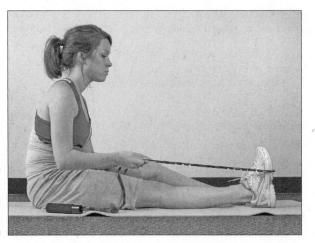

Figure 14-11:
The AIS Calf Stretch.

Doing the PNF Hamstring Stretch

In PNF, you tighten a muscle before stretching it. This particular move stretches your rear thigh muscles. For the PNF Hamstring Stretch, you should have a partner.

Lie on your back with your left knee bent, foot flat on the floor, and your right heel resting on your partner's shoulder, with the right leg as straight as you can comfortably tolerate (this will vary depending on your flexibility). To tire your hamstrings, press your heel into your partner's shoulder as she pushes her shoulder into your heel. Hold for 5 to 10 seconds and then relax and have your partner gently push your straight right leg back towards your head to stretch your hamstring for about 15 seconds. Repeat 3 or 4 times, and then perform the same sequence with your left leg.

To try this stretch solo, lie in the same position and wrap a towel, rope, or belt around your ankle, holding an end in each hand. Getting quite the same level of stretch doing it on your own can be challenging, but the stretch can still be quite effective. This solo stretch looks very much like the AIS Hamstring Stretch; refer to Figure 14-9 for a look.

Chapter 15

Finding Your Balance

● ●

In This Chapter

▶ Testing your balance

▶ Choosing balance-training tools

▶ Performing balance exercises

● ●

*W*hen you're young, you think nothing of walking down a hill, stepping into a bathtub, or navigating around a branch that's fallen on a trail. But at some point — possibly around the time you start appreciating early-bird dinner specials — you may notice that movements like these are becoming more challenging, even worrisome. That's because as you age, your sense of balance declines.

Loss of balance is no small concern. Each year, U.S. hospitals admit 300,000 patients with broken hips, injuries that often lead to permanent disability. Falling due to poor balance is a leading cause of these fractures. The happy news: By regularly performing a few basic exercises, you can improve your sense of balance almost immediately, even in your eighties.

But don't wait that long! In fact, we recommend balance training for teens and twentysomethings. Even when you're a whippersnapper who could navigate a room full of marbles on roller skates, improved balance will make you a better athlete, help you move more gracefully, and prevent unnecessary falls. Tripping on a curb may not be life-threatening when you're young and have strong bones, but who wants to end up in the emergency room with a torn ligament? In this chapter, we offer simple balance tests, along with several exercises for training this important aspect of fitness. Plus, we introduce you to nifty gadgets that make balance training fun.

Balance: Use It or Lose It

The fact that you don't stumble over every crack in a sidewalk is due to an amazing combination of bodily systems and skills that work in harmony: your inner ears, vision, *proprioception* (your body's remarkable ability to under-stand where it is in space), flexibility, strength, and brain function. If any one of these systems were to fail, you would bob and weave as if you'd had one too many glasses of wine.

Though all the components of balance naturally decline with age, you can do plenty to stave off the decline, especially in the areas of flexibility, strength, and proprioception. You can train your *vestibular function* (the sensory apparatus of the inner ear) to some extent; astronauts spend months in special vestibular chambers, which are specially designed to train the tiny ear canals that send balance information to your brain, preparing for the disorientation of space flight. But unless you have your sights set on visiting Mars, that's not where we'd recommend investing your time.

Instead, boost your flexibility and strength by stretching your muscles and challenging them with resistance, as we explain in Parts III and IV. And by the way, we mean *all* your muscles, not just your legs. Every part of your body is involved in balance. Even an imbalance between your abdominal and lower-back muscles can significantly compromise your balance.

As for proprioception, the exercises in this chapter can help you keep this important system humming.

Evaluating Your Balance

The first step is to see how your balance skills rate. Take the balance tests described in the next section, and then use the guidelines for interpreting the results to develop a balance-training plan.

Taking four simple tests

Do this four-part balance evaluation while standing in front of a stable chair. If it turns out that your balance isn't stellar, you can always sit back into the chair to save yourself from a fall. We also recommend having another chair to your side so that you can grab it for support if necessary.

Now, stand tall with your feet placed as wide as your hips and with your arms at your sides. Use this starting position for all four tests.

✔ **Test 1:** Lift your right foot off the floor a few inches in front of you, and hold it there for a slow count of 10. Notice how much you wobble around. Now try the same test lifting your left foot off the floor. Note any differences between your two sides. If you can do this test for a full 10 count without losing your balance or feeling like you're about to tumble off the edge of a cliff, move onto Test 2. Otherwise, go directly to the next section in this chapter.

✔ **Test 2:** Close your eyes, and lift your right foot off the floor a few inches. Hold this position for a slow count of 10. Notice how much more you wobble than when your eyes are open. Repeat with your left foot lifted. Take note of any differences between your two sides. If you're able to keep your foot lifted the entire time without feeling like someone has snuck up and pulled the rug out from under you, move onto Test 3. Otherwise, skip ahead to the next section.

✔ **Test 3:** Lift your right foot, and gently place the sole of your foot, toe pointing down, on the inside of your calf so that your knee is bent and pressed out to the side as much as is comfortable. Raise your arms overhead, and press your palms together. Hold for 10 slow counts. Notice how much you wobble and how many times you step out of the position because of loss of balance. Repeat on the other side, and take note of the differences. If you lasted the full 10 seconds on both sides, proceed to the final test.

✔ **Test 4:** Lean forward until your torso is about 1 foot above and parallel to the floor, and lift your right leg behind you so that your foot is about 6 inches off the floor. Keep your back and right leg straight, and soften your left knee slightly. Hold this position for 10 slow counts, noticing how much you wobble and twist and how many times you have to place your foot back on the floor to avoid falling. Repeat with the other leg and compare notes.

Interpreting your test results

If you had trouble with Test 1, your balance needs significant work. Before attempting the exercises in this chapter, perform the test moves several times a day for a few weeks. Also consider hiring a physical therapist or experienced personal trainer to take you through a more thorough balance-training program than we offer here. Improving your strength and flexibility should help, too.

If you maxed out at Test 2, you have some balance skills but can do better. Practices Tests 1 and 2 several times a day, and add the four basic exercises in this chapter. You may also be a good candidate for physical therapy or a few sessions with a personal trainer.

If you made it to Test 3 but struggled with Test 4, we recommend doing the four exercises in this chapter several times each day. Taking up yoga or Pilates will improve your balance as well. In fact, the "tree" position used in Test 4 is borrowed from yoga. Also, consider buying a balance tool such as a physioball, balance board, or Wii Balance Board, all described later in this chapter.

If you aced Test 4, you're a balance champ. But don't rest on your laurels. Balance requires life-long practice and nurturing. In addition to practicing the moves in this chapter, incorporate balance elements into your strength and cardio workouts. For example, lie on a physioball instead of a weight bench for your incline flies. Stand on a BOSU, rather than the floor, for your biceps curls. Yoga and Pilates will introduce you to poses and exercises that require a mind-boggling amount of balance. (Not to worry; the moves can easily be adjusted for beginners.) Take up martial arts, cycling, hiking, or trail running, all activities that require quick reactions on the move.

Trying Nifty Tools for Training Your Balance

Sure, you can train your balance by walking along the edge of a pool or using a curb as a balance beam — go for it. But you may find the balance-training gadgets listed here to be a bit safer and more convenient to use in your living room. The nice thing about balance paraphernalia is that it isn't super expensive; some of the options we give you actually cost nothing.

- **Physioball:** Who knew a glorified beach ball could be so versatile? A *physioball,* also known as a *stability ball* or *balance ball,* can add an element of balance to virtually any strength exercise by providing an unstable surface. We talk more about this piece of equipment in Chapters 12 and 26.

- **BOSU:** A *BOSU ball* looks like a physioball that's been sliced in half and then glued to a thick platter. The idea is that standing, leaning, sitting, or placing your hands on the ball makes you shaky — in a good way. It's the same principle as standing on a small boat in choppy water: The ground moves unpredictably beneath you, and you have to make constant small adjustments with every muscle in your body.

With one hand on a partner, try a basic squat perched atop a BOSU. This movement gets amped up about six levels because it's so challenging to squat down and stand up without sliding over the side of the BOSU. We especially like using the BOSU for push-ups. The "easy" version involves placing your hands on the ball as you push up. A more challenging version involves turning over the BOSU and placing your hands on the sides of the platform. If you really want to test your balance, place your feet on the dome and try doing a push-up!

- **Balance pods:** Never mind that these devices looks like shrunken BOSU balls with the mumps. *Balance pods* are the go-to tool for fine-tuning balance, coordination, and body awareness. You place them either randomly or in patterns on the floor and then walk, step, or hop from one to another. Or simply stand on one foot on top of one and try to balance. We love these pods because they're so versatile and inexpensive, costing about $30. Look in catalogs such as Flaghouse, Gaiam, and Spri for their versions of this tool.

✔ **Wii Balance Board:** This high-tech approach to balance isn't for everyone (if you have trouble operating your TV remote, it's probably not for you). But if you are gadget-minded, the *Wii Balance Board* may keep you motivated for balance training. The board looks something like a bathroom scale with the numbers removed. As you stand on the board, it provides feedback to the Wii console (and thus your TV) on how much you wobble, which leg is stronger, and how many times you do an exercise correctly.

✔ **Balance podcasts:** We're big fans of podcasts. To find useful balance workouts, log onto iTunes and search the podcast section for balance exercises. (They change weekly.) Some are audio only, and some also contain video. They can be as short as 3 minutes or as long as a half hour, leading you through a series of exercises. Choose a reliable source, such as a reputable organization, physician, physical therapist, or certified trainer. (See Chapter 4 for guidance on who's reputable.)

✔ **DIY balance tools:** Maintaining your balance doesn't require cash and fancy gizmos. A paper plate works just fine: While standing, place it under your right foot, and make circles with your foot about the size of a cereal bowl. This will strengthen your hips, thighs, and calves. Duct tape taped along a floor can be used as a "balance beam."

Use your imagination! Just don't get carried away and start trying to balance things like the Cat in the Hat. Safety first.

Doing Four Balance Exercises

The balance exercises here range from basic to moderately challenging and are not fancy. We believe that balance moves need not be complicated to be effective and that the Cirque-du-Soleil-level balance moves that some trainers are promoting are overkill. For example, we have a DVD created by a famous trainer who has people kneeling on top of a physioball while holding one dumbbell in an extended arm and performing a dumbbell shoulder press with the other. Impressive? Yes. Practical? No.

Even if you have good balance, we recommend doing the basic moves we describe here. Some people, especially young, fit people, will find them ridiculously easy to do. But that's not the point. You still can learn something by taking a simple everyday movement and thinking about it. For example, the first move — standing up out of a chair and walking forward — sounds easy, right? Most people do that a hundred times a day without any conscious awareness of doing so. But by focusing, you may notice that you push down on your thighs with your hands to work up the momentum to stand up (a sign of weakness in the thighs and lower back) or that you twist to one side and then stand up (a sign of muscle imbalances from left to right). Compensating this way may work for you now, but could be a sign of difficulties to come.

Correcting these very basic movement patterns requires flexibility, strength, and, yes, good balance. You see the problem in older people who have trouble getting up from a chair. They're often shaky getting to their feet and then stumble a bit on the first few steps forward. It's wise to work on these issues before they become problems.

We recommend incorporating these exercises into your strength routine two or three times a week. Or if you're really focusing on improving your balance, practice the moves daily. Do two or three sets of each.

Sit to Stand

This exercise works on the balance needed to go from a sitting position to standing, and vice versa, without much momentum, twisting, or loss of movement control. Here's how to do it:

Find a stable chair with arm rests, and stand tall in front of it with your feet comfortably apart and your arms at your sides. The distance you stand from the chair should allow you to sit down comfortably with your rear squarely on the seat, not on the edge or too far back.

Without placing your hands on the armrests, slowly sit back into the chair, controlling the movement rather than just plopping down. Take two slow counts to sit, and then stand back up without using your hands. Press your weight evenly into both feet, and avoid folding your torso too far forward. Try not to twist to one side or use much momentum to stand. As soon as you're standing, walk several steps with a focus on keeping your posture tall and without lurching to one side. Try this five to ten times.

Easier version: Assist yourself with the armrests, or have someone guide you through the parts of the range of motion that are tough for you.

Harder version: Use a chair without armrests, an overstuffed chair, or a couch that you really sink into. Finally, try it with a chair that has wheels on it — as long as there's no chance it'll glide across the room and leave you on your butt.

Hopping

Stand tall with your hands on your hips and your feet placed hip-width apart. Lift your right foot off the floor, knee slightly bent and foot held straight out in front of you just a few inches off the floor (see Figure 15-1). Take a small hop to the right. Focus on landing softly and with as little wobble or torque as possible. Then lift your left foot, and take a small hop to the left. Pause between each hop. Do 8 to 15 repetitions each side.

Easier version: Step, rather than hop, to the side.

Harder version: Take a longer hop, or hop forward, backward, or on the diagonal.

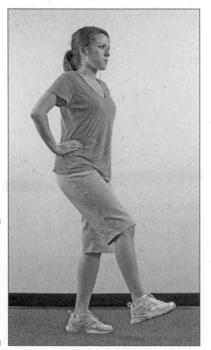

Figure 15-1: Hop to the side to improve balance when landing.

Balance-Beam Walk

Tape 6 to 12 feet of duct tape or masking tape on the floor in a straight line. Stand at one end of the line, and place one foot directly in front of the other, walking as steadily as possible (see Figure 15-2). If you "fall off" your line, simply get back on and continue from that point. Aim to make three back-and-forth trips.

Easier version: Extend your arms out to the side, but only as much as is necessary.

Harder version: Try this on a low balance beam or along the edge of a curb. Make sure you choose a platform low enough to avoid injury if you fall. A spotter is a good idea too, especially if your skills are in the development stage.

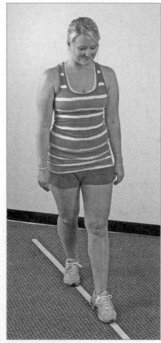

Figure 15-2: Practice walking in a straight line.

Pick-Ups

Crumple up four pieces of scrap paper, place them in a pile, and then stand about 3 inches behind the pile. Lift your right foot about 3 inches off the floor in front of you, keeping your knee bent comfortably. Gently flex your foot, and place your right hand on your hip. Soften your left knee. Slowly tip forward and down, and pick up one wad of paper (see Figure 15-3). Slowly stand back up. Focus on keeping your abs tight and your posture tall; don't round forward as you lean down. Hold at the top, and then dip down for the second piece of paper. Repeat to the other side to pick up the remaining two pieces.

Easier version: Extend your right arm out to help balance. Or, go halfway down and, for now, don't pick up the paper.

Harder version: Pick up a heavier object, like a book or a can of veggies. When you get really good, pick up a 3- to 5-pound dumbbell.

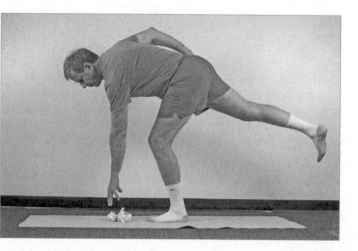

Figure 15-3:
Stand on one foot and bend forward to pick up a wad of paper.

Balance training for busy people

Don't have time during your workout to devote to balance training? Try multitasking while you're living life.

✔ While standing in line at the supermarket, balance on one foot. For a greater challenge, hold your cantaloupe, or your grocery basket, in one hand.

✔ While standing on a street corner waiting for the light to change, lift one foot forward and dangle it over the curb. Just watch out for traffic!

✔ While on an up escalator, stand on the edge of the step, lift one foot up, and lift the other heel up and down. Hold onto the rail lightly if necessary.

✔ While standing in a moving train or subway car, try to "subway surf": Don't hold onto any safety bars or seats (or companions!) and keep as still as possible. Just make sure you have a bar or seat within reach in case the train lurches suddenly. Don't try this on a crowded train, when you risk annoying other passengers.

✔ While watching TV, stand up and rock back on your heels and try to stay steady for five to ten counts. Repeat on the balls of your feet.

Chapter 16

All about Yoga

. . . .

In This Chapter

▶ Understanding asanas, or poses

▶ Appreciating the benefits of yoga

▶ Exploring the different forms of yoga

▶ Finding yoga classes and getting started

▶ Looking at a yoga workout

. . . .

*H*ere in the West, people tend to view exercise as a way to improve your body — to strengthen your heart, tone your muscles, and make your joints more flexible. Only in the past few decades has the mainstream fitness community come to accept what many other cultures have known for thousands of years: Exercise can also be good for your mind.

This realization has spawned a popular fitness catchphrase — *mind-body exercise* — and yoga is at the forefront. We think everyone can benefit from adding yoga to their exercise repertoire. Yoga takes you away from the typical pump and grind and sweat and gets you to focus on how your body moves and feels. Some studies show that just eight weeks of yoga practice can change the brain so you are calmer and more focused, have a better memory, and can learn more easily. This chapter explains what yoga entails, helps you choose a style and a class that suits you, and shows you a few moves.

Of course, yoga does a body good, too. Suzanne took a class from an older man who pranced around the room with enviable grace and agility. Suzanne was shocked to discover that the instructor was 80 years old!

Understanding Yoga: Knowing Your Asana from Your Elbows

Developed in India more than 5,000 years ago, *yoga,* which means "unite," consists of a series of poses (known as *asanas*) that you hold from a few seconds to several minutes, depending on the style of yoga you're doing. The moves — a blend of strength, flexibility, balance, and body-awareness exercises — are intended to promote the union of the mind, body, and spirit. Most forms of yoga focus on relaxation and deep breathing as you perform and hold the poses.

Yoga classes have a different feel from the usual Western workouts, some-times including a spiritual element such as chanting or burning candles or incense. However, many classes these days dispense with the traditional Indian touches and just get right down to the business of kicking your butt. You tend to see the more traditional classes at studios devoted specifically to yoga.

The most common misconception about yoga is that you have to be as flexible as Gumby to do it. In the wrong instructor's hands this is true, and if you're inflexible or a beginner, yoga will not be a comfortable experience for you. However, yoga has many, many variations in the poses, and a good teacher can teach you to do them in a way that accommodates your level of flexibility. As you improve, you'll need fewer modifications.

Looking at What Yoga Can Do for Your Body

Celebrity yoga disciples such as Jennifer Aniston, Madonna, and Gwyneth Paltrow wear their yoga bodies like badges of honor — as well they should. Clearly, yoga can shape your muscles; a yoga practice also helps you develop balance, strength, and coordination.

And here's something interesting: Some studies suggest that yoga can be useful for weight loss, even though a typical yoga class burns only about 240 calories in 45 minutes, no more than a relatively slow walk. Because yoga enhances the skill of mindfulness — the ability to be present in the moment and consider what you're doing in a very thoughtful and nonjudgmental way — it appears that people who practice yoga tend to be more mindful about their food choices and portions.

Many athletes supplement their main sports or workout routines with yoga to balance out their fitness and help avoid injury. Liz knows a world-ranked double-Ironman triathlete who, between 240-mile cycling workouts and 50-mile trail runs, religiously practices yoga to avoid injury.

You can substitute yoga workouts for your regular program once or twice a week. For example, instead of lifting weights or doing a traditional stretching workout, do a session of yoga. Some mind-body classes are intensely demanding on the muscles, so make sure that you don't overload your workout schedule. For example, some yoga classes call for intense moves like handstands and one-legged balance poses — great for the body but every bit as hard on you as doing squat with heavy weights or walking lunges. Resting your body between yoga workouts is important.

Finding a Yoga Style That's Right for You

There are many forms of yoga. Most include the same fundamental poses but differ in terms of how quickly you move, how long you hold each pose, how much breathing is emphasized, and how much of a spiritual aspect there is. Some styles offer more modifications to the really bendy and twisty moves, so they're more accessible to new exercisers and the flexibility-challenged. Others are for people who can already touch their toes with their tongue. If you find that you dig yoga, experiment with some of the different styles. You may find you like one more than the others.

Here's a brief look at the main yoga options.

- ✔ **Anusara:** Anusara, a relatively new form of yoga, has a deep spiritual element and a heavy focus on good posture and body alignment.

- ✔ **Astanga:** Astanga, sometimes called Power Yoga, is one of the most physically demanding forms of yoga in terms of flexibility, strength, and stamina. You move from one posture to another without a break, so we don't recommend this style for beginners.

- ✔ **Bikram:** Bikram, an intensely physical style of yoga, includes a lot of breathing exercises. The same 26 poses are performed in the same order during 90-minute classes that are usually conducted in a room heated to 100 degrees. (The heat is intended to make it easier to stretch.)

If you have high blood pressure, are at high risk for developing heart disease, or already have heart disease, get your doctor's permission before taking a class conducted in a room at a high temperature.

- **Hatha:** This is like a slow, easy, basic stretching class with an emphasis placed on breathing. The poses are basic, and sometimes the instructor includes a simple meditation. This is perhaps one of the most Westernized approaches to yoga.

- **Integral:** Integral classes involve lots of meditation and chanting. However, integral yoga is one of the easier forms to learn because the postures are relatively simple with plenty of modifications offered for the flexibility-challenged.

- **Iyengar:** Iyengar yoga instructors must complete a rigorous two- to five-year training program for certification, so the quality of teaching tends to be consistently good. Iyengar yoga involves props such as foam blocks and stretching belts. Instructors pay close attention to body alignment.

- **Kripalu:** Kripalu, a less physical and more meditative style of yoga, emphasizes body alignment and breath and movement coordination. There are three stages in kripalu yoga. Stage One focuses on learning the postures and exploring your body's limits of strength and flexibility. Stage Two involves holding the postures for an extended time, developing concentration and inner awareness. Stage Three involves moving from one posture to another without rest.

- **Kundalini:** Kundalini yoga was one of the first Westernized forms of yoga. Because it's designed to release energy in the body, it involves a lot of intense breathing exercises. Most of the poses are classic flexibility exercises.

- **Sivananda:** This classic style of yoga is one of the most widely followed in the world and follows well-known poses, with an emphasis on relaxation and breathing.

- **Vinyasa:** Often referred to as "vinyasa flow," vinyasa classes take you through numerous poses with little rest, though instructors tend to move at a manageable pace and encourage novices to try easier variations. Vinyasa is typically chant-free and excellent for developing flexibility and balance.

Getting Started

If you don't know downward-facing dog from walking your dog, taking your first yoga class can be daunting. Don't shy away! You'll quickly find that plenty of your classmates are new, too. To make your entry into the yoga world easier, following are tips on choosing a class, dressing like a yoga regular, and surviving your first session.

Taking yoga classes

Most health clubs offer yoga classes at no additional charge. You can find a wider variety of styles and techniques at yoga-only studios, which charge $8 to $25 per class. You'll likely also find classes aimed at different experience levels.

If you're a yoga novice, make sure you take a beginning class, and don't try to keep up with anyone else. Yoga can be extremely demanding, both in terms of flexibility and strength. Even if you can bench-press a heavy load in the gym, you may find yourself lacking the strength to hold a yoga pose for even 30 seconds. Yoga requires a different type of strength than weight-lifting does. For instance, many yoga poses require you to call upon the strength of your core and dozens of small spinal muscles that don't get much action in a weight-machine workout.

There's no national yoga certification, so we can't list certain credentials to look for in a teacher. In the yoga world, it usually means a lot if you've studied with a certain yogi master, but most people have trouble evaluating this type of credential. Rely on your own judgment and word-of-mouth recommendations. A good yoga instructor wanders around the room, gently correcting class members' techniques and offering variations that allow less-flexible people to accomplish all the poses.

Some yoga instructors don't take into account individual differences in fitness and flexibility, so it's up to you to know your own limits. Suzanne learned this lesson the hard way when her sister, Jennifer, a longtime yoga devotee, dragged her to an advanced yoga class. The 2-hour session included demanding hamstring stretches that made Suzanne so sore that she couldn't ride her bike for four days.

Some classes may be too spiritual for you and that's your call. Liz once took a class in which the instructor asked students to reveal their innermost fears. Liz didn't feel like sharing that bit of information with a group of strangers sitting around the room with their legs twisted around their necks.

Wrapping up a yoga session

Yoga offers an active timeout to energize your body and calm your mind. Most yoga classes end with several minutes of lying facedown on the floor. This *come-down time,* called *shivasana,* is low-key enough to make some people fall asleep, but after you get up, you feel recharged. Following shivasana, the instructor and class members typically sit with legs crossed and palms together at heart level. The instructor bows her head and says, "Namaste" (pronounced *na-mah-stay*), a Sanskrit term meaning, "I bow to you," and the class bows and responds, "Namaste." This ritual is used as a sign of respect and mutual gratitude.

Looking at yoga equipment and clothing

Yoga doesn't require a large commitment of clothing and equipment. Just make sure you wear something comfortable that lets you move freely in all directions without riding up or falling down. You may be most comfortable in clothing that's close fitting (but not oppressively tight) so that it stays close to your body while you have your legs apart and torso inverted. You can spend plenty on stylish yoga outfits or just wear any old stretchy shirt and shorts or tights.

Unlike most other fitness activities that require a major investment in footwear, yoga is generally practiced barefoot.

The one piece of equipment you absolutely do need is a *yoga mat,* one that's sticky or tacky (that is, nonslip), as opposed to smooth or slippery. Look for a mat that's at least 68 inches long by 24 inches wide. Look for a yoga mat at your local sporting goods store, yoga specialty shop, gym, yoga studio, or at online shops (search for "yoga mat" online). Many studios and gyms also have a variety of foam blocks, straps, and ropes to help you with your stretches, as well as blankets to use during meditations. You can also purchase these at the same place you buy mats.

Following yoga tips for beginners

In Chapter 21 we offer general advice for surviving a new exercise class with both your body and ego intact. Here are additional tips that pertain to yoga specifically:

- ✔ **Watch the instructor, not other classmates.** Yes, this goes for all classes, but it's particularly important for yoga because yoga tends to include a lot of balance work. When you're standing on one foot with the other in the air and your arms intertwined like plant vines, it's better to keep your eye on the person most likely to stay upright.

- ✔ **If a pose feels uncomfortable to you, skip it.** In a class Suzanne regularly takes, one pose makes her feel as if her lower legs are about to be twisted off at the knee. While the rest of the class does this pose, Suzanne kneels in child's pose (which we introduce later in this chapter) and contemplates how terrific her knees feel.

- ✔ **Bail if the instructor confuses you.** Keep auditioning instructors, and you'll find one you click with. Some offer just the right amount of instruction about how to get into position and what it should feel like, and others stuff your brain with so much information that you start to feel that performing downward-facing dog is more complicated than flying a 747 jet. Some instructors do the workout with you, whereas others wander around the room and teach the entire class verbally.

✔ **Bring a water bottle.** Many yoga classes are surprisingly demanding or lengthy, and a couple of sips mid-class may make the experience much more pleasant.

Trying a Yoga Routine

The following sections describe several basic yoga poses. Depending on the class, sometimes you simply move through them and sometimes you hold them for several seconds. These poses also allow for many modifications and adjustments, so you may want to peruse a Web site, pick up a book, watch a DVD or listen to a podcast, or take a class to get guidance on how these may best fit into your yoga practice.

Here are a few helpful DVD resources:

✔ *Rodney Yee's Yoga for Beginners* includes a great basic yoga tutorial. This DVD has three audio extras and is by one of the masters of the yoga video world.

✔ *Basic Yoga Workout For Dummies,* led by Sara Ivanhoe, teaches 12 basic poses and additional modifications to those poses. *Beyond Basic Yoga For Dummies,* another video led by Sara Ivanhoe, builds on the first video with additional poses and challenges.

✔ *Bendigirl Yoga* with Kristin McGee, an inspiring yoga instructor, is a terrific DVD series for teens and tween girls.

Downward-Facing Dog

Downward-Facing Dog, also known as *Down Dog,* is the quintessential yoga move. In a typical yoga class, you may come back to down dog 50 times (or maybe it just seems like 50 times). Down Dog is an awesome stretch that spreads through the whole body but is especially effective for the lower legs, shoulders, arms, and lower back. Here's how to do it:

1. **Start on your hands and knees.**

   Sit or kneel on the floor on your hands and knees with your knees directly below your hips and your hands slightly in front of your shoulders. See Figure 16-1a.

2. **Exhale, and start to straighten your legs.**

   Lift your knees away from the floor, keeping your knees slightly bent and your heels lifted. Lengthen your tailbone upward so your body forms an upside-down V shape.

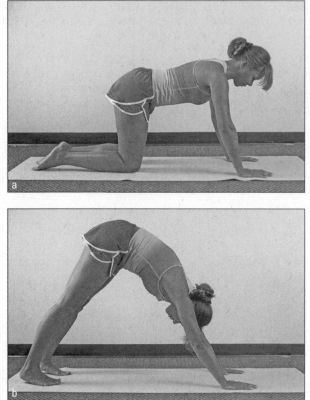

Figure 16-1:
Downward-
Facing Dog.

3. **Exhale, and push your top thighs back, stretching your heels onto or toward the floor — whatever your flexibility allows (see Figure 16-1b).**

   Straighten your knees but do not lock them. Firm your outer thighs and roll your upper thighs inward slightly.

4. **Firm your outer arms and shoulder blades. Hold the position before bending your knees and either returning to the start or moving into the next pose, or asana.**

Forward Bend

The Forward Bend can be extremely relaxing, because you stretch your back and legs. Here's how you do it:

1. Start in a sitting position, with your legs out in front of you in a V (whatever width of V is comfortable for you), toes pointed up toward the ceiling.

2. Pull up on your butt so that you're resting on your pelvic bone.

3. Stretch your arms straight up, trying to lengthen your spine as you stretch, and inhale (see Figure 16-2a).

4. As you exhale, lean your chest forward, keeping your back straight.

5. Point your chin toward your shins and your chest toward your thighs, as shown in Figure 16-2b.

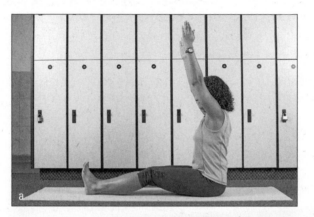

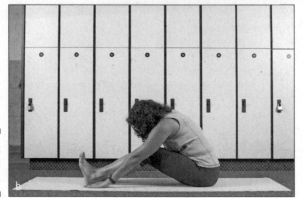

Figure 16-2:
Forward
Bend.

Child's Pose

This move stretches your lower back and arms and relaxes your entire body. If you have knee problems, lower yourself into position with extra care. Here's what to do:

1. **Start in a kneeling position.**

2. **Drop your butt toward your heels as you stretch the rest of your body down and forward.**

3. **In the fully stretched position, rest your arms in a relaxed position along the floor, rest your stomach comfortably on top of your thighs, and rest your forehead on the mat (see Figure 16-3).**

   You should feel a mild stretch in your shoulders and buttocks and down the length of your spine and arms.

Ease into this stretch by keeping your shoulders and neck relaxed. Don't force your derriere to move any closer to your heels than is comfortable.

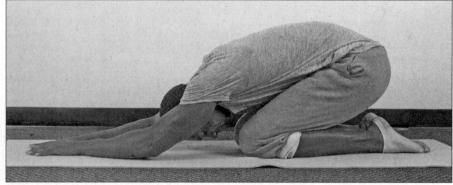

Figure 16-3:
Child's
Pose.

Modified Sage Twist

This unique pose rotates the spine from left to right, toning and relaxing as you go. Here's what to do:

1. **Start in a sitting position and extend both legs forward.**

2. **Bend your right knee and place your right foot on the floor, next to your inside left thigh.**

3. Place your right hand on the floor behind you, palm down.

4. Take your left palm or fingertips and wrap around the outside of your right knee.

5. Inhale, extending and lifting your spine upward; exhale and twist your torso and head to your right side (see Figure 16-4).

6. Repeat with the left leg bent, twisting to the other side.

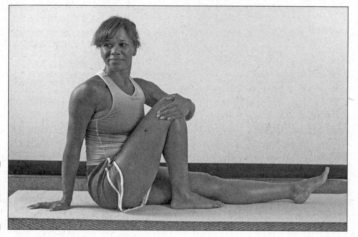

Figure 16-4:
Sage Twist
with a twist.

Cat Pose

The Cat Pose elongates your spine and eases tension in your back. Try it by following these steps:

1. Rest on your hands and knees, with your belly facing the floor.

2. Inhale deeply.

3. Exhale and pull in your abdominal muscles, tailbone, and butt.

4. Pressing down on your hands, press your back toward the ceiling so your spine rounds, as in Figure 16-5.

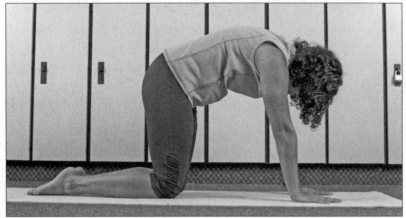

Figure 16-5:
Cat Pose.

Triangle Pose

Moving from a sitting or lying position to standing, the Triangle Pose stretches your spine and abdomen. Here's how you do it:

1. **Stand with your feet much wider than your shoulders, and place both arms straight out to the side, parallel to the floor, with palms facing up. See figure 16-6a.**

   Both feet can be flat on the floor, or you can point your left foot, keeping your heel off the floor.

2. **Inhale deeply.**

3. **Exhale and bend to the left, as in Figure 16-6b.**

   Keep your knees straight and your hips facing forward. Don't twist your lower body; simply bend at your waist.

4. **Slide your left arm down your left leg as you bend, and then hold your leg or ankle.**

5. **Hold this position, slowly breathing in and out several times.**

   If you're able to, lift your right leg off the floor, anywhere from 3 to 18 inches, keeping your knee straight.

6. **Repeat, bending to the other side.**

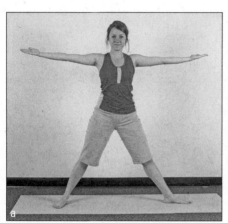
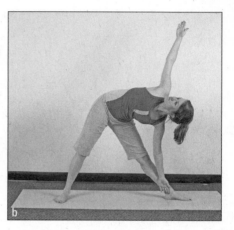

Figure 16-6:
Triangle
Pose.

Sun Salutation

This move stretches your abdominal, lower-back, front-hip, and thigh muscles. If you're prone to lower-back pain, make a special point of tightening your core, and don't arch your lower back. Here's how to do the Sun Salutation:

1. **Kneel on the floor; then bring your left leg forward so that your foot is flat on the floor, your knee is bent, and your thigh is parallel to the floor.**

2. **Lift your arms straight up with your palms facing in.**

3. **Pull your abdominals gently inward, and keep your shoulders down and back.**

4. **Look to the ceiling, and as you stretch upward with your upper body, push your weight slightly forward from your hips into your front thigh (see Figure 16-7).**

   You should feel this stretch travel through your torso and upper body, including your arms. You should also feel it at the very top of your back thigh.

5. **Repeat with your right leg forward.**

Keep in mind the following tips as you perform the Sun Salutation:

✔ Hold on to something solid, like a sturdy chair, with one hand if you have trouble maintaining balance.

✔ Don't lean so far forward that your front knee moves in front of your toes.

✔ Don't arch your lower back.

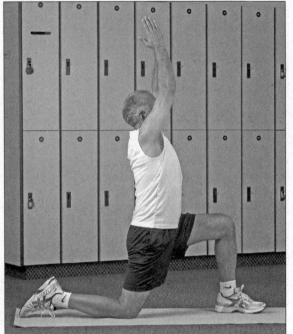

Figure 16-7:
Sun
Salutation.

Chapter 17

Getting the Lowdown on Pilates

For several years now, Pilates has been a top choice for celebrities, career women, moms-to-be, and every other kind of mom, thanks to the proliferation of Pilates studios, classes, and DVDs. Even pro football players and other athletes have gotten into the act, using Pilates to polish their athletic prowess.

But this system — a stellar way to improve posture and tone your muscles, particularly your core — has been around since the 1920s. Pilates is named after its inventor, Joseph Pilates, a former carpenter and gymnast. Many of the moves were inspired by yoga or patterned after the movements of zoo animals such as swans, seals, and big cats.

Even if you've never aspired to mimic a swan, you may find Pilates worth a try; it may even become your new favorite form of exercise. This chapter explains what Pilates can do for your body, helps you find a quality Pilates class or digital workout, and shows you a quick Pilates routine.

Understanding Pilates

First things first: This form of exercise is not pronounced *pie-lates* but rather *pih-lah-teez*. So rather than sounding like a strawberry-rhubarb dessert, it sounds like a fancy coffee drink. Of course, by now Pilates is so popular that you probably already knew that. In the following sections, we explain something you may not know: what Pilates entails and what it can do for your body.

How Pilates works

You do some Pilates exercises on a mat, and you do others using special Pilates machines (see "Two ways to practice Pilates: Choosing your type of workout"). Many of the Pilates positions are similar to yoga poses, but you perform them more quickly and in a more dynamic fashion. You don't hold still a lot in Pilates. In fact, a big part of the challenge is seamlessly melding one move into the other.

Pilates moves require you to engage virtually your whole body. At times, you may try to strengthen one muscle while stretching another, a job that requires plenty of concentration and coordination. You can't simply go through the motions like you can (but shouldn't) on gym equipment. Consider a move called Rolling Like a Ball (see Figure 17-2): You balance on your rear end, roll backward, and then roll back up into the balanced position. This move requires a good balance of abdominal and lower-back strength and is deceptively tough. Liz has seen massive bodybuilders taken down by this move — and this is one of the simpler exercises to execute.

Some of the standard sections of a Pilates workout, particularly those that focus on core muscles, are absolutely killer. Many beginners need to stop and take breaks. And that's okay. One of the things we love best about Pilates is the fact that any basic move has variations to make it progressively harder or easier. (We offer variations for the moves that we show later in this chapter.)

Pilates values technique and body positioning above going for the burn. The philosophy is that it's much better to do a move once correctly than eight times with mediocre form. This makes Pilates an excellent way to improve posture, core strength, and coordination, but it also makes the technique difficult to learn. In fact, you can spend years at what's essentially the most basic level.

How Pilates benefits even beginners

Though Pilates is a challenge to learn — did we mention that? — novices actually can see and feel benefits almost immediately. For instance, because of the focus on body mechanics, you stand and sit taller and walk more gracefully. Liz always leaves her Pilates classes feeling a few inches taller. Considering her petite stature, that alone makes taking the class worthwhile.

After a few months of regular Pilates sessions, you stand up straighter, walk more gracefully, and pull your abs in naturally, so even if you don't lose a pound, people may start asking which diet you're on. And if you actually do drop a few pounds, you notice some nice definition, especially around your middle, shoulders, back, and arms. Pilates does an especially good job of reaching deep into the core muscles that may be neglected in other forms of exercise, including strength training.

Runners, cyclists, computer users, and TV watchers are great candidates for Pilates because the technique helps counteract their tendency to hunch forward. It also develops a stronger core and greater sense of full body coordination.

As you may have deduced, Pilates may not be the best workout for someone who likes to master athletic activities quickly. Like dance, yoga, and all other mind-body disciplines, Pilates requires a long-term learning process.

Fitting Pilates into Your Workout Program

We are aware that if you incorporated every activity, technique, and sport we describe in this book you'd have to quit your job, leave your family, and skip at least two meals a day. So, no, we're not insisting that you do Pilates on top of everything else. Instead, we recommend the mix-and-match approach.

Pilates can serve as a substitute to strength training once or twice a week. Some people alternate yoga with Pilates and strength training, which is a good way to toss a variety of challenges at your body. However, in our experience, most people end up favoring either yoga or Pilates. Although the goals of both disciplines are similar — they aim to improve flexibility, balance, strength, and other aspects of mind/body fitness — and many of the moves are similar, the approach and tempo of the workouts are so different that they often appeal to different personality types.

We don't recommend dropping traditional strength training altogether in order to fit in Pilates (or yoga). As much as we love Pilates, it doesn't emphasize all parts of the body equally — the core gets a good workout but the arms don't always. And though a Pilates workout can move at a fast pace, it's not a substitute for cardio exercise.

Exploring Your Pilates Workout Options

Pilates can be mighty expensive. Private lessons set you back $40 to $200 a session. Yes, you read correctly: Some instructors charge $200 for a single session. That's because there are many more personal trainers who don't have a Pilates specialization than do, and when the Pilates specialists get a following, their prices tend to skyrocket.

Fortunately, private lessons aren't the only way to get a high-quality Pilates workout. In the following sections, we explain how to find a Pilates workout that suits your budget, interests, and goals.

Two ways to practice Pilates: Choosing your type of workout

Though every Pilates workout is a bit different, depending on the instructor, there are essentially two ways to practice Pilates. Here's a look at both.

Mat workouts

Mat workouts (whether live or on DVD or podcast) involve specialized exercises, typically following the same pattern. Some instructors mix things up, but traditional teachers tend to stick with the same order of exercises set out by Joseph Pilates himself. That doesn't mean the workout doesn't get more challenging as time goes on; each basic move has multiple variations. Many teachers follow the classic exercise series and then end with a series of moves that have a specific focus, such as engaging your abs or working on spine placement while standing. Most Pilates mat classes are done without music so the teacher can hear your breathing and you can hear the hand clapping that accompanies some of the moves to help you move at a certain beat.

Mat classes are a relative bargain, running from $12 to $25 per session at most studios and clubs, but that's still more than some monthly gym memberships. Some gyms offer Pilates classes to members at no additional charge and offer private instruction at a discount.

Machine workouts

You can take private or semi-private lessons on a series of machines with exotic names such as the Cadillac and the Reformer. Versions of these machines are also sold for home use. The Cadillac, with its array of springs, straps, poles, and bars, looks like a bed that the Marquis de Sade would've enjoyed. The Reformer looks like a weight bench souped up with assorted springs, straps, and pads. Many of the moves are exactly the same as those done in the mat class, but the straps and bands help you position yourself even more precisely or extend your body that much farther.

To the uninitiated, the first few sessions with Pilates equipment may feel weird. You pull on the straps with your arms and suddenly your entire body slides forward. Or you find yourself suspended from straps and belts several feet in the air above a thick pad. After your brain and body get the hang of it and you know the breathing and movement patterns, you begin to see how good it all is for your body.

If you can afford it, we recommend taking a private session or two on the machines. It's both an enlightening and humbling experience — enlightening because you discover that your body can move in ways you never imagined, and humbling because you discover ways in which your body should be able to move but can't.

Finding a qualified Pilates instructor

Spotting a well-educated Pilates instructor isn't always easy. No certification is required for teaching Pilates, and there's no standardized definition of Pilates. Ever since a 2000 court ruling, Pilates has been considered a generic term; anyone is free to call their teaching method Pilates. (Prior to this ruling, one person claimed to own the name and method and would sue anyone else who used it or charge them exorbitant fees.)

This ruling was a victory to both instructors and students. Still, anyone can set up a lemonade stand and call it Pilates, so as a consumer, you have to do your homework. More than a dozen Pilates certifications are offered, but unlike in the personal-training world (see Chapter 20), there's no movement afoot to standardize and accredit these certifications. Many specialty studios require instructors to possess a particular certification, but many gyms do not.

Some certifications involve weekend courses that teach the basics of the mat class; participants take an exam and those who pass receive a frameable certification. Other certifications are much more rigorous, requiring the instructor to complete one or more years of study, regular private lessons, and several hundred hours of internship that involve both teaching and observing mat and machine work.

Naturally, working with a teacher who has gone through intensive training will probably give you a better experience, so ask your instructor which certification he or she has and what he or she had to go through to get it. We like the Stott Pilates certification method, Balanced Body, and Re:Ab, but that's mainly because we've worked with teachers who've gone through their training and we've had good experiences. There are certainly other good certifications. To find a good Pilates instructor, you ultimately have to rely on your own judgment and recommendations from people you trust.

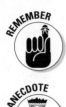

Certification does not magically turn an instructor into a gifted teacher; communication skills are an important part of the package. The best Pilates instructors, like the best trainers, use what they know and apply it to you personally.

Suzanne did a Pilates session with an instructor who was highly qualified but also highly impatient with Suzanne's inability to follow proper breathing technique. Clearly, that wasn't the day for Suzanne to focus on her breathing; she might've been less flustered working through the positions and gaining comfort with the exercise sequence.

In theory, anyone should be able to walk into any Pilates class and work at his or her level; you typically don't find classes labeled *beginner* or *advanced*. But in reality, certain classes tend to attract people at the same level. Whether it's because the students started together or because the teacher has a certain way of explaining things, it's likely that a given class will be aimed at beginners or Pilates pros. You can decide whether you want to venture into a class that isn't at your level. Even for Pilates veterans, taking a "beginner's" class every once in a while is a good refresher.

Doing Pilates at home

If you can't find a Pilates class or appealing instructor near you, or if you find the price of in-person instruction off the charts, you have plenty of alternative ways to participate in Pilates. Here are digital resources for learning the technique:

- ✔ **Pilates DVDs:** New Pilates DVDs hit the market on a monthly basis. Terrific instructors such as Mari Winsor, Linda Farrell, Jennifer Kries, and the team of Elisabeth Halfpapp and Fred DeVito produce DVDs with instruction so good that you feel you have a teacher in the room with you. Naturally, we also recommend *Pilates Workout For Dummies* (Wiley), a workout DVD by Michelle Dozios that not only demonstrates Pilates techniques for beginners but also offers challenging workouts as you advance.

- ✔ **Cable and Internet Pilates workouts:** You may find a good Pilates workout on your local cable on-demand fitness channel. Also check sources such as YouTube and iTunes for free downloads. We recommend you stick to the tried-and-true sources, such as the instructors we mention, until you have the ability to separate good Pilates from bad.

If you prefer books, you can pick up a copy of *Pilates For Dummies* by Ellie Herman (Wiley). It covers everything from basic Pilates to super-advanced exercises.

As for equipment, Gaiam (www.gaiam.com) sells a line of Pilates tools and machines at reasonable prices. You can master the tools, such as a bendy metal or plastic ring you squeeze between your legs, with the help of a good DVD workout or even a book. (Rings, balls, and bands start as low as $20 and go up to a few hundred.) We think that many of these tools are good quality. We even like the home versions of the Pilates machines (prices range from $600 to $3,000), but we hesitate to recommend them for beginners. Figuring out how to use a Pilates machine really is best done one-on-one with a live instructor.

Performing Some Pilates Exercises

Pilates includes more than 500 movements and exercises (and many have numerous steps), and different combinations of these moves make up a Pilates workout. We're showing a small sampling here so you can try them in your living room before shelling out the big bucks for classes and/or equipment. As with all Pilates moves, you can make these harder or easier. Here we offer you the basic versions along with suggestions for modifying them.

You may require several sessions to become comfortable with these and other Pilates moves and several months to become skilled at them. Pilates is a challenging activity, but it's one that pays off handsomely if you stick with it.

The Hundred

The Hundred is usually one of the first exercises in the traditional Pilates series of exercises designed by Joseph Pilates and followed by most instructors today. This exercise is frequently used as a dynamic warm-up for the abdominals and to get the lungs and the blood pumping. It requires you to coordinate your breath and movement while lengthening your body and holding everything still, except your pumping arms.

The exercise

Lie on your back and bring your knees toward your chest so your knees form 90-degree angles with your inner thighs. Extend your arms along your sides with your palms facing down. Pull your belly button toward your spine, and inhale through your nose. See Figure 17-1a.

As you exhale through your mouth, lift your chin toward your chest, and lift your arms about 3 inches off the floor (see Figure 17-1b). Keeping your arms straight and rigid, begin pumping them up and down so that they go a few inches above your body and end at the lower point, level with your sides. As you pump, breathe in for 5 pumps and out for 5 pumps, until you reach 100 counts total. Keep your eyes focused on your belly button and the rest of your body still.

When you're finished with the 100 pumps, bend your knees into your chest and lower your body to the floor.

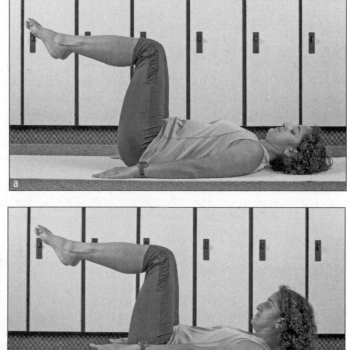

Figure 17-1:
The Hundred warms up your abs and gets your blood pumping.

Modifying the move

To make the move easier, try these options: Keep your knees bent as you hold them up, lift only one leg off the floor, or reduce the number of pumps as much as needed. To make this move more challenging, lower your legs closer to the floor.

Rolling Like a Ball

Rolling Like a Ball looks like a breeze but is actually a deceptively complex move. It requires the synchronized use of all your core muscles, plus good posture and decent flexibility to balance yourself on your tailbone.

The exercise

Sit up tall and hug your knees into your chest. Drop your chin to your chest, pull your abs in, and round your back a bit to create a hollowed out *C* shape with your spine. Point your toes and lift your feet an inch or so off the floor so that you're balanced evenly on the center of your tailbone. See Figure 17-2a.

Now pull your abs in even more to gently shift your weight backward (see Figure 17-2b). Roll back as far as your shoulder blades (see Figure 17-2c). Tighten your abs once again to shift your weight forward, and roll back up into the balanced position. Hold the position for a moment before rolling back again.

Remember to control the movement with your abdominals, not with momentum. You know you're doing this move correctly if you roll easily up into the balanced position and are able to hold it without a lot of additional body shifting. Do 3 to 8 repetitions.

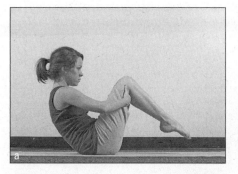

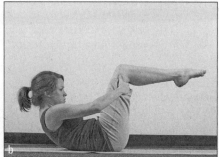

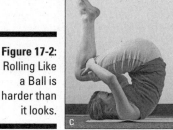

Figure 17-2:
Rolling Like a Ball is harder than it looks.

Modifying the move

To make this move easier, hold on to your shins just underneath your knees so you don't form quite as tight a ball. To make it harder, hold your hands out in front of your ankles without actually grasping them. This way, you don't have the benefit of your hands to help you maintain your ball shape.

Single Leg Pull

The Single Leg Pull is from the very challenging abdominal series. It works the core quite deeply, as well as the hips and thighs, and it enhances coordination and balance. Transitioning into this move from Rolling Like a Ball is common, but even on its own, this exercise is a real challenge.

The exercise

Lie on your back and draw your right knee into your chest as you extend your left leg. Lift your head off the floor, pull your belly button into your spine, and fix your eyes on your navel. Grasp your right ankle with your right hand and place your left hand on top of your right knee. See Figure 17-3.

Inhale and give your right leg two quick, short tugs toward your face, focusing on stretching and lengthening your left leg as much as possible. As you exhale, switch sides so that your left knee is now bent inward, your left hand is on top of the ankle, and your right hand is on top of your knee. Again, give two short, quick tugs inward. Continue tugging and switching in this pattern 5 to 7 times on each side.

Figure 17-3:
The Single Leg Pull works your core muscles and stretches your gluts and hip flexor.

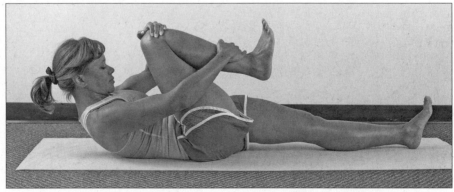

Modifying the move

To make this easier, keep your extended leg higher off the ground. If your flexibility is limited, you may also have to keep the leg slightly bent, though always aim for the straightest leg possible. To make the move harder, simply lower your leg.

Spinal Stretch Forward

We love the Spinal Stretch Forward because it's such an antidote to sitting hunched over a desk all day or lugging around a heavy child or two. It stretches the entire length of the spine, broadens the shoulders, and tones the core. It's also an excellent way to open up the lungs so you can breathe more deeply.

The exercise

Sit up tall on the floor with your legs straight, placed slightly wider than your hips. Roll your shoulders back and down. Flex your feet and sit up as tall as you're able, trying to get your spine completely perpendicular to the floor. Engage your core and lift from your breastbone. You're now sitting up as tall as you can without feeling discomfort. Extend your arms out straight with palms facing downward. See Figure 17-4a.

Exhale. Curl your chin toward your chest, and reach your fingertips straight out in front of you as you hollow out your center and reach forward to create a *C* shape with your body. If your flexibility and core strength allow it, extend your hands over your toes as shown in Figure 17-4b.

Inhale and uncurl slowly through your spine and return to perfect posture; in fact, try to sit up even straighter than when you first started. Repeat 5 to 7 times.

Modifying the move

To make this easier, maintain a slight bend in the knees or don't lower as far. To make the move harder, aim to reach even farther than your toes.

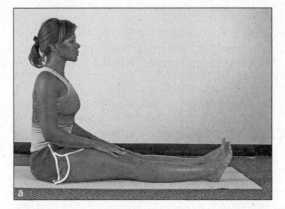

Figure 17-4:
Try the
Spinal
Stretch
Forward
if you sit
hunched
over a desk
all day.

Part V
Getting Fit in Health Clubs and Home Gyms

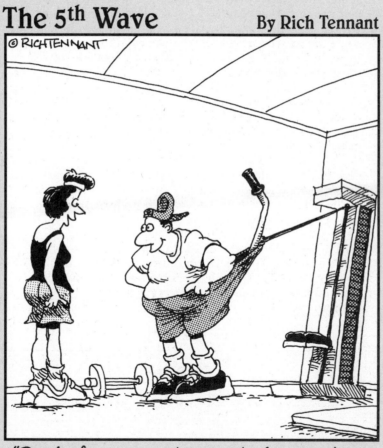

The 5th Wave   By Rich Tennant

"Ready for our next upper-body exercise?
Let's continue with the brain."

In this part . . .

We prepare you to take the health-club plunge — or create the best home gym for your budget, living space, and goals. Chapter 18 explains how to choose the best gym for you and how to recognize slimy sales tactics. We also update you on the latest health-club trends and share the unwritten rules of the gym: what to say, what to wear, and what to do about that pool of sweat you left on the leg-press machine.

To create your own home gym, take a look at Chapter 19, which covers where to shop for equipment, how to get a good deal, and where to put your devices so they don't just gather dust.

Chapter 20 explains why you may want to hire a fitness trainer and how to find a qualified trainer whose motivational style works for you. It also covers how to hold up your end of the deal by being a responsible client.

In Chapter 21, we fill you in on choosing an exercise class, either with a real, live instructor or with one who motivates you from your TV or computer screen. We run down the most popular classes available, from spinning to boot camp to Latin dance, and tell you what to expect from an instructor.

Chapter 18

Choosing and Using a Gym

In This Chapter

▶ Deciding whether to join a gym

▶ Evaluating a health club

▶ Going it alone in the gym

▶ Asking Miss Manners: Health club etiquette

*W*hen it comes to health clubs, gyms, and fitness facilities, we're biased: We like 'em. The good ones give you access to great equipment, phenomenal staff, and the freshest exercise programs around. There's always someone on the premises to give you help and encouragement. You also can get a much wider variety of workout choices than you would in your living room.

Of course, to reap the benefits of paying for a gym, it has to be decent. Plus, you actually have to show up. The reality is that most people don't. If every member worked out regularly, the place probably would look like the floor of the New York Stock Exchange. About half the people who join a club quit exercising within two months, and less than 20 percent work out three times a week.

To boost your odds of becoming a regular, it's important to choose a facility that suits your schedule, your goals, and your personality. This chapter covers the latest trends in health clubs and helps you choose the right club for you. And to make sure you pay a fair price, we explain some of the sneaky sales tactics and hidden costs you may encounter. Finally, we fill you in on health-club etiquette.

Should You Join a Health Club?

A fitness center isn't for everybody. Before you shop around, consider whether you're the sort of person who will thrive at a gym. This may save you plenty of money and guilt in the long run. If you decide that a gym isn't for you, there are other places to get fit (see Chapters 9 and 19 for ideas).

Four reasons to sign up

We can think of, oh, about three dozen reasons to sign up for a gym, but here are our top four.

- ✔ **You need inspiration.** At home you can always drum up an excuse not to exercise, even if it means dusting off your bread maker or reprogramming your TV's universal remote. But at the gym, what else is there to do but exercise? While you're at it, you may even strike up some interesting conversations and end up with a workout partner or a referral for a plumbing contractor. Even if you never talk to a soul, you can feed off the energy of those around you.

- ✔ **You want variety.** Even if you can afford $10,000 to build an elaborate home gym, you can still find more options at a health club. At home, you may have a stationary bike, a treadmill, or an elliptical trainer. At a gym, you have all three and more. The same goes for weights. You can strengthen your triceps just fine with a pair of dumbbells in your living room, but at a gym you also have the option of using machines, barbells, and cable pulleys. Gyms frequently update their equipment — most do so at least every year and the bigger ones do every few months — so you can try strength and aerobic machines that haven't yet hit the home market or are still too expensive.

    You can also choose from a long list of classes. The schedule refreshes three to four times a year, so just when you're about to get bored, along comes the latest class you read about on the Web and have been wanting to check out.

- ✔ **You have a passion for a particular sport or pastime.** Do you have the space and the cash to build a rock wall in your living room? Can you forfeit your bedroom for a boxing ring? No? Neither can we. But many gyms can accommodate special interests like these. Chelsea Piers, a large gym in New York City, isn't terribly convenient for a lot of people, yet they come from all over to use the largest indoor climbing wall on the eastern seaboard. In Miami, serious boxers head to the Normandy. And anyone who loves a racquet sport will feel like they've died and gone to heaven when they wander into Red Lerille's in Lafayette, Louisiana. If you have a passion for a sport or pastime, joining a gym that has the specialty equipment, the skilled staff, and like-minded people is the way to go.

- ✔ **You want expert advice.** At a good gym, a trainer is always on hand to help you figure out the chest machine or tell you how to firm up your butt. You also have a room full of other exercisers to watch, although they may or may not be good instructors to learn from. Many gyms now employ other sorts of pros too, such as physical therapists, acupuncturists, and nutritionists, so you have a one-stop shop for reshaping your body and getting healthy.

Four reasons to say, "No thanks"

Some people collect gym memberships. They figure that if they keep join-ing, one of these days they may actually go, but inevitably the relationship is short-lived. Don't bother buying a membership if you have no serious inten-tion of using it. If you fit the following categories, you're better off finding an alternative way to work out:

- ✔ **You want to exercise alone.** If you can't bear the thought of working out in public just yet, start off at home and consider a gym again in a few months when you feel more confident. If you're someone who simply prefers solitude, don't waste your money on a health-club membership. Or if you like to blast your TV on the highest volume or crank up the stereo, you probably ought to stay at home and annoy just the neigh-bors rather than an entire building full of gym members.

  Of course, if you find a health club intimidating simply because you've never been to one, don't let that stop you. Ask about some free passes or a trial membership, and follow the tips in "Braving the Gym for the First Time."

- ✔ **Your schedule won't allow time.** If you don't have the time to drive to a club or if you can't find one to accommodate your work hours, don't force the issue. Exercising at home makes more sense. Know, however, that 24-hour gyms are becoming more popular. (Even West Shokan, New York, near Liz's hometown, has had one for years — and the place doesn't even have a corner store.)

- ✔ **You hate exercising indoors.** If indoor workouts make you feel like a hamster on a wheel, head outside and walk, run, skate, or cycle (see Chapter 9). Keep in mind that you have to be pretty creative to get a great strength-training workout outdoors, but if you use your body weight (push-ups, pull-ups), benches, outdoor circuit-training, fitness courses, and so on, you can put together a pretty decent strength workout.

- ✔ **You prefer not to rock the boat.** If you enjoy your home exercise pro-gram and don't feel like you've been left out of the party because you haven't tried the latest treadmill-elliptical hybrid, it may simply not be worth your time and money to invest in a monthly gym membership.

Knowing How to Judge a Gym

Don't join a club simply because your accountant goes there or because the club is promoting a special discount. Shopping around before you part with any money is important. Here are some factors to consider (some may matter to you; others won't) when judging a gym.

Location and hours

Location is probably the most important consideration when choosing a gym. If your gym is on the other side of town, you won't go — even if it's the Taj Mahal of health clubs. Ideally, join a club within a ten-minute walk or 2-mile drive from your home or office.

The only exception may be a gym with special facilities that the nearest club doesn't have, such as a rock wall or a pool. But if you're a beginner who hasn't yet made exercise a habit, you may still be better off at a nearby club that doesn't have all the amenities.

Also, check your club's hours, particularly on weekends, when most gyms close earlier. Generally, the larger the club, the longer the hours. There are 24-hour gyms and gyms that close at 8 p.m.

Size

One of the big trends in gyms is the super-club. You can find low prices, an enormous selection of equipment and classes, plenty of energy, and a large staff of trainers. For an experienced exerciser, a super-club can be as fun as an amusement park; you can never get bored, roving from the golf clinic to the climbing wall to the Middle Eastern belly dancing class.

Super-clubs tend to take a "jack-of-all-trades, master-of-none" approach. These clubs may have a small yoga room, a limited boxing program, and a small climbing wall that would bore you after a week. If you're trying to familiarize yourself with a specific skill or technique, a mega-club isn't the place to get in-depth knowledge. Yoga, for example, is best learned at a studio that teaches only yoga. But if you want a smorgasbord of activities, a super-club is the place to be. And in all fairness, many super-clubs have fantastic classes and superb facilities. The Equinox chain, for example, does a good job of walking the line between super-club and high-quality offerings.

Some larger health clubs tend to take a no-frills approach, which means you may not have a spa, daycare center, pool, and 20 different types of workout classes, but you do have cardio and strength equipment, plus a locker room in which to change and shower. If no-frills is appropriate for you, you'll pay far less than at a health club that offers all the amenities.

If you're a beginner, mega-clubs can be overwhelming. In that case, another trend in gyms may be for you: a smaller, cozier, independent gym. You can get to know the entire staff on a personal basis, and they may even notice if you don't show up for a while. Smaller niche clubs come in all shapes and sizes, from the local club owned by a trainer who's passionate about fitness to the tiny but fancy studios aimed at people who want to pay more for great service and a lot of attention.

Cost

Membership fees vary greatly. Large clubs often charge less than small ones because they have more members. Consider these money matters when you choose a gym:

- **Hidden costs:** The monthly membership may be reasonable, but will you pay out the wazoo in extras? A few years ago, Suzanne checked out a club that cost $25 a month. What the sales guy didn't happen to mention was the $1.35 daily parking fee. If Suzanne went to the gym five days a week, she would've paid more per month in parking — $27 — than in membership fees. She ultimately found a gym with free parking (a prized commodity in Los Angeles). And Liz went to a yoga specialty studio that charged separately for the class, the mat, and locker room usage!

  Some gyms charge extra for specialty classes, such as boxing or Pilates. Other clubs don't have membership dues but charge hefty fees for trainers; the catch is that you can't use the club without one. This type of club could run you $10,000 a year. On the other hand, you're bound to get plenty of attention. Other clubs, like those found in apartment buildings or condo complexes, may be free with the price built into your rent or common charges.

- **Initiation fees:** In addition to the monthly membership fee, many clubs require an initiation fee. At least, they claim to require it. If you insist strongly enough, many clubs waive this fee. Or clubs use this initiation fee as a marketing ploy — something they don't really intend for you to pay. Some salesperson may say, "Just because you seem like a terrific person, and I really want you to get in shape, I'll waive the initiation fee. But shh — don't tell my boss. He'll kill me." Initiation fees can range from $25 to $1,500.

- **Length of the commitment:** Some clubs lead you to believe that you're joining for only a month when you're actually paying by the month and joining for a year. This is why you need to read your contract.

  Don't even think about a long-term membership. You don't know where you're going to be in three years (although some club chains do allow you to transfer your membership) — or whether the club will even be in business. One club in New York was selling lifetime memberships until the day before it closed its doors. Never sign up for more than one year.

  Suzanne's husband signed up for an 18-month membership at a club that was offering a screaming deal. A month later, he realized he didn't actually like working out at the gym because he didn't want to shower there on the way to work. Now he jogs in the neighborhood and showers at home, where Suzanne hopes he thinks long and hard about all the money he flushed down the toilet.

  If you're unsure about the club, ask for a free trial period or several free passes before joining. You may even want to sign up on a month-to-month basis if the club allows it; you'll probably pay more, but you give yourself an out if the club doesn't suit you. If you choose to pay by the month, we recommend using your credit card or an electronic transfer system instead of writing a check. The credit-card company or your bank can protect you from incorrect charges or help you put a stop to the fees if you no longer want to belong to the gym.

- **Cancellation policies:** Salespeople don't always tell you this, but in most states, the law requires a three-day cooling-off period. In other words, if you change your mind within three days, the club must refund your money in full. If the club won't, get your lawyer to shoot off a letter; that should do the trick. Also, ask what happens if you quit three months after joining. Some clubs will refund your money for any reason. But most will offer a refund only if one of the following applies:

  - You move more than 25 miles from the club.

  - You can prove that you have a medical condition that will prevent you from exercising for several months.

  - The club stops offering the services promised in the contract (although many even have a way around this).

Many clubs make special deals if you ask. The best time to ask is during slow periods like summer or the end of the month and during a slow economy, when clubs are hungrier for sales. You may also get a break if you join with a family member or friend. If you have friends who are already members, ask what they paid; if the sales rep cites you a higher fee, don't be afraid to say, "My friend Jane Smith paid $30 a month, and I'd like the same deal."

The dollar figure doesn't mean everything. Fifty bucks a month may seem outrageous for a small neighborhood club with old equipment; on the other hand, if the club is half a mile from your house, it's a bargain because you may actually go. It's a much better investment than a $30-a-month club that's 20 minutes away.

Equipment

You may not consider yourself qualified to judge the equipment at a gym, but even a novice can make some important assessments. If you wouldn't know a hamstring machine even if you were sitting on one, ask your tour guide specifically about the following factors:

- **Variety:** Do you want three varieties of bikes, or will you settle for one? Some clubs have 10-, 15-, and 20-pound dumbbells; at other clubs, you also find 12-pounders, 17½-pounders, and 22½-pounders. Some gyms have a single back machine; others have four so you can work these muscles standing, sitting, leaning forward, or lying face-down.

- **Quantity:** Is there enough equipment to support the membership? You don't want your wait for the treadmill to be like the line at the department of motor vehicles. Take a tour at the same time of day you plan to work out, and notice whether the machines are overbooked. Many gyms enforce a rush-hour policy that limits you to 20 to 30 minutes on the cardio equipment if others are waiting. This restriction can be frustrating if you've planned a longer workout that day. Or if you're third in line.

✔ **Quality, cleanliness, and upkeep:** Is the place in a state of disrepair? Is the stuffing coming out of the weight benches? Lots of duct tape is not a good sign. Get on a couple of weight machines and see how smoothly the weight stacks work. Pick up a few free weights and see whether the ends are loose. Listen to the cardio equipment: Are the treadmills loud and whiny? That noise means that the motors need a tune-up. Don't be afraid to test-drive a good portion of the equipment — or to ask other members whether they feel the machinery is well-maintained. Also, follow your nose. If the gym smells overly musty or dirty, follow your nose right out the door.

✔ **Equipment turnover:** Is the equipment older than dinosaur fossils? Or does the club have a new fleet of stationary bikes with built-in 500-channel televisions? Most gyms can't afford to replace all their equipment every year, but at least 10 to 30 percent of the machines should be new.

Group exercise classes

Make sure that the club offers what you want, whether it's the latest and greatest, such as boot camp, Zumba, iron yoga, or triathlon training, or more basic strength-training and traditional classes. (Some no-frills clubs don't offer any classes.) See whether the classes meet at convenient times. To assess whether classes are any good, ask whether you can sample a few before joining. Also, ask other members for their opinions. For more on qualities to look for in specific classes, and to read about trends in fitness classes, see Chapter 21.

Staff

If you're inexperienced, the staff is going to play an important role in your success. Ask the same questions you'd ask when hiring a personal trainer (see Chapter 20). Are the trainers in the club certified by a reputable organization? Are they experienced? Do they allow you to bring in outside trainers, or is everyone employed directly by the club? Look around: Are the staff members sitting around telling jokes to each other while some poor guy is pinned under a barbell? Is the only visible trainer updating his Facebook page at the front desk? Does anyone acknowledge your existence when you walk through the door?

Liz walked into a gym recently where the front desk person was on the phone. Not only didn't she say hello or acknowledge Liz in any way, but she actually turned her back so as not to interrupt her conversation. That does not set up a good tone for any sort of business, gyms included.

When you're taken on a tour of the club, notice whether your tour guide actually answers your questions instead of spewing fitness jargon in hopes of impressing you. Suzanne was pedaling on the recumbent bicycle at her gym when one of the sales staff came by with a prospective member. "These are the recumbent bikes," the sales guy said, to which the woman replied, "What's the difference between these bikes and the other ones?" The sales guy's response: "These are different because they're recumbent." Ideally, staff members should be able to provide a wee bit more information. (To find out what a recumbent bike actually is, see Chapter 8.)

Members

If you're new to a club, you may initially be intimidated by some of the other members. Our friend John recalls his second day at his new club: "I was in the locker room when this guy with the most perfect body — the biceps, the abs, the whole thing — walked up to the scale and weighed himself. He must have weighed an ounce over what he wanted because he went into a complete rage, punched the wall, and then walked away. I looked down at my body and thought, 'Oh, man. I'm going to be the wimpiest guy at this gym.'"

Fortunately, John didn't give up his membership. He soon found out that there are all types at his gym and that the narcissists are easy to avoid. So don't be too judgmental about the members of your gym. Sure, you may feel more comfortable at some clubs than others; some gyms cater to people over 40, and others attract bodybuilders who could open a door from the hinged side. But people are people, and most of them are nice, even if they look like underwear models. Don't give the membership factor too much weight, unless you're joining a gym primarily to socialize or you're looking for a gym with like-minded people (rock climbers, tennis players, or yogis for example).

Besides, you may be surprised by who becomes your friend. "The members I was most intimidated by ended up being just regular guys," says one friend of ours. "One guy had his head shaved except for a rat tail in the back. He looked really mean and scary, but he was a doll when you talked to him. It turned out he was a nurse."

If you're a woman and prefer to work out without men around, consider joining a Curves club. Many of the clubs are small so that they can be located in small towns and still turn a profit, but they offer a 30-minute total-fitness program in an environment that's often quite comfortable and encouraging for women, especially novices and those who are at their less-than-ideal weight. At Curves, you do a circuit that alternates strength machines with walking or jogging in place. The fixed, efficient nature of the workout appeals to many people — you don't have to create your own routine; however, others may find it constricting.

We know a woman in Missouri who joined Curves after being diagnosed with diabetes. "I used to say, 'Phooey on exercise,'" she told us. "I was just not an exercise person." But she enjoyed the company of her fellow Curves members so much that she started working out daily and within eight months had lost 50 pounds and was no longer diabetic. In general, Curves seems to work especially well for women who are intimidated by the typical health-club atmosphere.

Cleanliness

Is the place clean and well-ventilated? Pay special attention to the locker rooms: Are the bathrooms spotless, or is it foot-fungus city? Open the shower curtains and check the floor, the soap dish, and the walls for gunk and mold. If a club isn't clean, don't join — it's not worth the health risk. Ask how often the cleaning crew makes its rounds. And take a gander at the air vents to see whether they're dirty or full of mildew. Use all your senses, including your nose.

One club in Florida has banned soap, shampoo, and shaving cream in the showers to stem the tide of lawsuits filed by members who claimed to have slipped and fallen. Although we sympathize with the management, we do wonder what sort of odors emanate from the club.

Extra amenities

Competition is forcing many clubs to offer more than a Jacuzzi, towel service, and juice bar. A club may organize hikes, ski trips, and softball teams for singles. Or it may offer stress-management workshops and seminars on training for a marathon. Many clubs offer a wide variety of nonfitness programs such as cooking classes, book clubs, flower arranging seminars, and wine tastings. Often these are offered free to members and guests as a way to attract and build loyalty toward the club. We discuss some other extra amenities in the sections that follow.

Spa services

Many clubs offer a whole array of spa services. You can treat yourself to a massage, facial, mud wrap, salt scrub, aromatherapy bath, or *power shower* (a super-strong shower that we personally find a little scary). Prices for these services vary greatly, as does the quality of the services. ***Remember:*** Make sure that your massage therapist is properly licensed. (See Chapter 26 for more tips about massage.)

Programs for kids

A number of clubs have gone way beyond day care, building full-fledged kid gyms with tyke-sized weight machines and cardio equipment. The machines are obviously smaller and shorter with a host of safety devices to prevent kids from hurting themselves. This is great. It's never too early to get kids into the habit of exercising (see Chapter 23), as long as you don't force your 5-year-old into an Olympic training regimen. Some clubs offer exercise classes that the whole family can do together, as well as programs such as teen-only exercise classes. The most cleverly named of these we saw was called "Hoppy Hour."

Nutritional counseling

Another popular service is nutritional counseling, including weight-loss support groups, computerized diet analysis, and heart-disease prevention seminars. Prices vary widely, from $250 to over $1,000 for a package of three to ten sessions.

As with trainers, anyone can call himself a nutritionist, so make sure that you're dealing with a registered dietitian (someone with an RD after his name) or a certified clinical nutritionist (CCN). This lesser-known credential has stringent educational and training requirements plus a killer exam. It's just gaining wide acceptance among professionals. Most personal trainers don't have an RD, even though they may consider themselves nutritional specialists, especially if they have a "weight management certification." We don't think anyone but a registered dietitian or certified clinical nutritionist should dispense dietary advice, and that includes chiropractors — giving this kind of advice may even be against the law in your state. Don't let your "nutritionist" hard-sell you any products, including expensive supplements or prepackaged wonder foods that have been designed "especially for your body chemistry." If they offer to do a hair analysis to determine your body's mineral status, run the other way and don't look back.

Medical services

At many clubs, you can find medical and rehabilitation services, including sports-medicine doctors, chiropractors, physical therapists, acupuncturists, and sports psychologists.

Be aware that many of these health professionals may not actually be affiliated with the club; they may simply rent office space on the premises. This arrangement helps the health professionals attract more business, and it gives the club added cachet. However, you need to check out the credentials and reputations of the doctors and therapists as thoroughly as you would any others. Don't assume that the club has chosen the most-qualified health professionals; it may simply have picked those who will pay the highest rent.

Eco-friendliness

Many gyms are becoming greener these days, and if this is important to you, find out what the club's green policy is. Some gyms post their policies at the club or display them on their Web sites, but if you can't readily find the information, just ask. Green policies can include the basics, like recycling and using eco-friendly cleaning products, or they can go far beyond that.

Liz worked with one company famous for its commitment to sustainability. In building the gym, the company used sustainable flooring materials and low-fume paint, created systems for recycling water, and even had its furniture crafted from recycled materials that normally end up in landfills. When choosing exercise equipment, the company considered everything from the materials used to how the equipment needed to be shipped. Not only is the facility among the most eco-friendly in the country, it is also among the most beautiful. We wish more of the industry would make this type of commitment to the environment.

Braving the Gym for the First Time

Going to the gym for the first time can be stressful, especially if you're new to working out. But at some point, you have to take a deep breath and dive in. Being prepared helps, so in the following sections, we suggest what to pack and give you tips on making your visit as stress-free as possible. (If you're worried about breaching some kind of etiquette, see the later section "Health-Club Etiquette: The Unwritten Rules.")

Packing the perfect gym bag

You'll feel a lot more comfortable at the gym if you come prepared. Using 17 paper towels to dry yourself off after a shower is no fun, not to mention extremely eco-unfriendly. Some gyms provide towels, cosmetics, even workout clothes. Check with your gym so you don't overpack.

Here's a list of gym-bag essentials. A bag with lots of zipper pockets helps.

- ✔ Membership card, key fob, or ID (although many gyms are switching to thumb and finger identification)
- ✔ Water bottle
- ✔ Small towel to wipe sweat off the machines; consider using alcohol wipes to kill super germs
- ✔ Large towel for the shower (some gyms provide small towels for free but charge for large ones)
- ✔ Padlock for locker; many gyms now have programmable digital locks so you don't have to bring your own
- ✔ Gym clothes (shoes, socks, shorts, tights, sweats, T-shirt, sports bra or jock)
- ✔ Separate bag for wet, dirty clothes

- Toiletries (soap, shampoo, deodorant, and foot deodorant for sneakers)
- Sweat band, ponytail holder, or whatever you need to keep sweat from dripping into your eyes
- Shower sandals
- Post-workout snack, especially if you have a long drive home

These items aren't vital, but we highly recommend them:

- Weight-lifting gloves
- An iPod or MP3 player, book reader, or headphones — anything that allows you to access entertainment while you're working out
- Reading material
- Heart-rate monitor or a tracking device like an armband or shoe chip

Making yourself more comfortable

Here are strategies for feeling at ease in your gym:

- **Take a friend.** Going to the gym with a buddy can make you feel more comfortable and less self-conscious. You two can pretend to discuss the stock market while you figure out how to start up the elliptical trainer.

- **Go at off-peak hours.** This way, no one will be breathing down your neck to use a machine, and you'll have more attention from the staff if you need some reminders. Most gyms are busiest from 5:30 to 8:30 a.m., 11 a.m. to 2 p.m., and 5 to 8 p.m. (But some that cater to stay-at-home moms and retired folks are packed at 9 a.m., after school drop-off and morning coffee get-togethers.) If you can't go during off-peak hours, choose the morning, because most gyms aren't as packed as they are in the evening, and the morning crowds tend to be fairly regular. You'll get to know other faces, and they'll get to know yours.

  Monday is always the busiest day in any gym — everyone's trying to atone for sins they committed over the weekend, like eating too many chocolate snack cakes. Things trail off by Thursday or Friday (but don't wait until then to work out).

- **Don't feel embarrassed if you can't lift much weight.** Hey, you're a beginner. Besides, using only one plate on a weight machine doesn't mean you're lifting nothing. Plates weigh anywhere from 5 to 20 pounds.

- **Don't overdo it.** If you push too hard, you may feel so sore that you won't want to come back. The morning after your first few workouts, you should wake up feeling a little achy and tender but not so sore that you can't stand upright. The discomfort usually is at its worst about 48 hours after your workout, a phenomenon known as *delayed onset muscle* *soreness.* Don't be alarmed: Most people are sore after their first work-outs, even if they're careful. This is because your muscles aren't used to the extra work.

Delayed onset muscle soreness is caused by microscopic tears in the muscles that you exercise. These tears fill up with fluids and waste products, and until the muscles recover, you're going to be in a little pain. The good news is that after the muscles repair themselves, they're stronger and harder to tear. So after a few weeks of working out, you won't get really sore except after especially tough workouts.

✔ **Don't expect to master the equipment right away.** You can't learn Italian in a week, right? It takes a while to become proficient with the vocabulary, customs, and nuances of exercise as well. Even if you've spent several sessions with a trainer, you're not likely to remember how to use each and every machine. Refer to your notes or ask a member of the gym staff for help.

✔ **Make friends.** Knowing other members can give you more encourage-ment. One good way to meet someone is to ask for a spot — in other words, ask somebody to assist you while you do a weight-lifting exer-cise. Smile and look approachable. Someone may ask you to spot him. For instructions on how to spot and be spotted, see Chapter 12.

In general, when you talk to people at the gym, stick to topics related to working out. Ask whether they're done using a particular machine or bench. Ask how to do a certain exercise. The worst approach is to go up to people in the locker room when they're naked, stick your hand out, and introduce yourself.

✔ **Don't worry about people staring at you.** Most people are far too absorbed in their own workout to pay attention to anyone else — or they're just as self-conscious as you are and are praying you aren't being overly critical of them. But if you really want to block out your fellow gym members, wear headphones or ear buds; you don't even need to turn them on. Just make sure the wires don't get caught in any weight machines.

✔ **Wear comfortable clothes.** Go for maximum comfort and minimum embarrassment, but don't wear anything so baggy that it impedes your movement or can possibly get caught in some moving part. Don't wear something that exposes you to the world when you climb on some strange contraption. You may end up spreading your legs in front of 30 strangers, none of whom is your gynecologist or proctologist.

✔ **Ask for help if you need it.** Liz knew a guy who was pretty proud of him-self for finally making it to the gym. He got through his first workout only to slice his Achilles tendon on the shower door. He lay there in agony for quite a while before calling for help because he was so embarrassed, not to mention naked. The injury required six stitches, and the guy hobbled around on crutches for six weeks. It took several weeks after that for the staff to coax him back to the gym. He finally returned, although he now takes his showers at home.

Health-Club Etiquette: The Unwritten Rules

Every type of club has its own customs, like the secret handshake you and your buddies used back in fourth grade. Health clubs don't have secret code words, of course, but you may feel more at home if you know a few of the unwritten rules.

The must-do's

Here are some tips on how to act in certain situations at the health club:

- ✔ **If someone's using the weight machine that you want:** Ask whether you can *work in.* That's a term for alternating sets with another person. Asking to work in is perfectly legitimate; no one has the right to camp out at one weight machine for a half-hour or hog three machines simultaneously.

    Working in with someone is convenient if all you have to do is switch the pin in the weight stack. But it's awkward if you have to readjust the seat or add or subtract weight plates. In those cases, waiting until the person is done is a better choice.

- ✔ **If someone is standing over your shoulder waiting to use the machine that you're on:** Kindly ask that person to work in with you. Or tell the person how much longer you plan to use the machine. Say something like, "This is my last set. Then it's all yours." Many facilities have time limits for the cardio equipment; even if they don't, try not to hog a piece if there's obviously a crowd milling about waiting for a treadmill.

- ✔ **If you need help adjusting a machine or you forget how to use it:** Turn to a staffer or a gym member with a kind face and say, "I'm new here. Can you help me?"

- ✔ **If someone's doing an exercise that you want to learn:** Find an appropriate break in that person's workout and ask him to show you the exercise. Most people are happy to help — in fact, they'll probably be flattered that you asked.

- ✔ **If you're done with a piece of equipment:** Wipe off all your sweat so the next person doesn't slide off or become overly familiar with your bodily fluids. Don't be afraid to politely ask the person before you to wipe down as well, on the off chance he forgets.

- ✔ **If you aren't 100 percent sure that you can safely complete your repetitions:** Ask someone to spot you.

Suzanne used to work out at a gym that featured a photo of a guy who lost control while doing a squat (an exercise we explain in Chapter 13). He dumped his barbell forward, and the barbell landed on the weight rack — with the guy's neck sandwiched in between. Fortunately, his two spotters came to the rescue, and he survived unscathed. Chances are this isn't going to happen to you; after all, the guy was squatting 992 pounds. But the point is to be careful out there.

✔ **If someone's hitting on you and the feeling isn't mutual:** Heck, we don't know. You're on your own here.

Major no-no's

Most of the following rules are common sense, but they're violated so frequently that we feel compelled to mention them.

✔ **Don't forget your towel.** No one likes to sit down in a pool of sweat. Always wipe off your equipment after you finish.

✔ **Don't fill up your entire water bottle when someone else is waiting for the drinking fountain.** Let the other guy get his drink and then resume filling up your bottle.

✔ **Don't leave your dumbbells on the floor.** Always put weights back on the rack and in the right order. Don't stick the 15-pound dumbbells where the 10-pounders are supposed to go.

✔ **Don't leave barbells or machines loaded up with weight plates.** You can't assume the next person can or wants to lift the exact same weight you just lifted. Some men leave the bench press loaded up with a 45-pound plate on each side of the 45-pound bar — as if the minimum any human being would bench-press would be 135 pounds. If you see someone do this, you have every right to ask him to remove the weights.

✔ **Don't sit on a machine or bench that you're not actually using.** Between sets, allow others to work in. And don't block the aisles between machines, either.

✔ **Don't drop your weights from 3 feet in the air.** Always place them gently on the ground so as not to simulate an earthquake or crush someone's toes.

Now and again, Liz sees a guy who performs a bizarre lift: He sets a very heavy dumbbell on the floor, bends over with locked knees, and snatches the barbell into the air while screaming at the top of his lungs. When the dumbbell is above his head, he lets go of the weight. Needless to say, this is very dangerous and distracting behavior.

- ✔ **Don't interrupt a staff member who is obviously helping or spotting someone else.** You'd want the trainer's full attention if you were the one being helped.

- ✔ **Don't violate anyone else's personal space.** If someone seems to be jamming through a workout, that's not the time to tap him on the shoulder and ask his opinion on school prayer. This rule applies to the locker room, too.

- ✔ **Don't "borrow" a gym's equipment for use at home.** Nothing is more aggravating to gym members than looking for a jump rope or weight collar that has mysteriously disappeared.

- ✔ **Don't hog the cardio machines if you've exceeded the posted time limit.** We've seen people surreptitiously cover the console with a towel while they reprogram the machine, hoping that other people won't notice their time is up. That's rude.

Locker-room rules

The stories we could tell about bathroom misbehavior could fill an entire book. We've seen a guy get naked and blow-dry his private parts. We've seen people cut themselves shaving and leave a pool of blood for the next person who comes to the sink. We've seen people mistake the shower for a restroom.

Remember that you're sharing this space with a lot of other people, so have some consideration! Here are a few rules that should be obvious but, based on our experience, seem to bear mentioning anyway:

- ✔ Don't take a marathon shower if people are waiting. Don't leave hair clogging the drain, and don't leave empty shampoo bottles in the stall.

- ✔ Don't use more than one locker or leave things in a locker overnight if your gym has a policy against it.

- ✔ Don't hog the mirror or the blow-dryer.

- ✔ Don't shake baby powder all over the floor.

- ✔ Throw your garbage in those cylindrical and rectangular objects known as trash cans. Would you really just toss your empty pantyhose package on the floor if you were at home? Okay, even so, don't do it at the gym.

- ✔ Limit the number of towels you use, especially during busy hours, when the club is likely to run out. Liz supervised at a gym where one guy would use up to a dozen towels per session, leaving a shortage for everyone who came in after him.

Chapter 19

Designing Your Home Gym

Some celebrities spend as much on their home gyms as many other people spend on their homes, but don't get the wrong idea. A home gym doesn't have to be a palace with high ceilings, racks of shiny weights, and space-age machinery in order to house really effective workout equipment. A complete home gym can consist of a rubber tube, a step, a ball, and a few DVDs — equipment that a student on a budget can fit into a small apartment.

In fact, in our cost-conscious climate, home fitness equipment is plenty popular, as many people view a one-time equipment purchase as a better deal than paying monthly gym dues. Besides the economics, you can't beat the commute to your living room, and you can work out at 3 a.m. on Sunday while stark naked if you really want to. You won't encounter hidden fees, $5 bottles of water at the snack bar, or wannabe bodybuilders admiring themselves in the mirrors (well, unless you happen to live with one). Plus, you don't have to wait in line for the shower or deal with any unidentified biological matter that doesn't contain your own DNA.

Yet, despite all the convenience, home exercisers have a high dropout rate. The novelty wears off, the bike breaks down, or the 5-pound dumbbell gets used as a doorstop. You can avoid this scenario and the accompanying guilt by designing your home gym carefully. This chapter shows you how.

Planning Your Exercise Space

The inspiration to exercise may have come to you suddenly, but don't make any rash decisions when you buy equipment. The last thing you want to do is give your credit card a workout based on dubious claims about what some piece of plastic attached to some springs can do for your body. You can save yourself time, aggravation, and money by putting thought into your purchases. Before you even set foot in a fitness store, visit a fitness-equipment seller's Web site, or speed dial Home Shopping Network, size up your goals, your budget, and your available space. Here are some specifics to consider before you go shopping.

Looking at the big picture: What you want to work on

Think seriously about your goals, and consider what type of equipment you need to succeed in the four areas of fitness: aerobic fitness, strength, flexibility, and balance. Don't just say, "I'll start with an elliptical trainer, and maybe eventually I'll buy some weights." If you plan to get your cardio exercise outdoors — walking, jogging, or skating, for example — then, sure, spend your entire home-gym budget on strength equipment. Just make sure you have a cardio plan for the winter. Flexibility and balance gadgets aren't essential, but most are so inexpensive and take up so little space that we think they're worth the investment.

Choosing an inviting spot for your equipment

Where you park your exercise bike can make all the difference between using it to get fit and simply using it as an extra chair for your Academy Awards parties. Here are some tips on choosing a spot for your exercise equipment:

- ✔ **Entertainment:** Put your equipment near entertaining distractions such as the TV or your MP3 docking station (or away from them, if you want to be away from other family members).

- ✔ **Comfort:** Make sure your workout spot has adequate ventilation, space, lighting, and climate control; there's a reason that only spiders hang out in cold, damp basement corners.

> ✔ **Convenience and visibility:** If you're lucky enough to have a spare
> room, consider reserving it exclusively for your gym. If you don't have
> an extra room, at least try to keep all your gadgets and equipment near
> one another. Don't store your dumbbells in the bedroom, your treadmill
> in the basement, and your stretching mat in the coat closet. Also, plan to
> keep your equipment within reach. You don't want to hunt through ten
> drawers to find your favorite exercise DVD. And chances are anything
> you store under your bed will stay there — permanently.

Consider installing a mirror, preferably in the area where you plan to lift
weights. A mirror enables you to keep an eye on your form so you know you're
doing everything right.

Taking careful measurements

Before you buy a major piece of equipment, carefully measure the length,
width, and height of your available space. You don't want your dumbbells
smashing that new mirror when you raise your arms out to the side. You
don't want to bump your head against the ceiling when you press the incline
button on your new treadmill. Keep in mind that many equipment stores
have high ceilings to accommodate tall equipment.

Measure your door to make sure that you can get your new machinery into
the house. Liz ruined a brand-new stationary bicycle when she pounded on
the handles with a rubber mallet in an attempt to squeeze the bike through
a doorway that was too narrow. One of the handles broke off, which served
her right.

Thinking about flooring

Avoid tile or cement floors for your exercise space. If you use exercise DVDs
or iPod or on-demand workouts, place your DVD player in a room with carpeting. The extra padding provided by carpeting helps protect your joints when
you jump up and down or step on and off equipment. Plus, there's less danger
of slipping. Don't pump iron on a tile floor, either. If you drop a weight, you'll
crack the tile.

If you have the luxury of an extra room just for your home gym (and lots of
money to spare), consider a rubberized floor. They can run as high as $3,000.
A cheaper solution is a series of strategically placed thick mats, which will
run you only a few hundred dollars and can double as a stretching area. If
you're creating an exercise room from scratch, an eco-friendly and durable
flooring option is Marmoleum, a natural product made from renewable
resources, including wood flour, tree rosins, and linseed oil.

Whatever type of floor you have, we recommend putting rubberized mats ($50 to $100) underneath your cardiovascular equipment. This reduces vibration and keeps your floor from getting stained by your sweat and the globs of oil and other junk that inevitably drip from the underside of a treadmill or other equipment. If you choose rubberized flooring, you can skip the mats.

Equipment Shopping Tips

After you select and measure your space, you're ready to shop. The following tips apply to home equipment in general. Check out the sections "Investing in Cardio Equipment" and "Buying Strength Equipment" for suggestions that are specific to cardio equipment and strength machines.

Shopping around

Prices vary widely, so by all means, bargain-hunt. But remember: A machine isn't a bargain if it collapses with you on it or gives you a hernia. Here are some sources to check out:

- **Stores:** For fancy equipment with lots of moving parts — treadmills, elliptical trainers, rowers, weight machines, and the like — stick with exercise equipment specialty stores. They tend to sell sturdier, more reliable, and better-designed machines. For simpler equipment like dumbbells, ankle weights, steps, and jump ropes, department stores, sporting goods stores, and online ordering are fine. In fact, even small dealers now offer online ordering.

- **Manufacturers:** If you know the exact make and model you want, you may save money by calling the manufacturer directly. Some manufacturers let you buy direct — in fact, some may require you to buy direct — and others refer you to a local dealer. But do your homework. Sometimes you can get a better deal from the manufacturer. Other times, going through the dealer is cheaper. You can often save a couple hundred bucks by making a few phone calls or surfing the Web.

- **Online (and television) retailers:** Now that mainstream manufacturers have set up large retail Web sites, clicking on the shopping basket is less risky, even on big-ticket items such as treadmills and bikes. However, you do need to be extra careful when buying exercise equipment off TV or the Internet. The picture and real-time video may look fabulous, but when the gizmo arrives at your doorstep, it may be a useless plastic piece of junk.

Buy from the Internet only after you research the product, know exactly which make and model you want, and know that the online dealer is reputable. Reputable dealers are typically larger, nationally established brands and are sometimes associated with brick-and-mortar retail shops. Gym Source (www.gymsource.com) is a good example of an extensive online store with multiple, nationwide locations; it sells high-quality equipment and has an excellent reputation.

✔ **People offering used equipment:** Buying used equipment at a garage sale or on eBay or Craigslist is fine if you stick to gadgets without motors or complicated designs. Freecycle (www.freecycle.org), where people post items they're giving away rather than selling, is another good place to look for free weights and other basic, nonmotorized equipment. We also think buying higher-end equipment used is okay if you go through an authorized dealer that gives you a warranty. *Tip:* No matter what type of used equipment you buy or whom you buy from, ask for a trial period and get all the instruction manuals.

✔ **Trainers:** A knowledgeable trainer can save you a lot of research time and may be able to help you purchase equipment. Trainers often get discounts from equipment dealers because they recommend and buy equipment on a regular basis. But ask your trainer whether he receives a commission from the dealer or whether he'll be charging you a commission; this may eat away at any potential savings. In other cases, a dealer may give you a discount on top of the trainer's commission.

Taking a test drive

You wouldn't buy a car without taking it for a spin. The same rule applies to exercise machines. Be sure to test every feature. Pull every handle and push every bar. Make sure that a stationary bike pedals smoothly at several tension levels. Try a treadmill on the flat setting and on the incline setting. If the salesperson won't let you give the machine a whirl, say adios.

We realize that following this rule gets tricky if you shop for your equipment on the Internet. As tempting as it is to order your home gym equipment with the click of a mouse, we still recommend going to a store or trying a friend's before you buy. If you have absolutely no way of taking a test drive, at the very least read the reviews from consumer-advocate sources such as *Consumer Reports* or on the various exercise equipment review Web sites. One caveat: Glowing reviews are sometimes planted by the sellers themselves. Review the return policy and costs very carefully before you click on "check out."

Looking for safety features

We highly recommend buying equipment with safety features, especially if you have children. For example, to start some treadmills, you must punch in a code or use a special magnet attached to a string that you wrap around your waist or finger. If you happen to fall, the magnet breaks the connection with the treadmill, and the machine automatically shuts off.

Keeping your kids away from the equipment, whether it's in use or not, is really important. Some of the very features intended to ensure safety can have deadly consequences in the wrong circumstances. For example, children have been killed when treadmill safety cords became wrapped around their necks.

Asking for a discount

High-tech cardio machines and strength machines tend to be marked up about 40 percent above wholesale, so your salesperson probably has some leeway. Asking for a 10 percent discount is perfectly appropriate. You may not get it, but it never hurts to ask. Also, if you're buying several items, ask the salesperson to throw in a complimentary accessory, such as a rubber floor mat to place underneath your equipment. Depending on the square footage, a mat can cost $50 to $200. Some stores will cut your mat to size.

Also ask about interest-free payment plans. They can make a big-ticket purchase a lot more affordable if you don't happen to have wads of cash stuffed in your savings account. Just remember to mark that one-year date on your calendar; if you pay it off even one minute late, suddenly your treadmill may cost more than your minivan did.

Checking out warranty and service plans

If you're choosing between two similar machines, take the one with the better warranty, even if it costs a bit more. Both cardio and weight machines should have at least a minimum one-year warranty on all parts. Find out who's responsible for repairs and maintenance: A good warranty is worthless if no one within 3,000 miles can fix the darn thing. Extended warranties usually aren't worth it, though.

If you buy a machine from an equipment specialty store, chances are someone from the store will come to your house and fix it. When the elliptical trainer in Suzanne's basement started screeching like a car with 20-year-old brake pads, Suzanne was pleased to discover that the machine was still under warranty, even though it was three years old. A friendly repairman showed up pronto and replaced several parts at no cost. Now Suzanne doesn't have to blast the volume on her TV to drown out the squeaking.

Some equipment manufacturers have repair personnel on call throughout the country. If you buy from a discount sporting goods store or a TV offer or over the Internet, you may be out of luck — but maybe not. In response to consumer complaints, some of the larger online sellers have set up extensive repair networks.

Investing in Cardio Equipment

Home cardiovascular machines have gotten pretty fancy, and the array of choices can be mind-blowing. Should you go with the elliptical trainer? The rower? The elliptical-rower? The elliptical-rower–stair-climber–treadmill–automatic slicer–microwave oven?

Actually, although the choices are many, we're pleased to report that your chances of buying a high-quality machine are better than ever. Since the first edition of this book was published in 1996, the frenzy to market gimmicky cardio machines — riders, gliders, and such — has slowed markedly. (Infomercial producers and home shopping networks seem to have switched from hawking schlocky cardio contraptions to hawking schlocky toning gadgets and bogus weight-loss supplements.)

Which type of home cardio machine is the best? Our answer hasn't changed: The best machine is the one you'll use. That's why testing several machines before you bring one home is so important. You don't want to end up with a space-eating, dust-collecting monster that you can't wait to unload in your next garage sale. This chapter helps you sort through the different options. After you buy your equipment, read Chapter 8, which describes how to use good form on each type of cardio machine. Also, as we explain in Chapters 8 and 9, you don't need fancy or expensive equipment to get in shape.

Two cardiovascular bargains

Yes, you can improve your stamina with equipment that costs less than $100 — even less than $50. Here are two dirt-cheap yet very effective aerobic conditioning gadgets.

A step

Though essentially nothing more than a glorified milk crate, a step can whip you into shape. Most steps are rectangular, hard plastic platforms; some are springy wood. Good steps have some sort of rubber covering on the top to prevent your feet from slipping. Look for Lego-type inserts called *risers* that snap on underneath to increase the height of the step. Reebok and The Step Company make sturdy steps. Steps are typically under $100.

A jump rope

Jump ropes may remind you of pony-tailed little girls in schoolyards, but don't be fooled: Skipping rope offers some very real, very adult fitness benefits. It strengthens your cardiovascular system, improves your agility, burns up to 15 calories per minute, and tones your thighs, calves, abdominals, back, chest, and shoulders. You can take your rope with you anywhere, and using it doesn't require any more space than a small coffee table takes up.

Many ropes are now made of tough, molded plastic; metal wire coated in acrylic; or space-age polymers with names we can't pronounce, let alone spell. These materials make for ropes that turn faster and more smoothly. Look for features like soft foam or rubber handles, which prevent callusing, and ball-bearing-like swivel action between the cord and handles.

You can get a perfectly good jump rope at a sporting goods store or department store for as little as $2, although you may want to spend $40 to $50 for the fancy features. To size your rope correctly, stand on the center of the cord and pull the ends straight up along your sides. The handles should just reach your armpits.

Use a light rope if your aim is to work on skill and agility and to jump fast. Fat, weighted ropes (¼ to ½ pound) work well for building upper-body muscular endurance, but using them for fancy footwork or special tricks is a bit like asking a Clydesdale to run the Kentucky Derby. Buy one of each, and you can mix up your workouts. With weighted ropes, the weight should be in the cord, not the handles; otherwise, you just wind up with very sore, tired wrists.

If you're the type who gets motivated by knowing your numbers, you may like ropes with small computerized counters attached to or built into the handles; these gizmos count your jumps, track time, and estimate calorie burn. We've also tried a computerized ropeless "rope." You simply jump and the handles spin around as if the line were invisible. We felt pretty silly and couldn't help feeling this "rope" was missing the point. To us, half the benefit of jump roping comes from learning the coordination skills of jumping over the rope. We prefer to "skip" this trend, so to speak.

When you jump, keep your arms relaxed and slightly bent, and keep your upper-body movements to a minimum. Instead of turning your arms in big circles, simply let your wrists swivel slightly. (This is especially important when using a heavy rope; otherwise, you're in for sore shoulders.) Start with a few short sets — about 30 jumps for a light rope, 5 to 10 turns for a heavy rope. Rest by marching in place between sets. Gradually increase the number of sets and jumps per set while decreasing the time you spend marching. Eventually, you'll be able to jump 10 minutes or more continuously (probably less with a heavy rope). Humming the theme song from *Rocky* helps. Building up to long periods of jumping rope is tough, because it's a very intense activity. Jumping rope is best used as a cross-training workout or between strength-training exercises while circuit training (explained in Chapter 13).

Treadmills

Treadmill prices have dropped considerably in the past few years, while the quality of some lower-priced models has improved. You can now buy a decent treadmill for under $1,000. These models work in a household with one or two lightweight walkers who use it several times a week. However, if you have even one person who runs at least 5 miles more than three days a week in your home, you probably need to spend closer to $3,000 for a more substantial model, which usually has more bells and whistles. And if you weigh more than 150 pounds or are a real clomper, you also need something in this higher-end range. (Liz, though on the light side, pounds the treadmill like a team of horses; she opted for a super sturdy mill at home.)

Important treadmill features

Treadmills used to be large, noisy, cumbersome contraptions. Now most of them are smooth, streamlined, and relatively quiet, though they're still not going to fit in any non-celebrity's closet. (That said, there are a couple of decent foldable ones.) We do recommend thoroughly inspecting any treadmill before you buy it, so here's what to look for:

- ✔ **A motor to move the walking belt:** Make sure that the belt moves fluidly.

  We think that self-powered treadmills, the ones without motors, are a waste of money. You typically can't get the walking belt moving unless you incline the machine, but that makes the exercise too challenging for many beginners. Running on these treadmills is impossible — you need an even steeper incline, and the belt tends to stick.

- ✔ **Safety features:** Don't look twice at any model that doesn't have an emergency stop button and an automatic slow-start speed. A front hand rail is helpful for maintaining balance and is probably safer than side rails, which may actually disrupt your balance if they impede your arm swing.

  If you have young children, choose a machine that requires a security code or special magnet to make it go. We like the magnet feature for adults, too: If you lose your balance, a magnet that's connected to the treadmill's console pulls off the display panel, causing the machine to automatically shut off.

- ✔ **Feedback:** Your machine should display the time, distance, speed, and calories burned. Many treadmills also come with a set of preprogrammed workouts and a heart-monitor hookup. (If the heart-rate monitor isn't built into the handrails, you can wear a chest monitor, and your heart rate will appear on the display screen.) You may be able to find a treadmill display with motivating graphics of people exercising at your pace. Many treadmills now also have USB ports or some other method of downloading workouts into the treadmill and, conversely, uploading your workout information out of the treadmill and into a program that slices and dices your information.

✔ **An incline capability:** Walking uphill adds intensity and variety to your workouts. With most machines, you either turn a crank or press a button to simulate hills.

Beware of treadmills that create an incline with hydraulic pistons. These models, often found in department stores, are not likely to support your weight through continued use and tend to break easily and often. If you look at the front of the treadmill on either side and see a metal bar that resembles a bicycle pump (that's the hydraulic piston you're looking at), pass on the machine.

✔ **Entertainment:** Given the entertainment options available on home treadmills nowadays, you'd be hard pressed to use boredom as an excuse not to exercise. Many reasonably priced models have consoles with flat-screen televisions, audio ports and high-end speakers, wireless Internet connectivity, iPod docking stations, and special downloadable and uploadable workout cards. You may want to avoid the built-in TV and opt to mount your TV on the wall or directly onto the machine using a special bracket. With some models you have no choice but to take the built-in screen, which typically can be popped out and replaced if it goes bust. But you may wait a few days for the repairperson to show up.

Our favorite treadmills

NordicTrack and Icon used to be bottom-of-the-barrel brands, but both companies now make treadmills starting in the $1,000 range that are worth considering. These companies seem to be leading the home "exertainment" revolution, offering more choices for built-in entertainment than most other manufacturers. We also like True, Star Trac, Precor, Life Fitness, and Cybex, brands that are popular in commercial gyms, too. Their models are significantly pricier but are well-built, have great warranties, and hold up well even with high usage.

Incline trainers

Incline trainers are a new breed of treadmill with a slightly wider belt than a traditional treadmill. Most of the models only go up to 5 or 6 mph, but they have monster motors that allow them to incline up to 40 degrees, which makes you feel like you are trudging up the Himalayas. The manufacturers claim that compared to walking on a flat setting, exercising on an incline trainer burns three to five times the number of calories. Although many of the studies have been done by the manufacturers themselves, we tend to believe the claims based on other well-established information regarding hill climbing in general.

We like these machines for people who want a tough workout but don't do well with the pounding and grinding on their joints brought on by high-impact workouts such as running. If you're training for hiking or for a walk or run in a very hilly area, if you're focused on toning your butt and thighs, or if you just want to burn lots of calories, an incline trainer is a good tool. However, if you're a serious runner or aim to be one, this machine isn't for you. Also, if you don't have good uphill walking form or your joints aren't compatible with uphill walking, these machines may overstress your knees, ankles, or lower back.

These machines tend to have a smaller footprint than many conventional treadmills. So they're good for spaces that are short on, well, space. This is because you swing your arms as you march upward, but you don't need as much room to spread out your stride because these machines aren't intended for faster running paces. Brands we like are Icon, Bowflex, and NordicTrack. They have a lot of the fun extras, such as an insertable workout DVD and downloadable and uploadable workout port. They're also surprisingly sturdy for the money. They start as low as $1,000 and run up to $4,000.

Elliptical trainers

Part stair-climber, part treadmill, part stationary cycle, *elliptical trainers* are still one of the hottest trends in cardio machines. Your legs travel in an elongated circular movement, and on some models, you pump poles back and forth for an upper-body workout. On other models, you place your feet in two basket-like pedals and swing your legs in a wide arc back and forth. On the best models, you feel like you're doing a sort of rhythmic glide; on the worst, you feel like you're stumbling downhill on your tiptoes or you're deliberately ripping your hips out of their sockets.

Many of the home elliptical trainers, especially those under $500, aren't as smooth or as comfortable as the more expensive gym-quality models. Home units tend to have a stride length that's too short, too deep, too choppy, or a combination of all three problems. And many of them are so flimsy that we were able to loosen the bolts from the frame and rock them from side to side while taking a test run. This doesn't bode well for durability. Many home elliptical trainers with arm poles are useless because they offer no resistance at all.

However, we do recommend a few brands, especially Icon and NordicTrack. NordicTrack, in particular, offers a high-quality home elliptical with a surprising number of fancy options, such as TV screens and built-in fans. The company even offers a self-powered elliptical that requires no electricity, so you can feel good about exercising your body without harming the earth. (You still have to factor in manufacturing pollution and energy use.) Many of its models come in at under $1,000. Check out www.nordictrack.com on a regular basis, because the company often runs sales on all its equipment, but its elliptical in particular. For higher-end models, in the $1,500 to $2,000 range, we like Precor elliptical, which is the original and still the best.

Stationary bikes

Stationary biking is a no-brainer: Park your butt on the seat, plant your feet on the pedals, and away you go, so to speak. You can spend up to $4,000 on a fully-loaded, high-tech super cycle — or $400 for a sturdy, no-frills workhorse. Just keep in mind that every cool feature you opt for jacks up the price.

Before you buy, test-drive upright, recumbent, and studio bikes:

- ✔ **Upright:** Upright bikes are the original stationary bikes. Many people prefer to sit upright as they ride, and you do get a slightly greater calorie burn in this position compared to recumbent bikes when riding at the same perceived intensity level.

- ✔ **Recumbent:** Recumbents provide back support, a feature you may appreciate if you have lower-back discomfort or a spare tire. On a recumbent bike you pedal straight out in front of you; this position targets your butt and rear thigh muscles at a different angle than upright bikes.

- ✔ **Studio:** Studio bikes, more commonly called Spin bikes, have a weighted flywheel in the front and a saddle and pedal position that allows these bikes to imitate the feel of an outdoor bicycle. When you tighten the resistance knob directly in front of the saddle, you feel as if you're grinding up a steep hill. Spin-style bikes are made of stronger steel than other stationary bikes and are built for the rider to come out of the saddle (partially stand) and pump down hard on the pedals. These bikes aren't computerized, but many models now have small feedback monitors to provide information and motivation.

Whichever style you prefer, don't buy a bike from a department store, because quality isn't normally a big consideration in the designs of these products. Some cheap bike seats have been known to collapse with a rider mid-workout. You don't want to know where the seat pole winds up. Besides, specialty stores carry plenty of inexpensive models, and you can get decent models from the Internet, especially from the sites of large dealers and well-established manufacturers.

Important bike features

Two stationary bikes that look similar may feel very different to your derriere and offer different electronic options. So test-ride every bike and do a thorough check of the features:

- ✔ **A comfortable, sturdy seat:** Whatever seat you prefer, it should lock securely into place. Some people like a seat that's hard and narrow; others prefer one that's wider and softer. Don't assume that a wide, cushy seat is going to be more comfortable. Extra padding under your rear end is nice to have when you watch TV, but when you exercise, the extra surface area can cause chafing and discomfort.

   Some people's butts don't match up with any cycle seat (Liz is one of these people), in which case placing a gel pad on top of the seat may help. A pad costs about $40. You may have to test out a few different gel seats to find one that you feel is tush-compatible. Suzanne finds that wearing padded cycling shorts makes any bike seat more comfortable.

- ✔ **Seat and handlebar adjustments:** Make sure that when you sit on the seat, your leg is almost straight at the bottom of the pedal stroke. The handlebars and width of the pedal straps should be adjustable, too. (For details about stationary-bike adjustments, see Chapter 8.)

- ✔ **Feedback:** You can pay extra for fun features such as preset workout programs, a heart-rate monitor, and games that let you race against the computer. But at the very least, your bike should have a speedometer that displays revolutions per minute (rpm) and miles per hour (mph), an odometer to measure distance, and a timer to keep track of those minutes as they fly by. Even some Spin bikes now offer a small feedback monitor.

- ✔ **A way to indicate the level of difficulty:** Look for a knob or button that indicates resistance levels, such as 1 through 12. This way you can accurately measure every workout and track your progress. If 10 minutes on Level 1 used to wear you out but now you can breeze through 20 minutes on Level 3, you know you've come a long way. Because Spin bikes aren't computerized, they don't allow for such flashy or precise measuring, although some models have hash marks or numbers on the knob so that you can reproduce the same amount of resistance from one workout to the next. This is a helpful feature. Many use heart-rate monitoring features to track intensity levels.

Our favorite bike brands

Here's a brief list of our favorites, but be sure to test-ride any model you're considering to make sure it's comfortable for you:

- ✔ **Non-computerized uprights, or "ergometers" ($1,000 or more):** Monarch and Bodyguard

- ✔ **Computerized uprights ($900–$4,000):** LifeCycle, Cybex, Precor, NordicTrack, Icon, Star Trac, and CatEye

- ✔ **Computerized recumbents ($100–$3,000):** Precor, Life Fitness, NordicTrack, Icon, Star Trac and LifeCycle

- ✔ **Spinning-type uprights ($600–$2,000):** Star Trac ($900–$1,700), Spinner ($600–$1,500), LeMond ($1300– $2,000), and Reebok ($700–$1,500)

Rowing machines

The best breed of rowing machine has a chain or cable that wraps around a flywheel. The chain is attached to a handle that you pull in a smooth movement toward your chest as you straighten your legs and slide the seat backward. These new rowers do a much better job of capturing the feel of rowing on the water.

Forget the rowers with two arms that you pull toward you as you slide the seat backward. You can never get the tension in the arms quite even, and the entire rowing movement feels sticky and unnatural. If you already have one of these, we're betting it's the most expensive coat hanger you own.

Concept2 (www.concept2.com) makes an excellent rower that's available through dealers around the country and directly through the company. This machine is so good that the U.S. Olympic Rowing Team trains on it during the off-season. And being under $1,000, it gets a best-buy rating from us. Among all the categories and brands of equipment, Concept2 has held its dominance possibly longer than any other. And the machine continues to improve. Compared to earlier models, it now folds more easily, breaks down less often, rows more quietly, and provides better feedback. We don't know of any other standout rowing machine.

Stair-climbers

Stair-climbers, also called *steppers,* have two foot plates that you pump up and down to mimic the action of climbing stairs. These machines usually have front or side rails that you hold onto for balance. Their consoles display time, distance, steps per minute (spm), number of flights climbed, and calories burned. Stair-climbers used to be much more popular, but they've all but faded from the workout scene since elliptical trainers came into fashion. However, some people still like home steppers because when done right, they offer an intense workout.

Most steppers have an *independent action;* that is, the movement of one pedal is not affected by the other. With dependent models, the act of straightening one leg to lower the step causes the other pedal to rise. This isn't just a technical detail: Usually, you like the feel of one and hate the other.

Almost all steppers in the $200 to $1,200 range use hydraulic pistons or air pressure to power the pedals. These cheaper steppers are nowhere near as smooth as the stair machines people line up for at the gym. Some people don't mind the way they feel, but do stay away from the $200 models, and look for one that doesn't wobble from side to side as you climb. Precor, Star Trac and Cybex make decent ones in the $1,000 to $5,000 end of the price scale; you pay for near-institutional quality design and build.

The basics of buying TV fitness gadgets

In general, try to avoid buying fitness products from TV. Though we admit that we've seen a few good products, including exercise DVDs, advertised in infomercials, TV offers no way to judge the quality of a machine, pill, or gadget. Here are some tips to keep in mind as you watch fitness product advertising:

✔ Don't be suckered by the infomercial audience or "real people" offering testimonials. Those wholesome folks who whip themselves into a frenzy at the mere mention of the product at hand are usually paid. Ditto for celebrity endorsements. Athletes and celebs know that fame can be short-lived, and at some point their name may be their only asset. "There's a lot you can talk yourself into," one athlete told us. "You figure, I've gotta make a living. If the public's dumb enough to buy this stuff, that's their problem." Beware, too, of health and fitness "experts" with fancy titles they may have invented.

✔ Beware of the phrase "guaranteed or your money back." Read the fine print: The manufacturers may promise that you'll lose 4 inches in one month — if you stick to a low-fat diet and a far more extensive exercise program.

✔ Don't be impressed by references to Europe, ancient China, or 3,000-year-old secrets. Bogus fitness products use European research much the same way that "reality" TV shows use Peruvian religious miracles as examples of amazing phenomena: They're too far away for the average person to check out carefully.

✔ Beware of phrases like "three easy payments," and watch shipping costs. One gadget claims to cost "Not $60! Not $50!" but "just two easy payments of $19.95." Add in exorbitant (and nonrefundable) shipping and handling costs, and it costs $66.85.

✔ Don't be awed by the fact that a product was "awarded a U.S. patent." You could patent a nose-hair clipper for mice if you wanted to. To get a patent, you need to have an original idea or process, not necessarily a good one.

✔ Beware of the term "proven." Many companies cite scientific research without telling you where the studies were conducted.

✔ Hide your credit card between midnight and 4 a.m. At that hour, everything kinda looks good. Go to bed. If you're tempted to buy an infomercial product, jot down the number and wait before ordering.

Buying Strength Equipment

There's no shortage of great gadgets to help you build your muscles at home. There's also, regrettably, no shortage of junk. This chapter covers all your legitimate strength-training options — from $3 rubber tubes to sophisticated, gym-quality machinery. We introduce you to some innovative new products and help you decide which type of equipment is best for your home and your budget.

If you're going to lift weights at home, read Chapters 11 through 13. In those chapters, we explain how to use all types of strength equipment and how to design a strength-training program that'll get you results.

Just as a $3,000 machine isn't needed to put one foot in front of the other and raise your heart rate, neither is a fancy piece of equipment a requirement for strengthening and toning your muscles. However, it can be fun and inspiring to have something shiny and steel or rubber or plastic to push against or pull to help you build strength. If you'd rather rely on body resistance to strengthen up, we offer plenty of effective suggestions in Chapters 12 and 13. If, however, you like a piece of equipment or a gadget, here you go.

Exercise bands and tubes

Rubber bands and tubes are the absolute cheapest way to strengthen your muscles — you can buy three or four bands for $15 or $20. They're also extremely versatile and great for traveling. Even if you own weight machines or an extensive set of free weights, we recommend throwing in a few bands for variety. (Just know that bands and tubes have their limitations, which we explain in Chapter 12.)

Bands are flat latex strips about 6 inches wide and about 3 feet long; you hold onto each end or tie the ends around something sturdy, like the leg of your sofa. Tubes come in a variety of sizes and are shaped like very flexible garden hoses, usually with plastic or rubber handles attached. You'll probably like bands for some exercises and tubes for others; you just have to experiment. Because bands and tubes are so inexpensive, it pays to get a variety.

For a few dollars more, you can buy bands or tubes with plastic or rubber handles — a real plus for getting a firm grip on an exercise. Some bands or tubes have built-in ankle and thigh straps. SPRI, Gaiam, and Lifeline make nifty band kits that come with a travel bag and several door and bar attachments, priced from $30 to $60. They also make platforms for less than $200 that allow you to attach the band in a variety of positions and heights. Dyna-Band also makes quality bands.

Because some bands don't come with instructions, we recommend buying a couple of DVDs with band workouts. The following series and instructors are just a few that offer excellent band workouts: *10 Minute Solutions, Exhale: Core Fusion,* Tamilee Webb, and Cathe Friedrich. You can also find a ton of free demos on YouTube and the other social media video sites, though you do need to be careful about the hit-or-miss nature of the instruction. Live Strong offers reliably safe and accurate exercise demos.

You also can buy band loops with little foam circles of padding, but you don't really need them. You can just tie your regular band in a circle, which is even more versatile because you can control the diameter of the circle. The smaller the circle, the tighter the tension. You can use a circle to do a number of leg exercises and a few upper-body exercises, too. Some brands offer products with three brands braided together; these are very sturdy and do offer a different feel when you pull on them.

Free weights

Free weights — dumbbells and barbells — are excellent investments: They're simple, versatile, and relatively inexpensive. (They do, however, have the highest accident potential — see Chapter 12 for details.) You won't compromise safety by buying the cheap weights sold at department and sporting goods stores. Weight is weight. There's not much difference between one brand and another. Free weights are usually sold by the pound. You can pay up to $5 a pound for shiny chrome or rubber-coated dumbbells and bars. Gray or black steel will run you $0.45 to $1.50 per pound.

Dumbbells

For a beginner, *dumbbells* (the short weights that you can lift with one hand) should be a higher priority than *barbells* (the long ones that require both hands). Dumbbells give you more exercise options, and they force each side of your body to pull its own weight. Plus, they take up a lot less space than barbells.

When it comes to buying dumbbells, you have a few options:

- ✓ **Multiple sets of dumbbells:** The best, most convenient option is to buy several pairs of dumbbells — 5-pound weights, 10-pounders, 12-pounders, 15-pounders, and so on. Get eight or nine different pairs. Owning a whole array of dumbbells saves you lots of time, because all you have to do is put down the 5s and pick up the 15s when you want to change weights.

Although some people use the 10-pound dumbbells for every exercise, this isn't a good idea. A weight that's heavy enough to challenge your back muscles is much too heavy for your arm muscles; a weight that's just right for your shoulders is too light to do your chest any good. If you want to see results, you need to give each muscle the right challenge

For most beginning women, we recommend buying dumbbells weighing 2, 3, 5, 8, 10, 12, 15, and 20 pounds. Even if you can't use the 15s and 20s right away, you'll grow into them pretty fast. The whole set costs between $60 and $150. For beginning men, start off with 8, 12, 15, 20, 25, 30, 35, 40, 45, and 50 pounds. This set runs $200 to $1,000.

✔ **An adjustable dumbbell kit:** A kit comes with two handles and several weight plates that you clamp onto each end of the handles with a clip or screw-type mechanism called a *collar.* These kits sell for $30 to $200, depending on the quality and the number of weight plates included, so it's the cheap choice. Adjustable sets also take up far less room than a full complement of weights.

However, with adjustable dumbbells, you constantly have to remove the collar and add or subtract weight plates, which is a huge pain. Also, locking the weights on securely can be difficult; they can jiggle around or, worse, slide off in the middle of your workout.

✔ **Nesting dumbbells:** If you don't have the space for a whole array of dumbbells but don't want to fiddle with dumbbell kits, either, try nesting dumbbells. The two most established brands in this category are ProBell and PowerBlocks. One pair of ProBells gives you the same versatility as six pairs of dumbbells, ranging from 5 pounds to 30 pounds in 5-pound increments. Instead of sliding weight plates on and off, you turn a dial to indicate how much weight you want to lift. Through a feat of engineering, the ProBell picks up the requested number of plates.

PowerBlocks consist of a series of rectangular, weighted, metal frames, each one nesting inside a slightly larger frame. A series of holes runs along the outside of the frames; you insert a pin inside a hole to select the number of frames you want to pick up. You can buy a set of blocks that go from 5 pounds to 90 pounds in 5-pound increments and change the weight instantly. PowerBlocks come with an optional stand and take up about the same amount of room as a small nightstand. A 45-pound set sells for about $240; the 85-pound set sells for just under $700. PowerBlocks rattle around a bit more than ProBells, and their shape is more cumbersome, but PowerBlocks allow you to lift up to 90 pounds with each hand, whereas ProBells go only up to 30 pounds.

Just note that ingenuity and space savings come at a price. The steel ProBell set costs $199 — about twice the cost of six pairs of no-frills steel dumbbells. But you can save money on the higher end: The $249 chrome ProBell costs less than a set of six shiny chrome dumbbells. The ProBell stand costs an additional $149. See www.probell.com.

Shop around and try out different brands of dumbbells. Some have contoured handles that may feel more comfortable than straight ones. Some dumbbells have foam grips; others are coated in rubber. Dumbbells with hexagonal ends are great because they don't roll away. A dumbbell rack is also a good idea. A rack can cost $200 or more but will keep your weights organized and your home gym looking tidy.

Barbells

Most people can get along just fine with an array of dumbbells, but you can't beat barbells for power lifts like bench pressing and squatting (see Chapter 13). Plus, barbells add even more variety to your workout.

We recommend buying a single bar with a number of weight plates, because buying a whole assortment of bars is expensive. Bars typically run between $25 and $300, depending on the type of steel and where you buy the bar. Bars tend to cost more at specialty shops than at sporting goods stores. Plus, if you live in a small space, you may not have the wall width to use a bar without denting the walls or smashing into a lamp.

Bars are typically 4 to 7 feet long and come in two sizes: the skinnier *Standard* (about 25 pounds) and the thicker *Olympic* (about 45 pounds). *Plates* (the round weights that you slide onto the bars) and *collars* (the clips that secure the plates) are designed to fit one bar size or the other, so make sure that you buy plates and collars that match your bar. We prefer Olympic bars because they're more comfortable to wrap your hands around — they're also the standard in most gyms.

Purchasing a rack with your barbell is a good idea. Upright racks take up less room than horizontal ones. A one-bar rack can cost as little as $100.

As an alternative to traditional barbells, you can buy a series of lighter bars from 9 pounds to 27 pounds covered with comfortable rubber padding. One popular brand is Body Bar (www.bodybars.com). Although these bars don't allow you to clip on weights and are a bit pricey, they're good for beginners. They allow you to figure out how to do barbell exercises without having to use the heavier Standard or Olympic bars.

Weight benches

When you buy dumbbells and/or barbells, buy a bench, too. A bench lets you do many exercises that you couldn't do otherwise. For instance, doing free-weight exercises while lying on your back on the floor is difficult; your elbows may hit the ground before you complete the movement. You also can do several exercises while sitting or kneeling on a bench.

If you're lifting dumbbells lighter than 30 pounds, a plastic step platform rather than a full-fledged weight bench is fine. With two sets of risers placed underneath, the platform is high enough and sturdy enough for light dumbbell exercises, but you may want to pad the step with a towel to provide cushioning on your back.

If you're lifting heavier dumbbells or using barbells, buy a real weight bench. A bench is higher off the ground and more stable. We recommend benches that can be easily adjusted to incline or decline so you can challenge your muscles at different angles.

Look for a bench with a thick foam pad covered with Naugahyde or imitation leather. The pad should be sturdily bolted to a steel frame and legs. A bench should be at least a few feet high and shouldn't wobble when you get on and off. A basic flat bench goes for $50 to $500, depending on the quality and thickness of the padding, frame, and legs. We recommend paying a bit more for one that can be set at various inclines because it gives you the ability to vary your exercises. York and Hoist make good ones, but we really love TuffStuff benches (from $150 to $500) because they both incline and decline, so you can work your muscles from a variety of angles, and you have the versatility of positioning to do different exercises. Most benches do one or the other, in which case a bench that inclines is more versatile than one that declines. One product that does a great job acting as a bench, a step bench, and a storage unit is called the Reebok Deck. For less than $100, this bench goes from flat to incline and decline and has a small cubby carved into the center for storing bands and small dumbbells. It's made of plastic but it's sturdy and workable. When you're done lifting, you can do a step workout on it.

Another inexpensive alternative is having your physioball double as a bench. A physioball is sort of a sturdy, oversized beach ball (see Chapter 12). You can lie on top of it to do incline flys or sit on top of it to do your arm curls and shoulder presses (with light weights). This is definitely cheap with benefits; because the ball has a tendency to roll around as you move your body parts, your core must engage in order to keep it still. You get a decent ab and lower-back workout thrown into the bargain.

Multi-gyms

Multi-gyms are those contraptions that look like a bunch of health-club weight machines welded to each other (see Figure 19-1). Multi-gyms take up a lot of room — usually more than a stereo wall unit — and most require at least 7 feet of vertical clearance space. But many people prefer multi-gyms to free weights or bands because they're so safe and easy to use. Most multi-gyms come with instructions — some even come with DVDs demonstrating all the different exercises you can do.

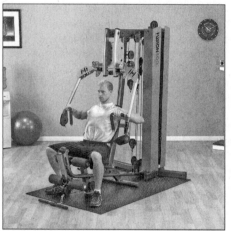

Figure 19-1:
Multi-gyms
are safe and
easy to use.

Courtesy of Body-Solid, Inc.

A basic unit has one 200-pound stack of weight plates in 5- to 10-pound increments. This means only one person can use the machine at a time. A basic multi-gym costs $800 to $1,500, whereas the really fancy ones with multiple weight stacks and lots of variations and adjustments go for $5,000 or more. If the whole family plans to work out together, you may want a multi-gym with two or three weight stacks, but these can run up to $10,000.

Expect to use up the same amount of space for one of these as two recliner chairs, even more for the larger, multi-stack models. Some multi-gyms are designed to wedge into a corner, helping you save space.

Good high-end brands include Paramount, TuffStuff, Cybex, and FreeMotion. For reliable less-expensive models, look at Hoist and Precor.

With the exception of the rather pricey Bowflex or Total Gym systems, which many people swear by and we think aren't a bad spend, we haven't yet found a multi-gym sold on TV or in a department store or discount warehouse that isn't cheaply made. They wobble and are poorly designed, and the resistance never moves as smoothly as a weight stack. Even some of the TV demonstrators can't help arching their backs on some of the moves. And sure, you may be able to do 52 exercises with one of these contraptions, but it'll take you about three hours just to make the adjustments, which will give you one more reason to blow off your workout.

Take your time shopping for a multi-gym. Try out a whole bunch of different machines, and pay attention to which exercises feel most comfortable. Multi-gyms that look the same sitting on the showroom floor may actually have important differences that you won't notice until you use them. For example, some multi-gyms come with a horizontal chest press; others come with a vertical chest press. You have to decide whether you prefer to lie on your back and press upward or sit up straight and press forward. Ask the equipment dealer to compare the different ways each multi-gym works each muscle group.

Here's a checklist to consult before you go shopping for a multi-gym. Inspect each machine carefully, and look for the following features:

- ✔ **At least the chest/shoulder press, high pulley, low pulley, leg extension, and leg curl exercise stations:** Depending on the brand and model, you may also get chest butterfly, chin/dip, leg press, and abdominal board attachments. If these attachments aren't included with the basic unit, they're usually available as extra-cost options. Keep in mind that most multi-gyms require you to unsnap and rehook cables or arm positions to switch between exercises; making all those adjustments can add extra minutes to your workout and interrupt the flow of your routine.

- ✔ **Free assembly:** Pass on any machine that the dealer doesn't put together for you, especially if it comes with an "easy-to-follow" video on how to build it yourself.

- ✔ **Weight stacks that move up and down smoothly:** Test several exercises in the store to check for sticking points and levers that don't allow you to fully straighten your arms and legs.

- ✔ **A frame made of thick tubular or rectangular steel:** The frame shouldn't shake or wobble when you lean against it. Also, the frame should be painted or powder-coated to prevent chipping and rusting.

- ✔ **Upholstery that's sewn on securely:** If you see corners that are curled at the edges, the upholstery probably will rip, tear, or unravel. The same goes for the rubberized padding around the foot rollers and other small parts. If it's made from cheap, thin foam, chances are it'll look chipped and beat-up after a few uses.

- ✔ **Plates and cables made of quality materials:** Avoid materials that look like they'll snap, fray, or crack.

- ✔ **Adjustable seats and arms:** If you can adjust the machine, the whole family can work out comfortably.

- ✔ **A good warranty:** The warranty should cover 10 years for the frame, 1 year for moving parts, and 90 days for upholstery. If you ask before you buy the machine, some dealers will give you an extended warranty at no cost. Don't *buy* an extended warranty, however. They tend to be expensive and not worth the money.

Check Craigslist and Freecycle (www.freecycle.org) for good bargains on home gyms. Liz knows someone who got a barely used weight machine on Freecycle from someone who was moving out of the area and didn't want to truck the machine across the country. Even if a multi-gym is not in tip-top shape, a good handyman can probably get the contraption into working condition.

Considering Flexibility Helpers

Most people get by just fine with fundamental stretching exercises that don't rely on anything but body positioning and gravity. But if a flexibility gadget gets you to stretch when you otherwise wouldn't, it's worth the money. (The same applies to balance gadgets, which we cover in Chapter 15.) Here's a look at some worthwhile investments on the flexibility front.

✔ **A stretching mat:** You can use a thick towel or blanket to pad a hard floor, but a mat is a more formal reminder to do your stretches, and you can use it for abdominal exercises and floor exercises, too. Just about any mat you come across will suffice. You can spend as little as $10 for one at Walmart or Target, and even a top-of-the-line mat — one that's cushiony and long enough so that your head isn't hitting your wood floor — shouldn't cost more than $100. Some can be folded in half for storage; others roll up.

✔ **A physioball:** In addition to doubling nicely in the balance and strengthening categories, a ball is a safe way to improve the flexibility of your lower back. You can drape your body over it forward, backward, or sideways. An oversized ball is also useful for abdominal and leg strengthening exercises. Expect to pay about $30 to $75.

The right fit is important. When you sit on the ball, your thighs should be roughly parallel to the floor. However, if you're somewhat inflexible, get a slightly bigger ball. You won't have to bend as far. Also, for stretching, don't inflate the ball all the way; it'll be softer, easier to mold your body to, and less likely to roll away.

✔ **Stretching strap or rope:** Use these nylon bands (Dynamic Stretching Strap or Stretch Out Strap) when using the Active Isolated method of stretching (see Chapter 14). For $15 to $30 (including a DVD), you may want to own one, especially if you're too stiff to get into certain stretching poses. For example, if you're sitting on the floor with one leg out and you can't reach your toes, you wrap the strap around your instep and hold a loop in each hand. After holding that position for a while, if you can stretch a little farther, you can let your hands creep up to the loop that's slightly closer to your toes. You can also buy a length of yachting rope at your local hardware store. Just buy a length twice your height.

Chapter 20

Hiring a Trainer

. . . .

In This Chapter

▶ Identifying good reasons to hire a trainer

▶ Screening potential trainers

▶ Knowing how much a trainer should cost

▶ Recognizing the signs of a quality trainer

▶ Being a good client

. . . .

*O*perating exercise equipment isn't nuclear physics, but neither is it something you can always figure out on your own. We recommend signing up with a trainer — for at least one session — to get yourself started on a fitness program suited to your goals. Even workout veterans have plenty to gain from periodic sessions with a fitness professional.

A trainer can teach you the subtleties of using exercise equipment: how to grip a barbell, how far to lean into a stretch, and how to adjust a stationary bike to fit your body — stuff that's tough to glean from a book or online. We know a woman who hired a trainer just to teach her how to use the new technology in her gym, such as the computerized weight machines, the wireless TV/radio headphones, and the fancy treadmill programs.

A good trainer can teach you all this and more and help you reach your goals much faster than you may on your own. But beware: The industry has its share of quacks. This chapter explains how you can benefit from a trainer and discusses how to find a qualified one.

Five Smart Reasons to Hire a Trainer

Trainers do a lot more than just whip wimpy actors into shape for their next action movie, and they don't all charge $400 an hour. (We tell you more about how much you should expect to pay in the "Appropriate trainer fees" section later in this chapter.) Consider hiring a trainer if you're in any of the following situations:

- ✔ **You're totally out of shape (or *deconditioned,* as the politically correct like to say).** If climbing the ropes in high school gym class was the last time you worked out, a personal trainer is a great way to bring you into the modern age. A lot has changed over the years, from the equipment to the lingo to proper stretching and strength-training techniques. A trainer can get you comfortable in your new environment and start you on a program that's appropriate for your fitness level; this way, your foray into fitness won't end a week later with a trip to the orthopedist and you won't embarrass yourself by trying to get a cup of coffee from the latest computerized chest-press machine. You don't need to sign up for life; just a few sessions can get you up and running.

- ✔ **You're training for a specific goal.** Say you want to run your first 5K race, but you aren't sure how long, how far, how often, or how hard to train. A qualified trainer can design a workout program that'll get you to the finish line. Look for a trainer who specializes in the area you want to work on, such as losing weight, building strength, or getting fit for ski season. We know a trainer who works only with runners, designing their running schedules and appropriate strength-training and stretching routines. Many of her clients are people who want to run their first marathon without getting injured.

- ✔ **You feel like you're in a rut.** Have you been doing your biceps curls with 5-pound dumbbells for the past three years? Do you always punch in 3.2 mph on the treadmill? If you feel like you could do your gym routine blindfolded and with both hands tied behind your back, it's time for a new challenge. A trainer can reevaluate a stagnant workout regimen, giving you a jump-start and putting you back on the path to improved fitness.

- ✔ **You're coming back from an injury or coping with a medical condition.** If you have a specific condition such as lower-back pain, or if you've just had surgery on your knee, a trainer can help you get back on your feet. A growing number of trainers specialize in conditions such as multiple sclerosis or breast cancer. Many trainers now take specialized certifications, attend specialized training courses, or participate in internships in medical facilities to gain experience in working with clients who have very specific needs.

  Check with your doctor; she may want you to visit a physical therapist first. Still, more and more physicians are giving the okay for trainers to participate in a patient's rehabilitation.

- ✔ **You need motivation.** If you won't exercise unless a trainer is standing there counting your repetitions, consider the money well spent.

Weeding Out the Poseurs

Few states have legal requirements for fitness trainers, and even those laws have loopholes. At the same time, a behind-the-scenes scramble is underway among the various professional organizations vying to be declared the official certifying body (see the nearby sidebar for details). The industry itself has taken steps to self-regulate, partly because it's the right thing to do but no doubt also to prevent the government from stepping in and taking control.

However, because being certified is not a legal requirement, anyone who can hoist a dumbbell and put up a Web site can call himself a personal trainer. That's why you need to screen a potential trainer with the same care that you use to screen a potential employee. The following sections tell you what to look for when investigating trainers.

We know one trainer with long, flowing dark hair and abs like a trampoline but sketchy education and knowledge. She often had her clients doing high-impact activities on cement floors and exercises that probably were not safe for her overweight and out-of-shape clients. Her clients loved her — until one of them developed a chronic foot injury from all the jumping. That was when the client discovered that the gorgeous trainer with the hot body was neither certified nor insured.

Certification

We think any trainer you work with should be certified — by a reputable organization. If you're skeptical, ask to see a copy of the actual certificate. Also, make sure that your trainer's certification is current; most expire after a year or two unless the trainer takes continuing education classes.

The following are among the organizations that certify trainers. Their Web sites can refer you to certified trainers in your area:

- ✔ **American College of Sports Medicine (ACSM):** The ACSM offers several certification levels. The certification we recommend is the Health/Fitness Specialist or the Personal Trainer certification. The HFS requires a bachelor's degree in an exercise-related degree, whereas the PT exam does not. Both tests are tougher than most certifications out there, so many trainers avoid them, but they're still the gold standard for personal trainers. Visit www.acsm.org.

- ✔ **American Council on Exercise (ACE):** This organization certifies both personal trainers and group fitness instructors (the type that teach classes); it also offers a higher-level exam for "certified exercise specialists" and a more basic exam for "certified lifestyle and weight loss coaches." We prefer the certification geared toward personal trainers.

The ACE Personal Trainer certification is the most popular in the industry, and although the test has a reputation of being easier than the ACSM HFS test, and you don't need a degree to take it, it's still plenty challenging. The certification is more practical than most, emphasizing the trainer's ability to design appropriate programs for a wide variety of fitness levels and medical conditions. Visit www.acefitness.org.

✔ **National Academy of Sports Medicine (NASM):** This group offers a practical Personal Trainer certification. Trainers must attend a workshop and pass an exam; trainers need strong physiology, anatomy, and biomechanics backgrounds going into the workshop, which provides the education, solutions, and tools needed by fitness professionals to systematically progress any client through specific phases of training in order to reach any goal. NASM trainers have a strong emphasis on understanding the in-depth workings of the body as a functional unit. Interestingly, this group also offers online college and graduate degrees in fields related to personal training. Check out www.nasm.org.

✔ **National Strength and Conditioning Association (NSCA):** This organization offers two tough certifications: the Certified Strength and Conditioning Specialist (CSCS), geared toward training high-level athletes in team sports, and the Certified Personal Trainer (CPT), designed for trainers who work in gyms. CSCS requires a four-year college degree; CPT does not. Trainers certified by the NSCA usually know a lot about strength training and conditioning; the NSCA asks candidates to identify every muscle involved in a particular exercise and requires them to know precisely what role each muscle is playing at which point in the movement. Visit the NSCA Certification Commission at www.nsca-cc.org.

✔ **Specialty certifications:** Some specialty fields, such as yoga (see Chapter 16), Pilates (see Chapter 17), and kickboxing (Chapter 21) do have certifications, though we consider them more education than certifications because they aren't standardized or accredited in any way. Other fields, such as boxing, don't offer certifications. Don't expect a specialty instructor who teaches spin or line dancing to have a bona fide accredited certification. But if he does have a diploma from one of the organizations we list, that's a plus.

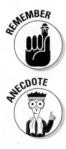

Remember that a certification is just a minimum. It lets you know that your trainer had enough basic knowledge to pass a test. It is by no means a guarantee of competence.

While proctoring a certification test before the advent of computerized testing, Liz asked one candidate to demonstrate a thigh stretch. He sat down on the floor and twisted one of his legs behind him, and then he began scooting himself forward on the floor. When Liz asked why he was doing that, the candidate explained that the maneuver shocks the muscle into stretching. He admitted that the stretch was indeed as painful as it looked, but said that was an unfortunate but necessary part of the exercise. No computer will ever catch that sort of nonsense or be able to gently set that sort of thinking straight.

How certification exams are improving

Currently there are more than 300 personal trainer certifications that come up on a Web search. Some organizations certify any breathing body. These schools are sometimes advertised on late-night TV or in the back of fitness magazines (alongside the ads for legitimate schools). Many of them require no more knowledge than how to enter your credit card for payment and how to work a printer to print out a certification.

In recent years, many of the major fitness organizations that represent gyms, personal trainers, and consumers have banded together to create the National Commission for Certifying Agencies (NCCA), an organization charged with accrediting certifications. This means that the certifications themselves go through a certification process of sorts.

The process overseen by the NCCA is designed to make sure the questions asked on a certification exam actually test the type of knowledge needed to be a competent personal trainer. Also, it ensures that the exams are scored correctly and independently from the organization that created the exam. As a result, certification exams have become more standardized and accurate, benefitting both professionals and consumers.

Currently, many organizations have put their certification exams through this rigorous process; these include the larger organizations, such as the American Council on Exercise (ACE), the American College of Sports Medicine (ACSM), the National Strength and Conditioning Association (NSCA), and the National Academy of Sports Medicine (NASM). You can obtain the full, continually updated list here: www. credentialingexcellence.org.

Some certifying groups have objected to this process, arguing that the accreditation process is too lengthy and too costly and does not allow them to match up their exams with their education process. But we feel it's a step in the right direction. And besides, there is precedent for this. Many professions — physical therapists, nurses, and registered dietitians, to name a few — have similar processes for their certifications. We applaud the effort to put personal trainers on par with the standards held by other health professionals.

Still, getting certified by quality organizations is a time-consuming, pain-in-the-butt process. Certified trainers have to study for at least a few months and then spend a few hours taking a test. At the very least, going through this process shows commitment: You know that the trainer isn't just doing this job because it pays better than her old job as a bike messenger. And by getting the certification, trainers surely pick up enough to have a basic level of competence.

Some professional fitness organizations that aren't accredited offer wonderful educational programs. And many colleges and universities offer their own extensive programs and versions of a certification exam. Also, some health clubs put their employees through rigorous training courses. Trainers who have been through these programs have points in their favor, especially if they go through a rigorous four-year program, but we still like to see trainers earn high-quality certifications. Indeed, many of these programs use one of the major certifications as their final exam.

University degrees

Many registered nurses and physical therapists are getting into the training business. They tend to know a lot about how muscles work; what's more, they may be able to accept insurance reimbursement if a doctor recommends training for treatment or rehab purposes.

Obviously, if your trainer has a master's degree or PhD in a field related to exercise and a ton of experience, you may consider letting her slide on the certification. But chances are such a person would be professional enough to have one, anyway.

Experience

Choose a trainer who has at least two years of experience at a club or on her own. Also consider your own needs: If you're looking to have a detailed program designed, you have medical conditions or injuries that require experience, or you have specific athletic goals you want to reach, look for someone with many years of experience.

In-home trainers these days often have some sort of promotional material to give you, or a Web site or Facebook fan page where you can check out their credentials, philosophy, and recommendations. You can actually find out a lot about how a trainer presents herself on her site or page. If you just want to tone up and you see that she brags about the grueling, two-hour boot camp she just put a client through, you may suspect she won't be your best match. Also, her information should clearly explain fees, payment schedules, and cancellation policies. Some trainers have you sign contracts and liability releases. Often these releases indemnify both parties from suing each other, but let's face it, if the trainer makes a real blunder (and, of course, you always hope this never happens) he'd likely still be on the hook for any damages.

Liability insurance

Make sure your trainer has insurance to cover any mishaps that may occur. Many trainers have you sign a release, but this doesn't absolve them from responsibility and from using safe and appropriate judgment, such as asking you to bench-press 250 pounds during your first workout. You should not work with a trainer who isn't covered by the club's insurance or his own.

Lawsuits against trainers are unusual but not unprecedented. The widower of a health-club member who died of a stroke filed a $40 million suit against his wife's trainer for giving dangerous nutritional advice. (The club was also named in the suit.) According to the suit, the trainer recommended ephedra, an herbal supplement that has been linked to dozens of deaths and should never be taken by people with high blood pressure. At the time, the woman was taking prescription medicine for hypertension. The widower eventually settled out of court, but the consensus was he would've won had it gone to trial.

Appropriate trainer fees

Fees vary from region to region and from big cities to small towns. In Des Moines, you may pay $30 an hour; in New York, the going rate is between $90 and $250 per hour, and trainers charging as much as $350 per hour are not uncommon.

Keeping trainer costs in check

Here's how to get your money's worth from a trainer:

✔ **Hire a trainer through your health club.** If you belong to a health club, you'll probably save money by hiring a trainer through the club. Many clubs now employ a "tiered system," with trainers who are working toward credentials costing a bit less than trainers who have a wall full of credentials. Actually, sometimes the lower-level trainers are better because they're often just starting out with all the enthusiasm someone new to the job can bring. Whatever the system, good gyms thoroughly screen their trainers and keep an eye on them. However, don't assume that the club hires trainers who are certified and experienced.

✔ **Sign up for joint sessions with a friend.** This has become more popular and acceptable over the past few years in both clubs and in home training. The trainer may charge slightly more than the regular hourly fee, but split two ways, your session is still a deal. You won't get quite as much attention from the trainer, but teaming up with a friend may make a session affordable. Try to choose a friend who's at the same fitness level as you or who has similar fitness goals. If you're training for a marathon and your friend is a linebacker getting ready for football season, the trainer is going to have a tough time serving both your needs at once.

✔ **Ask for help with weight-training only.** Do a half-hour of cardio exercise on your own (see Part II of this book) with a program designed but not supervised by your trainer, and then hook up with the trainer for a half-hour of weight training. This is a service primarily offered by gym trainers, as opposed to trainers who come to your home. This system has also become more popular in recent years. If you know what you're doing on the cardio side, it's a good deal.

✔ **Avoid overtime.** Ask whether your trainer charges by the hour or by the session. Typically, sessions last 45 to 90 minutes, including discussion and consultation time (not just workout time). If you're paying by the hour and your session runs over, you may wind up paying a lot more than you expected.

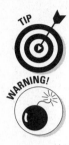

Charges depend on experience and popularity; the more experienced and popular a trainer, the higher the fee. Ask friends or call gyms to get a sense of rates in your area so you know whether a trainer's fees are way out of the ballpark.

On the off chance that someone is charging too little, watch out. Your so-called trainer may just be a pizza-delivery guy who happens to work out in his spare time and thinks he can make extra cash on the side.

Digging Deeper: Making Sure the Trainer You Choose Is Right for You

Choosing a trainer may not require as much homework as, say, choosing a hip surgeon. But do give the decision significant consideration, and don't be afraid to try someone new if you don't hit it off with the first trainer. It's your time, your money, and your health we're talking about.

Narrowing down your choices

After you know what to look for (see the earlier section "Weeding Out the Poseurs"), you're ready to refine your choice of trainers. The following sections cover a few ways to make sure a trainer is a good fit before you sign on the dotted line.

Get references

Be sure to check references. The best way to get the lowdown on a trainer is from other clients. You can ask around and try to find out by word-of-mouth or just come right out and ask the trainer for a list of references. Or, you can go completely 21st century and check out the trainer's Web site, blog, Facebook page, and Twitter feed to see what people are saying there. We recommend using a variety of methods to get the inside scoop on a prospective trainer.

Hold an interview

To make sure that you're compatible with your trainer, talk with him at length and ask questions before hiring him. A trainer may look good on paper but may not be able to speak in complete sentences. Or you may have a personality conflict — the trainer may have too much or too little enthusiasm for your taste. You also want your trainer to have good listening skills and at least a dash of empathy for those times when you're pushing through a last rep or struggling to understand which body part goes where during a stretch.

Considering the online trainer option

If you're not big on human contact, if you want to save money, or if you just can't get enough of technology, you may be interested in hiring an Internet trainer. You can find one by entering "online personal trainer," "workout programs," or "weight-training programs" into your Internet search engine.

We can't really call these "personal" trainers, because you never actually come face to face with a person, but many of these Web sites offer more individualized advice than you can get from a book or a DVD (or a lousy human trainer). The better ones ask you to perform some basic at-home fitness tests, similar to those we describe in Chapter 2, and then enter the results online. The really bad ones ask you for little more than your credit card number and then spit out automated programs.

After you plug in your info, your cybertrainer sends you a workout routine with suggested exercises, sets, and repetitions. Usually, you can download videos and/or printouts demonstrating how to perform each recommended exercise. You can print out the routine and take it with you to the gym or tack it up on the wall at home. If you plug in your workouts online, you get feedback — allegedly from an actual human being — but many programs are based on formulas that have little flexibility.

Some sites cost up to $500 for four months of cybertraining, whereas some pretty decent ones are actually free, offered by equipment manufacturers as a value-add to a piece of equipment you buy. *Tip:* Watch out for programs that charge $100 a session and those with exercise descriptions written in jargonese. Pay attention to the credentials of the trainers (or robots) who are supposed to have designed the routines.

Liz knows a woman who won't work with a particular trainer because the trainer laughs too loudly; she's afraid he'll draw too much attention to her when she already feels self-conscious about working out. After hearing the laugh, Liz tends to agree.

During the interview, ask what the trainer's specialty is and make sure it's in line with your goals. If you're hoping to run your first marathon, seek out a trainer who has taken several courses on running form, has trained other marathoners, and is perhaps a marathoner herself. Some trainers who specialize in weight loss have taken courses with doctors and scientists who study the field and so are up on the latest science of what works and what doesn't.

Don't judge your potential trainer by looks alone. Just because someone's a chiseled workout god doesn't mean he knows which exercises are best for you or even how to teach them to you. A great teacher can live in a less-than-god-like body. And conversely, we know some gorgeous creatures who can barely tell a push-up from a push-up bra.

Do a trial session

Before you commit to several sessions with a trainer, ask for a free or discounted trial workout. Also look for a money-back guarantee if you're not fully satisfied with your trainer or the session. Many trainers will comply in the hopes of getting a long-term client. Most gyms that offer personal training either offer a first session free or a discounted session before making you commit to a package of sessions.

Evaluating your trainer

Trainers have different philosophies and use a variety of techniques. Some come from the drill-sergeant school of motivation; others prefer the cheerleading approach. Still, there are some characteristics that all trainers should share. As you work with your trainer, make sure he

- ✔ **Assesses your fitness and goals:** Before anything else, your trainer should assess your current physical condition. (See Chapter 2 to find out what's included in a fitness evaluation.) Then your trainer should have a long talk with you about your expectations for the training sessions — your hopes, your dreams, and your specific goals. All this information is crucial: To really be of help to you, a trainer must know where you're starting from and where you want to go.

- ✔ **Gives you a balanced program:** Unless you specifically request otherwise, your sessions should include three or four components: cardiovascular exercise, strength training, flexibility, and (ideally) balance/coordination/agility exercises. Some trainers prefer that you do the cardiovascular portion on your own, but if you ask, your trainer should help you design a program and keep tabs on your workout and intensity. *Note:* Many trainers also skip the stretching and cool-down portions of a workout.

- ✔ **Watches you closely:** Your trainer should pay attention to your form and give you pointers throughout the session. On the other hand, you don't want a trainer who blabs incessantly. Your trainer also should *spot* you — in other words, stand poised to grab the weight and give you some help if your muscles give out.

- ✔ **Reassesses your goals and measures your progress:** A good trainer retests you after the first six weeks of training and, if you've been working out consistently, every two to three months thereafter. A trainer who is really on the ball also reassesses your goals periodically — often enough to keep you motivated and on track.

- ✔ **Listens to you:** If you mention that an exercise doesn't feel right, your trainer should figure out why and show you an alternative move for the same body part. There's no single exercise you absolutely must do. If you tell him you're feeling stagnant, overtrained, or underchallenged, he should alter your program.

✔ **Speaks English, not jargon:** Some trainers say things like, "Your patella edema is a limiting factor in increasing your volume of oxygen uptake." Translation: "You can't run faster because you have bad knees." If you can't understand what your trainer is saying, find someone new. You shouldn't expend extra energy just trying to figure out what the heck you're being asked to do. Trainers with jargonitis tend to be really insecure. Occasionally, however, a small dose of fitness verbiage is good for you; a trainer may be trying to teach you something that you actually should know, like where your triceps are. (By the way, if you don't know where your triceps are, read Chapter 11.)

✔ **Teaches you to be independent:** Ironically, good trainers train themselves out of a job by teaching you how to do everything on your own. After a few months, you should be able to set the correct amount of weight, adjust the machines, use proper form, and modify your routine as needed. Of course, if you'd never exercise by yourself, you're welcome to hire your trainer for life; she'll be glad to accommodate you. Regardless, you should know how to do everything on your own. This way, if you're out of town on business or vacation, you can keep up your workouts at a hotel or local gym. And if, heaven forbid, your trainer goes on vacation, you won't have an excuse to stop working out.

Getting the Most out of Your First Training Session

Even with the guidance of a trainer, your first session may be a little awkward. One friend of ours says she just had to swallow her pride while trying out the weight machines for the first time. "Here was this cute, young trainer helping me climb onto the hamstring machine," she remembers. "I felt like a 40-year-old woman trying to get on a horse for the first time. I'm lying on the bench with my butt in the air, and the trainer's saying, 'Keep your butt down.' And I'm saying, 'That's as far down as it goes. It's just big.'"

Having a good sense of humor can get you through a first workout session without any ego damage. So what if you sit backward on the shoulder machine? So what if you glide off the physioball like a slippery fish? Your trainer may as well earn his money showing you the right way to use the equipment.

Here are some tips to help ease your anxiety and make your first session a productive one:

- **Schedule the session at a time when the gym isn't busy (any time other than weekday mornings or evenings).** This way, you won't have 12 other members clamoring to use the arm-curl machine while the trainer teaches you to adjust the seat.

- **Take notes.** During the session, your trainer should keep track of your session in some way, whether it's a paper or electronic system, so he can remember what you've done from one session to the next and help monitor your progress. He may track things such as each exercise in your program, how much weight to lift, and how many sets and reps to do. You can also keep track of this information with your own notes — you may find it easier to remember what to do when you work out alone. For example, if your trainer writes "lat pulldown," you can add, "pull bar down to chest; strengthens back muscles; adjust seat to second notch." Some facilities number the machines to make them easier to remember and identify, too.

- **Ask lots of questions.** Don't be too intimidated to ask the trainer why he picked a particular chest exercise or for a reminder of where your delts are. No question is too stupid (unless you're asking what time the 3 p.m. boxing class starts).

- **Don't expect to absorb everything your trainer tells you on the first day.** Every time you work out, you'll pick up more information, such as how to adjust each machine and how to stretch each muscle group. You can make things easier on yourself by scheduling a second training appointment to reinforce what you found out on the first go-around. Some gyms charge for a second appointment; some don't. If you bring up the issue when you join the gym, some clubs may throw in a few extra training sessions.

Being the Best Client You Can Be

You have the right to demand a lot from your trainer, but your trainer can also expect a certain level of courtesy, attention, and effort from you. Keep in mind the following rules of client etiquette. Some of these tips apply just to home trainers; others apply to trainers at a gym.

- **Be ready to go.** Don't show up at the door in your pajamas. Your trainer shouldn't have to serve as your alarm clock or wait a half-hour for you to get your act together. Like you, the trainer has a schedule, and time is money. If you're late getting started, the trainer has every right to cut your session short or charge you extra.

✔ **Don't answer your doorbell or phone or check e-mail on your BlackBerry.** This just wastes the trainer's time and distracts you from your workout. Also, if you have kids, make sure that someone is watching them. Your trainer won't be happy if your 5-year-old runs into the room screaming, "Mommy! Mommy! My Barbie is sick!"

✔ **Schedule in advance.** You'll have a very happy trainer if you schedule a month in advance. (Just make sure that it's a schedule you can stick to.) At the very least, don't call in the morning and expect a session that afternoon.

If canceling or rescheduling, give your trainer as much time as possible. Many trainers have a 24-hour cancellation policy, which requires you to cancel or reschedule your session with at least 24 hours' notice. This allows your trainer time to adjust his schedule and possibly fit someone else into that spot. It also helps keep a positive rapport with your trainer.

✔ **Speak up.** Just because you've hired a trainer doesn't mean you've lost the power of speech. If something doesn't feel right, say so. Your trainer isn't a mind reader.

One woman we know severely pulled her inner-thigh muscles because a trainer went overboard on a stretch. Afterward, she said she felt pain for nearly a minute before she heard a loud pop. Why didn't she say anything? Because she didn't want to question the trainer. Granted, the trainer should have paid better attention, but he couldn't have been expected to know how the woman felt.

✔ **Keep the relationship professional.** Your trainer isn't your therapist. Inevitably, you'll get into personal stuff; after all, this is your personal trainer. But don't take your bad day out on your trainer, and don't expect your trainer to fix your life. And never make a pass at your trainer, just as he or she shouldn't be making a pass at you or making inappropriate comments.

Chapter 21

Choosing an Exercise Class or Digital Workout

*I*f you loved playing Simon says as a kid, you'll love group workouts, whether in a class or on a TV or computer screen. To burn fat, build muscles, and have fun, all you need to do is copy everything the instructor does (assuming you've chosen a good instructor).

Group exercise has experienced a creative explosion since the days when Richard Simmons still had hair. In addition to traditional classes like low-impact aerobics and step (which are getting harder and harder to find), you can try firefighter boot camp, Zumba, BodyPump, and Pilates. Many classes use equipment, such as dumbbells, balls, jump ropes, and even treadmills.

To explore your options, you can start by downloading a podcast of an exercise style, and if it's appealing to you, find a gym that offers the class. Or start with a live class and if you prefer privacy, download a streaming video or order a DVD. These days, geography doesn't hold you back.

This chapter covers most of the popular instructor-led offerings besides yoga and Pilates, which have become so popular that we devote an entire chapter to each (Chapters 16 and 17, respectively). For each class we describe in this chapter, we tell you how much you'll sweat, what you'll gain, and how you'll fare if you're a klutz.

Getting Through When You Haven't a Clue: Taking an Exercise Class

If you're new to exercise classes, you have plenty of company. Of all the latest creative offerings, group exercise is attracting many folks who traditionally have stayed away. Liz recently peeked into a group cycling class and noticed that every bike in the house was occupied by a man. A decade ago, most men avoided the group fitness studio like it was a pedicure salon. (Come to think of it, we see a lot of men having their toes done now, too.)

Don't fret, either, about getting injured. Exercise classes are much safer than they were in the Jane Fonda era of ultra-deep knee bends, jerky moves, and high kicks now considered criminal today. Most health clubs and studios require the instructors to have experience and, in certain instances, certification. Many clubs audition teachers, do regular evaluations, and pay attention to participant feedback.

Signing up

To make life easier for yourself when you're just starting out, choose classes with the words *beginner, introductory,* or *basic* in the title. You'll get a much different impression of boot camp from a slower, simplified beginner class than if you accidentally wander into an advanced class and hear, "Okay, the name of today's circuit is Last Man Standing!"

Class fees vary widely. Some health-club memberships include unlimited classes, and others charge up the wazoo for specialty classes. Specialty studios charge $10 to $40 per class, and they may charge extra to rent the equipment. At many clubs and studios, you can save money by buying a package of classes — say, ten at once — but be sure to find out whether you must use up the package by a certain date (some states have now made expiration dates illegal). Another option is to buy a month's worth of unlimited classes. Some clubs let you try out one or two classes for free. You also can seek out classes in places like community centers and churches.

Knowing what to expect from a live instructor

No matter what type of class you're taking, a teacher who is standing right in front of you should do the following (later in "Working Out with an On-Screen Instructor," we offer tips for evaluating instructors that lead you via your iPod or TV screen):

✔ **Ask questions at the beginning of the class:** Some examples include, "Any newcomers?" "Anyone with an injury I need to know about?" or "Is there anyone here who's never tried jump rope before?"

✔ **Include a warm-up and a cool-down period:** The cool-down should be followed by stretching exercises.

✔ **Give clear instructions so you always know where you are and what's coming next:** Your instructor may say, "Two steps right," and then point right with two fingers. She should cue the moves coming up next instead of springing a lunge on you at the last second.

✔ **Speak in plain language:** The really obnoxious instructors say things like "plantar flex at your ankle joint" rather than "point your foot." However, a good teacher should educate you. It's perfectly okay for an instructor to say, "Feel this move in your quadriceps — that is, your thigh."

✔ **Watch the class rather than gaze at himself in the mirror:** He should face the students at least some of the time and occasionally walk around adjusting everyone's form.

Liz once bailed on a step class because the instructor never turned around to acknowledge the existence of the class members, let alone check their form.

✔ **Make the class entertaining:** You don't want your instructor to take your classes so seriously that they become a chore or a bore.

✔ **Have an education:** It's a definite plus if your instructor is certified by one of the major national fitness organizations (see Chapter 20). However, some specialty fields, such as boxing and tai chi, don't have organized certifying bodies. Don't hold that against them, but do ask where your instructor was trained so you know she does indeed have some training.

Getting the most out of your classes

Before the class starts, tell the teacher you're a novice. A good instructor will keep an eye on you and correct your mistakes without making you feel like a doofus. If you don't mind the spotlight, stand in the front — the instructor will be more likely to notice and correct you. If you're shy and prefer to make your mistakes more privately, stand in the back or get lost in the middle. Throughout the class, keep your eye on the teacher rather than a fellow student. And don't compete with anyone. This isn't the time to give your ego a workout.

If you get tired, just march in place or dial down your intensity. Don't stop cold and walk out in the middle of a class — you risk nausea or even fainting. But don't be afraid to bail if the instructor is a lemon.

Oh, and one other tip: Don't lend any of your valuables to the instructor. Suzanne recently got trapped in a yoga class with a teacher who seemed to think she was auditioning for *Last Comic Standing*. Unfortunately, the painfully unfunny instructor had borrowed Suzanne's wristwatch, so Suzanne had to stay until the bitter end — either that or be willing to buy a new watch.

If the class is good, even if it leaves you feeling like a clod, come back for more. Skills and fitness take time to develop. You'll feel pretty darn good when you master a class that used to wipe you out.

Considering popular classes

Two classes that have the same name may be completely different. One body-sculpting class may use dumbbells; another may use rubber exercise tubes. And of course, no two teachers have the exact same style. Still, all body-sculpting classes, like other types of classes, have common characteristics. Here's a rundown of the most common classes around, roughly in order of their popularity.

A recent trend is quick fitness classes — 15- to 30-minute classes that help people sneak in a workout in the busiest of days. Some gyms tack these on the end of longer classes so you have the option of supplementing your first class or running into the classroom just to work your abs or your thighs.

Step and BOSU

Now one of the oldest staples on the group fitness schedule, *step* is a choreographed routine of stepping up and down on a rectangular platform (or in the case of BOSU, a domed, flexible apparatus). Many classes combine step with other types of workouts. Sometimes both apparatus are used in the same class; sometimes not.

What it does for you: Step aerobics or BOSU gets your heart and lungs in shape and tones your tush. Step is a terrific cross-training activity for runners, cyclists, and walkers. BOSU is also exceptional for developing balance and flexibility.

The difficulty factor: Difficulty depends on the choreography, the pace, and the height of your step. In some classes, you hold weights while you step. Higher-impact step and BOSU require major amounts of coordination — some instructors make you feel like you're auditioning for a Broadway musical. Women like step because it's such a great butt-and-thigh toner. However, if you have back, knee, or ankle problems, try another class or at least keep the platform very low.

What to wear: Shoe manufacturers such as Reebok, Nike, and New Balance make light cross-training shoes that work well for step. These shoes have ample ankle support, are a bit stiff along the sides, and have plenty of heel cushioning and flexibility at the ball. Reebok also offers good group-fitness shoes with similar features. Running shoes generally won't cut it. Plus you may stumble if the waffle pattern on the bottom of the shoe catches on the top of the platform.

Signs of a sharp instructor: Good instructors ask whether anyone has any back, knee, or ankle problems. They accommodate newcomers by going over the basics, such as how to place your foot on the platform. Instructors also should alert you before every *transition* — step jargon for any change in the routine, such as changing directions — and make sure that you don't lead with the same foot for more than a minute or two.

Tips for first-timers: No matter how fit you are, start with the lowest step — don't put any risers underneath. Don't feel intimidated if the guy next to you looks like he's stepping onto a coffee table. Also, if you find yourself getting confused or behind, forget about the arm movements and concentrate on the footwork, or simply march in place and watch for a while.

High- and low-impact classes

High- and low-impact classes are the original Jane Fonda-Richard Simmons–style classes that ushered in the era of group classes. Don't know who these people are? Doesn't matter. You still see these classes form the core of many large gyms' group fitness schedule. Fads and trends may come and go, but high- and low-impact classes remain like barnacles on the sides of a ship, albeit with name changes like Cardio Push, Let It Go Low, Get High, or Eighties Flashback.

What it does for you: You get in shape and burn calories.

The difficulty factor: Difficulty depends on the class. With *low-impact,* you always have one foot on the floor; you don't do any jumping or hopping. *High-impact* moves at a slower pace, but you jump around a lot. High/low combines the two types of routines.

Signs of a sharp instructor: Instructors should spell out the terminology, rather than just say, "grapevine left, grapevine right."

Tips for first-timers: Shop around for a teacher you like who plays music that inspires you; there's nothing like a little "Eye of the Tiger" to get you going in the morning.

Body sculpting or kettlebells

Body sculpting is a nonaerobic, muscle-toning class. Look for names like Total-Body Power or Hot Body Blast. Most sculpting classes use weight bars, exercise bands, dumbbells, or a combination of these gadgets. You perform traditional weight-training moves in a class setting. Some focus on one specific body part; core conditioning classes like Absession, Ab Lab, and 8-Pack Abs have become especially popular. Kettlebell classes, in which you swing ball-shaped weights with handles on them (see Chapter 13), also are very hot.

What it does for you: Body sculpting gives you strength and muscle tone and lowers your risk of bone loss but only if you lift heavy enough weights. Sculpting classes are ideal if you're interested in the fundamentals of weight training but don't have the bucks to throw down for a personal trainer, you're too shy to enter the weight room, or you're unmotivated to lift on your own.

The difficulty factor: Prepare to be sore if you're a novice or if you usually do different exercises. Almost anyone can do body-sculpting classes the first time out if they're taught well. Kettlebells are a little harder to get in the swing of (we couldn't resist the pun!), because you have to figure out how to control the weights and not send them flying through a window or into your neighbor.

Signs of a sharp instructor: Instructors should tell you to use moderately heavy weights so that you don't do more than 15 reps per set. (We define reps and sets in Chapter 13.) As we explain in Chapter 13, you don't develop much strength or tone if you do dozens of reps with very light weights. (BodyPump is one of the popular classes that involves up to 100 repetitions for some exercises; these classes are pre-choreographed and the instructor isn't supposed to vary the routine at all. We don't recommend this approach.) The instructor should correct your form and remind you where you should feel the exercise. Watch for a warm-up and cool-down, too.

Tips for first-timers: Prepare yourself for muscle soreness the day or two after your workout. First-time Kettlebellers should take a class designed for novices. A bit of technique is involved in the stance, swing, and selection of the correct weight for each exercise.

Circuit training and boot camp

Circuit training or boot camp is a fast-paced class in which you do a series of exercises, usually alternating sustained cardio exercise with weight training, boxing, or athletic movements. *Circuit training* is like a game of musical chairs: Everyone begins at a *station* (that is, a place where an exercise is done), and when the instructor yells "Time!" or some such phrase, everyone moves to the next free station. Some classes alternate an aerobic activity (like stepping or stationary cycling) with a muscle-strengthening activity (like using weight machines). *Boot-camp classes* are like circuit training classes on steroids; they're far more intense, and the exercises are typically more complex and challenging. If you watch *The Biggest Loser,* you see boot-camp-style workouts.

What it does for you: Both type of classes increase strength and cardio fitness and burn lots of calories. However, you don't get the same level of conditioning as you would from doing your cardio and strength training separately. If you take circuit classes, aim to get in an additional 20 minutes of straight aerobic exercise at least three days a week.

The difficulty factor: Moderate. Circuit training can be intense, but it's quite adaptable to the individual and requires minimal coordination. If your instructor is more interested in letting spit fly in your face than giving technique pointers, participant injury rates are likely to be high. Depending on the circuit and the moves, you may be stumbling over your feet or punching air when you should be smacking the punching bag. Stick with it, though, and you'll get the hang of it. If you have a short attention span and an adrenaline rush, this is the workout for you.

Signs of a sharp instructor: If an instructor swaggers in with a *Full Metal Jacket* attitude, we say: Get out quick! Good instructors are aware of each class member's level and modify the moves accordingly. They recognize that operating at a fast pace does not mean throwing caution and good technique to the wind.

Tips for first-timers: Pay attention to how you feel. Many people are surprised by how challenging this type of workout can be.

Boxing and martial-arts-inspired classes

A boxing or martial-arts-inspired class usually takes the training moves of a boxer, kickboxer, or martial artist and choreographs them to music. However, some instructors don't use music and instead choose to count or call out commands. You do some or all of the following: jump rope, shadowbox, do forward kicks, punch, and do the fancy footwork that boxers do in the ring and martial artists do in the movies.

What it does for you: This class develops power and endurance. These workouts also improve your coordination, strength, agility, and balance.

The difficulty factor: After one of these classes, you'll know why boxing athletes and martial artists are renowned for their fitness. Most classes are geared toward advanced exercisers, although some clubs offer beginner and multilevel classes, too. Many of the classes require decent coordination to master the footwork and handwork, but if you like to sweat and think at the same time, sign up.

What to wear: You can buy specialty boxing and martial-arts shoes, although medium-to-high-top cross-trainers are fine. Most gyms supply boxing gloves and other additional equipment needed.

Signs of a sharp instructor: We recommend classes taught by someone with good boxing and/or martial arts skills, rather than, say, a yoga instructor who's just futzing around with a jump rope. Most teachers don't have these certifications, because there really isn't any formal organizing body in these specialties, but some instructors do have degrees of belt or rankings of some sort. If they don't, it's best if they've at least attended some instructional seminars.

Tips for first-timers: Pay attention to how you feel, and skip or modify moves that feel too difficult or uncomfortable. Don't give up; boxing gets easier.

Dance-based workouts

A dance-based workout is a cardio routine with choreography borrowed from dance moves. Classes range from simple moves with a little attitude thrown in to what seems like a tryout for a dance competition. At many urban clubs, you find funk aerobics, hip-hop step, and even *salsa hip-hop,* a funky class spiced up with salsa dance moves. Look for names like Get Up and Groove, Cardio Jam, Jammin' Latin, and Zumba (a fusion of Latin and international music). Taking an actual dance class in, say, ballet, tap, or modern can also give you a mighty good workout, so don't overlook that option.

What it does for you: These classes develop heart and lung power and really improve your posture, body awareness, flexibility, coordination, and agility. You teach your body to move in complex ways and use muscles you didn't know you had.

The difficulty factor: Difficulty depends on the level of the class. Dance classes are so popular now, perhaps because of the popularity of reality-TV dance contests, so a class is out there for every level and every style. Even if you have two or even three left feet, you can find a class you can get through without feeling your joints were carved from wood. And secretly, who hasn't always wanted to feel light on their feet?

What to wear: You can wear your typical tights and T-shirt, but don't be surprised if you're the only one. Funk classes, for instance, tend to have their own style of dressing: high-top sneakers, off-the-shoulder tops, baggy shorts, sexy bras, oversized socks. In many classes, you slip your shoes off and leave them at the door.

Signs of a sharp instructor: Good instructors break down complicated moves into a series of smaller ones before putting them all together. They repeat, repeat, and repeat sequences until they're drilled into your brain.

Tips for first-timers: If your parents didn't pass down the funk gene in your DNA, start with a beginner class or something super basic like Zumba. Dance, more than any other style of class, can leave unprepared novices in the dust.

Cardio-machine classes

Cardio-machine classes are group classes taught on stationary bicycles, rowers, treadmills, or just about any other cardio machinery. These classes follow the same basic pattern: You pedal, walk, run, step, or row while the instructor talks you through a visualization of an outdoor workout. ("You're going up a long hill now — you can't see the top yet . . ."). During the class, you vary your pace and intensity, sometimes pushing yourself as fast as you can, other times cranking up the intensity and going slowly, and other times breezing in recovery mode.

By far, the most popular equipment class is *studio cycling,* which most people know as *spinning.* Treadmill classes go by names like Tread and Shred, Millwork, or Thrill Mill. Rowing classes are typically called IndoRow or Rowbics and are done on a piece of equipment called the Concept II Rower (which we describe in Chapter 8).

What it does for you: A cardio-machine class burns lots of calories, ratchets up your cardio fitness, strengthens your thigh and calf muscles, and — if you so desire — prepares you for the real outdoor deal.

The difficulty factor: Most equipment classes last 30 to 90 minutes and are geared toward all levels of exercisers, depending on which class you take. However, even beginner classes are a bit more challenging than novice classes of other breeds. You don't need much coordination, but you do need the wherewithal to push through even when you feel tired.

What to wear: For non-cycling machine classes, wear what you'd typically wear to exercise on that piece of equipment. For cycling classes, most studio-cycling bikes have the same hard, narrow seats as outdoor racing bikes, so a pair of padded bike shorts or a gel seat can help keep your fanny happy. Most bikes have water-bottle cages so you can stash your water within easy reach. Some studios such as Soul Cycle (in major cities like New York and Los Angeles) provide shoes, but if your club doesn't, wear stiff-soled shoes; walking and running shoes are too soft. Many bikes have clipless pedals so you can wear outdoor cycling shoes with cleats that click into the pedals.

Signs of a sharp instructor: Good instructors know all the nuances of the equipment and share all this insider info with the class. Rather than stay parked on their piece of machinery, they walk around and make technique adjustments.

Tips for first-timers: Show up early to your first class so you have plenty of time to make your equipment adjustments and familiarize yourself with all the buttons and knobs.

Specialty classes

Specialty classes are your flavor-of-the-month classes, though some have more staying power than others. Health clubs and studios dream up exotic routines like pole dancing, trapeze school, and stiletto strength (which prepares your body for walking in high heels) in an effort to attract people into the exercise studio. Often these classes are gone in three months, but if they've served their purpose, which is to get your butt off the couch and bouncing on a trampoline, they've done their job.

The difficulty factor: The skills required are all over the map, as is the quality of instruction and effectiveness of these workouts. But give 'em a try. Exercise in any way, shape, or form beats eating chips and channel-surfing any day of the week.

Signs of a sharp instructor: Often the instructor is the mad-genius inventor of the class or a loyal disciple. To this we say either "Great!" or "Good luck with that."

Tips for first-timers: Usually everyone's a first-timer, so you're in good company.

Working Out with an On-Screen Instructor

We love getting instruction any way we can, so if it comes in the form of a DVD, a podcast, a streaming video off YouTube, or a Wii Fit game, that's all great with us.

DVD, digital, and streaming workouts don't suit everyone. You may feel silly prancing around your living room alone or in front of your computer or iPod screen, mimicking an instructor who says, "You're doing great!" even though he can't see you. But if you're short on time, are self-conscious about your body, or are taking care of kids at home, a prerecorded workout may be a better option for you than a live class. You don't feel pressure to keep up with anyone else, and you can build an extensive workout library for less than one month's worth of gym membership dues. If you're really creative, you can probably do it for close to free. You may even get more imaginative routines than many health-club instructors can drum up.

Safety is an important consideration, especially when you don't have much exercise experience and you're working out in an unsupervised setting. Follow these safety tips:

- **Make sure that you clear adequate space in front of the TV or screen.** You don't want to bang your shins on anything or knock over any lamps.

- **For cardio and strength-training tapes, wear proper shoes instead of working out in bare feet or socks.** In any case, don't jump around on concrete floors. You may want to buy a board made of springy wood similar to what you find in good aerobics studios. These boards help absorb impact. Gerstung makes a 30-x-60-inch board for about $160 and a 30-x-30-inch board for about $80.

- **Even if the instructor doesn't do it on the video, gauge your intensity by checking your heart rate or taking the talk test during or immediately following an intense portion of the workout.** We explain these methods in Chapter 6.

- **Don't try to keep up with the instructors.** They practiced the routine for weeks before it was recorded. Look for someone in the video who goes at your pace. Many good videos feature demonstrators who exercise at different levels. At the start of the workout, the lead instructor should say something like, "If you're a beginner, keep your eye on Valerie." If you get winded, keep moving by marching in place or walking in a circle.

- **If you're just starting out, follow a workout that includes several short sessions rather than one long one.** The shorter workouts last 5 to 25 minutes as opposed to 30 to 90 minutes. They're usually programmed to include a warm-up and cool-down.

- **Gather all the equipment you need before your workout.** This way, you don't have to stop mid-workout and rummage through the closet for your jump rope or hand weights. Place your mat or chair or bench at a 45-degree angle to the screen so you get a good view of the instructor without having to crane your neck or compromise your technique.

- **Remember that your DVD player has a pause button.** Use it if you need to get water or you just need to catch your breath. Take advantage of all the extra features the DVD or workout has to offer, such as the ability to customize the music, the workout intensity, and the length of the workout.

If a workout is offered in a health club, you can find it on a disc, in a store, online, on iTunes, on TV, or in a game. You just have to know where to look. Here's a brief rundown on where to find your prerecorded group-fitness selections. (Keep in mind that the options change all the time.)

DVDs

Most workout DVDs aren't simply taped workouts you pop in and follow; you often select the type of music you want, the intensity, the length of your workout and even, to some extent, your preferred exercises. Some DVD workouts are sophisticated enough to work around injuries you may have. Manufacturers can now pack more than two hours of workouts on to a single disc, so with all the mixing and matching, you can go several months without doing the exact same workout. Often, the same can't be said when you go to a live class. Plus, you can pause, rewind, and freeze frame if you want to study a position or, heck, just stop and answer the phone.

Where can you find a good DVD? You can head to Walmart or Target or an online or brick-and-mortar bookstore. Or watch for special product promotions. For instance, one of the best-reviewed DVD instructors of all time, Jessica Smith, has a free workout DVD inside specially marked boxes of Special K at the time of writing.

We're big fans of Collage Video (www.collagevideo.com; 800-433-6769), a catalog that carries probably the widest selection of exercise DVDs anywhere. Each blurb tells you how tough the workout is, how long each segment lasts, what type of music it's set to, and what equipment you need. They even have a little video snippet of each DVD so you can get a feel for the instructor's style and the production values of the workout. Collage's prices aren't always the lowest, but the service is excellent, and the warehouse is well stocked.

Before you invest in a DVD, read the reviews posted on Collage, Amazon, or other sites. Another informative source is Video Fitness (www.videofitness.com), which posts reviews of specific DVDs and general critiques of instructors. Read multiple reviews for each workout, because as with any form of entertainment, opinions differ wildly.

Streaming and digital downloads

Many services, such as Netflix, iTunes, and ExerciseTV, feature video workouts. Exercise TV is both a cable channel with workout shows and a Web site (www.exercisetv.tv). It also has an on-demand channel where you can select video workouts; at any time, the channel offers about 100 workouts and offers instant downloads or streaming options. This means you don't have to wait for your disc to arrive in the mail, and in many cases, you don't have to wait the 6 minutes for your file to download. You simply load your credit card information and go. If you don't mind exercising in front of your computer, you can be waving your arms and lifting your knees in no time. And with TV and computer technology coming closer and closer to a full merge, there will be little difference between the two in a few years, anyway. Many of the same DVD titles that are available on the tangible disc are available to stream or download. For a low-tech freebie, head to the local library and rent a few DVD exercise titles.

On-demand TV and ExerciseTV

Many cable operators offer ExerciseTV either part- or full-time, and if they do, chances are they also offer on-demand; this means you can fire up a workout any time, day or night. Some of these workouts are actually the same as found on DVDs available for sale, whereas others are shot especially for on-demand; still others are episodes from ExerciseTV shows. Most are excellent. Just watch out for workouts taught by trainers known for their celebrity clients; these workouts tend to be loud and poorly instructed. There are a lot of categories to choose from, such as 10-minute workouts, cardio, toning, bridal blasts, and so on. If you're already paying for cable, the workouts are free.

Podcasts and YouTube

If you own an MP3 player or computer, here's a freebie tip: Flip to the podcast section of iTunes. Here you can find tons of free workout podcasts, both audio and video. Liz has learned meditation and some pretty decent yoga and running techniques in this way. She also sweated through two iPods before finally perfecting a system that keeps moisture from seeping into the seams of her device. (Two zipper-lock baggies and a safety pin; it ain't pretty, but it gets the job done.)

As for YouTube, you can also find some good workouts there, although you need more patience and persistence than with iTunes. Although YouTube is now the second-largest search engine after Google, it's still a bit like the Wild West; searches can yield surprising and frustrating results. You may search for abdominal exercises and wind up looking at ads for laundry detergent — presumably because of the washboard reference; but you may also stumble upon the most amazing Pilates class.

Video games

When your 12-year-old goes to school, you may want to snag his Wii or Xbox and try out one of the new Wii Fit games or one of its counterparts. Most of the Wii games require the Balance Board platform and some sort of handheld or strapped-on remote or sensor. The games range in price from $20 to well over $100; price doesn't necessarily relate to how well they're designed or how much fun they are.

The idea behind the Wii game is that the sensor tracks your repetitions and workout information and gives you feedback about your form. At this point, we can say the games are fun and engaging but are still in their infancy, so they're therefore a bit clunky. For example, running around a track is still, after all, just marching in place, and there's no way around this. But 3D effects are changing gaming, and sensors are being refined all the time, as are the graphics and other special effects. Liz learned how to snowboard on the new Shaun White game. With all the swooshes and spins down the mountain — or whatever kids are calling the moves these days — she came away with everything but frostbite. The improved special effects are a good direction for fitness, especially if they help young people rise up from their screens and flex their muscles for a few hours every day.

Part VI

Exercising for All Ages and Stages

The 5th Wave   By Rich Tennant

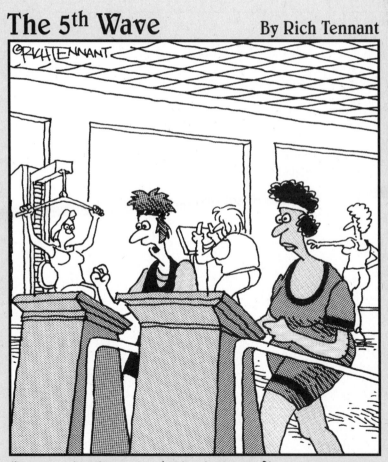

"I exercised so much during my first pregnancy that the baby was born with athlete's foot."

In this part . . .

Y ou discover that exercise isn't just for twenty-
something singles. Not by a long shot. In Chapter 21,
you see why pregnancy is one of the best times in life to
exercise — not just for your health but also for your
baby's. In Chapter 22, you find out how to make exercise
fun and exciting for kids of all ages, even tweens who
seem to be surgically attached to their video game consoles.
Chapter 23 helps you get and stay fit in your senior years
so you can keep up with your grandkids and maintain
good health, an active lifestyle, and a sharp mind.

Chapter 22

Fit Pregnancy: Exercising for Two

In generations past, the last place you'd find a pregnant woman was a health club or a running track. Back in the 1950s, doctors recommended that pregnant women walk no more than 1 mile a day — broken up into several sessions! Pregnancy was considered a time to rest in bed, not strengthen your hamstrings, because doctors worried that exercise would cause miscarriage or birth defects. But they were just guessing. Now that scientists have actually researched these issues, they know it's perfectly safe for most expectant moms to work out, as long as they exercise common sense and don't try to set a world record in the high hurdles. (Be sure to get your doctor's permission before embarking on a prenatal exercise program. Some high-risk conditions do rule out exercise during pregnancy.)

Not only is moderate prenatal exercise safe for the baby, but breaking a sweat also has tremendous benefits for Mom, including fewer aches and pains, more stamina, and a lower risk of developing gestational diabetes. In fact, in a development that may surprise the doctor who delivered you, researchers are finding that prenatal *in*activity — rather than exercise — is what puts moms-to-be and their babies at risk for serious health conditions.

In this chapter, we explain the benefits of prenatal exercise and offer pregnancy workout options along with important safety precautions. We also provide tips on sticking with exercise even when your feet are swollen to the size of bread loaves (that was Suzanne's experience) and you barely have the energy to answer the phone (yup, Liz — although she did roust herself up once a day for a jog until her ninth month).

Understanding the Benefits of an Active Pregnancy

One obstetrician we interviewed says his inactive patients tend to come to the hospital in labor petrified of the impending delivery, but his fit patients are fired up and ready for action. "For them, it's like the Super Bowl," the doctor says. "They say, 'Stand back, let me go. I'm going to push this sucker out!'"

Going into labor with confidence is just one of the many advantages enjoyed by active moms-to-be. See the forthcoming bulleted list to find out what else you'll be doing if you stay fit during your pregnancy.

Keep in mind that if you were overweight and sedentary when you conceived, the benefits described in this section apply to you, too. In the past, overweight women were practically told, "Don't move, don't even breathe," but new research shows that obese pregnant women can safely exercise during pregnancy and they enjoy the same benefits as leaner women.

- **Reducing back pain and soreness:** Your baby's growing size puts pressure on your hips, butt, and back, which can lead to stiffness and soreness. But exercise improves your posture and helps negate much of this achiness.

- **Avoiding excessive weight gain:** You absolutely need to gain weight during your pregnancy, because of the extra fat stores, body fluids, and blood your baby needs to grow properly; gaining too little weight can stunt a baby's growth. (See www.nationalacademies.org and type in "recommended weight gain for pregnancy" for specific weight-gain guidelines.) However, many women gain too much weight, increasing their risk of developing *gestational diabetes* (GDM), high blood sugar. Women with GDM deliver heavier babies who are at higher risk for obesity and diabetes years down the line, and the moms themselves have a 70 to 80 percent chance of developing type 2 diabetes after pregnancy.

    In addition, women who gain excess weight during pregnancy have higher odds of delivering via C-section because their babies are larger. They have more weight to lose after pregnancy and tend to retain more of their pregnancy weight than women who did prenatal exercise.

- **Having a leaner child:** Active moms-to-be have leaner but not excessively lean babies, and this leanness continues to age 5. This starts your baby off on the right foot, fitness-wise, from Day 1. See Chapter 23 for additional tips on helping kids get and stay fit.

- **Sleeping well:** If you're having trouble sleeping during your pregnancy — and that's just about everyone — exercise can help you sleep more soundly at night and feel more awake during the day.

✔ **Feeling groovy:** Even if you start the day feeling lousy and lethargic, exercise is likely to invigorate you. Plus, working out makes you feel more like a powerful, fit mama and less like a beached whale.

✔ **Staying fit in the future:** Fit women who work out during pregnancy appear to be fitter and healthier two decades later than women who were fit before pregnancy but temporarily quit exercising while pregnant. In one study that followed moms for 20 years, those who'd stuck with exercise throughout pregnancy had gained just 7.5 pounds in the two decades since, compared to nearly 22 pounds for those who quit working out while pregnant but resumed afterward. At age 48, the continuous exercisers had lower cholesterol levels and resting heart rates, and they could run 2 miles more than 2½ minutes faster than the moms who'd taken a break.

✔ **Reducing delivery complications:** Several studies show that women who exercise have fewer complications during delivery and generally need fewer drugs for pain relief. That makes sense. As one doctor told us, entering labor in poor physical condition is like running the Boston Marathon without training. It's wise to prepare your body for the mega-workout to come.

✔ **Reducing time spent in labor:** Some research suggests that fit women have shorter labors than unfit women and that they have a lower rate of C-section. But exercise doesn't guarantee you a free ride in the delivery room. Even if you swim or walk until the day you give birth, you still may have the labor from hell. Still, fit women do seem to bounce back from pregnancy (and labor) a lot faster than their inactive counterparts.

For an in-depth look at the research supporting prenatal exercise, we recommend *Fit Pregnancy For Dummies,* by Catherine Cram and Tere Stouffer Drenth (published by Wiley), along with *Exercising Through Your Pregnancy,* by James Clapp III, MD, a top prenatal exercise researcher and strong advocate of prenatal workouts.

Working with Healthcare Providers and Trainers

If you're pregnant, consult with your healthcare provider before starting an exercise program. Discuss your goals and the activities you plan to do, and get an okay from your physician or certified nurse-midwife before you get started. The health of your child is more important right now than your fitness goals, so if your healthcare provider tells you not to work out, heed his warnings.

So what about individual exercises? Is it safe to do lat pulldowns in your third trimester? Is it better to perform arm exercises while sitting or standing? These are questions you can ask a trainer with expertise in prenatal fitness, an increasingly popular subspecialty among personal trainers, according to the American Council on Exercise (ACE). ACE's newest certification, the Advanced Health and Fitness Specialist, includes training in prenatal and postnatal fitness. A session or two per trimester can help you stay motivated and modify your routine as your body changes. To find a qualified trainer, contact ACE at www.acefitness.org or 888-825-3636.

Great Activities to Consider during Pregnancy

Many of the activities listed throughout this book are safe to do during your pregnancy, including those in the following sections.

Whichever activities you choose, remember the following guidelines for staying cool and hydrated:

- ✔ **Don't exercise without a water bottle close at hand.** When you're responsible for someone else's life, too, it's especially important to stay healthfully hydrated. Dehydration is the number-one cause of cramps, particularly in your legs, and it can increase your blood pressure and heart rate, among other things. Always drink before you get thirsty — by the time your body demands, "Water, now!" you're already at a fluid deficit.

- ✔ **Keep your cool.** Exercise in a well-ventilated area and make sure you wear clothes that breathe. Try to work out in the early morning or in the evening when it's cooler, or opt for an indoor workout. As a pregnant woman, you do have a built-in mechanism that allows you to reduce exercise-related heat stress, and fit pregnant women tend to begin sweating at a lower temperature than inactive women. Still, this adaptation only works to a point, so use common sense. Extra-high body temperature irritates the fetus and can lead to premature labor. Keep drinking that water, which cools your body internally.

Walking this way

Some women walk for exercise until the day of delivery. Runners may want to switch to a walk-run program or an all-walk routine if they find that running is just too hard on their lower back and knees. Liz ran for eight months, but on the day the calendar flipped to her ninth, she stepped off a curb and felt her right knee go ping! This was from the joint loosening that many women experience during pregnancy. For the rest of her pregnancy, she was happy to walk.

Here are a few tips for walking for fitness while you're pregnant:

- ✔ **Pay special attention to your walking posture.** Stand tall, with a natural S-curve to your back and your shoulders back and down, not hunched. Lead with your chest. Keep your arms relaxed, and move them forward and back instead of swinging them across your body.

- ✔ **Wear supportive walking shoes.** Because you weigh more than usual, your joints are under extra stress, and they need all the shock absorption they can get. Your feet may swell to the point where you need shoes a half-size bigger than usual.

- ✔ **As your pregnancy progresses, avoid steep hills, which make your heart rate soar and may put more pressure on your lower back.** Listen to your body and really respect what it's telling you. Even if you were a macho ultra marathoner in your pre-pregnancy life, you may have to dial it down to a walk.

- ✔ **Pay attention to the weather.** Don't walk in very hot or humid weather, because your heart rate elevates more rapidly and your body overheats more quickly. (And always carry water, even if you never did before.) And don't walk when the ground is icy, because your sense of balance is not what it used to be.

- ✔ **Use the rails.** If the weather sends you indoors and onto a treadmill, hold on to the rails (but not with a death-grip). Treadmills require more balance than walking on the ground.

Getting into the swim of things

Some pregnant women find walking or other cardio workouts uncomfortable, particularly in the third trimester, so they switch to lower-impact activities such as swimming. In the water, you don't have to worry as much about your balance. The water supports your weight and the weight of your baby, too, taking the stress off your lower back, and reduces the effect of gravity, lessening pressure on your joints. Swimming can even help reduce pregnancy-related swelling.

Meanwhile, you can still get a great workout. You can run in the pool, swim laps, and tone your muscles with equipment like webbed gloves and foam dumbbells. As your pregnancy progresses, you may need to modify your water workouts.

Using a kickboard may become uncomfortable because it forces you to arch your back, which can trigger back pain. The frog kick (used in the breast-stroke) may also cause discomfort. Don't forget to drink water — you can get dehydrated even in the pool. And beware: When you step out of the pool, you may suddenly feel the weight of your pregnancy four times over, so exit slowly.

Despite her aversion to getting wet, Suzanne switched to water exercise at week 32 of her twin pregnancy. With her feet so swollen that a thumbprint would keep its shape for minutes, she abandoned her beloved elliptical trainer and joined a water-exercise class, where she was the youngest member by 30 years. She didn't mind; the pool was the only place where her feet didn't throb.

Taking prenatal exercise classes

Many health clubs and hospitals offer exercise classes specially designed for pregnant women and brand-new moms. Some classes stick to cardio work-outs; others include strength training, with gadgets such as exercise balls, free weights and bands, and even kettlebells (all equipment that we describe in Chapter 12). Naturally, the exercises are adapted to the limitations of a pregnant body — including the loss of balance, shifting center of gravity, increased joint laxity (looseness), and reduced stamina.

Participants love these classes because the atmosphere is so much more supportive than it tends to be in regular classes. You don't find a drill-sergeant instructor yelling, "Okay, today is plyometric-jumps-off-the-bench-day." And you don't find class members in dental-floss bikini outfits showing off their sculpted abs. Plus, prenatal exercise classes offer camaraderie and a chance to swap war stories about hemorrhoids, heartburn, and husbands who — try as they might — just don't get it.

Reading up on prenatal fitness

If you expect to stay fit when you're expecting, you can find no better source of information than *Fit Pregnancy,* the only magazine devoted to the concerns of pregnant women (and new moms) who exercise. Created by the editors of *Shape, Fit Pregnancy* (also at www.fitpregnancy.com) features great cardio, strength, yoga, and Pilates workouts; stylin'

prenatal exercise gear; reviews of prenatal exercise books and DVDs; and the latest news on prenatal fitness research.

Fit Pregnancy also offers fun pregnancy-related blogs and sound advice on prenatal diet and nutrition as well as sex and health issues such as genetic testing and infant vaccinations.

Trying prenatal yoga and Pilates

The poses and gentle movements involved in yoga are ideal for pregnancy, improving muscle tone, boosting energy and, especially, enhancing flexibility. During pregnancy, the hormone *relaxin* floods your body, loosening your pelvic joints in preparation for delivery. As a side benefit, all your joints become looser, and with careful stretches, you can capitalize on this window of opportunity. You may gain the greatest flexibility of your whole life when you're pregnant and retain that flexibility if you stick with yoga afterward.

For a mom-to-be, perhaps the most important benefit of yoga is the sense of calm that the practice fosters. As one instructor put it, "Yoga is about feeling, not thinking," and nothing could be more applicable to the birthing process.

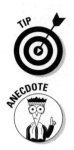

Just be sure to avoid exercises lying on your back (especially after your third month) or exaggerated twists, and don't do inversions like headstands and shoulder stands.

Yoga is not for every pregnant woman, as Liz found out. When Liz would move into one of the standing poses, her daughter would kick so hard that Liz would literally spin until she was facing another direction. Also, some women find their joints get too floppy to enjoy yoga without pain. Be sure your yoga teacher has the knowledge to teach a prenatal class. Some very fine yoga teachers aren't always schooled in some of the risks associated with certain positions and movements.

A growing trend, too, is Pilates classes for pregnant women. (We describe Pilates in depth in Chapter 17.) Here again, you need to make sure your teacher knows what he or she is doing. Many of the standard Pilates movements are off-limits to women after their first trimester, but teachers who are properly educated know how to modify them.

Lifting weights

If you've never lifted weights before, pregnancy isn't the time to start an unsupervised strength program. But if you know what you're doing in the weight room or you're experienced using dumbbells at home, you have no reason to quit your routine. And as long as you make the appropriate modifications, there are plenty of great reasons to stick with it. (We don't want to discourage novices from strength training during pregnancy, but you need to work with a trainer who's very experienced with pregnant women or join a supervised, prenatal weight-training class at a health club.)

Lifting weights during pregnancy not only keeps you looking terrific but helps cut down on general aches and pains and may even counteract some of the shoulder and back pain that can be caused by enlarged breasts and a growing uterus. Everyday activities won't take as great a toll, and when the big day comes, you'll have more strength to pick up your new bundle of joy (not to mention the diaper bag, stroller, and car seat you'll be lugging around).

You do need to adapt your weight-training program to your ever-changing body. You may prefer machines to free weights, because they offer more support and require less balance. Of course, some machines won't fit you anymore. Ask a trainer to show you more-practical alternatives to your regular routine.

Give special attention to the muscles that are bearing the brunt of your temporary burden, such as those in your knees, ankles, hips, and lower back. Your wrists may need some extra attention because many women develop carpal-tunnel syndrome during pregnancy — Liz did. Wrist strengtheners and stretches, combined with daily icing, helped ease the discomfort. But if any exercise starts to feel uncomfortable, stop doing it. Anytime that you feel dizziness, nausea, or a pulling in your abdomen, hips, pelvis, or elsewhere, choose a different exercise.

When you're pregnant, don't focus on sculpting your muscles or setting a personal best in the bench press. Instead, aim to maintain your strength and enjoy the movement. Your last few repetitions of each set should be somewhat challenging but shouldn't require all-out oomph. Expect to reduce the amount of weight you lift toward the end of your pregnancy, when you may have less energy. Breathe steadily and pay close attention to your form. Don't grip the handles too hard — gripping too hard raises your blood pressure, which shoots up anyway when you exercise.

Putting a prenatal spin on studio cycling

If you enjoy riding a bike outside, studio cycling, which most people refer to as *spinning* (described extensively in Chapter 8), is a great alternative during pregnancy. There's no impact and zero chance of falling or getting hit by a car, and you can hang with the group while exercising at your own pace.

As your belly grows, eliminate out-of-the-saddle (seat) movements, which can put excess pressure on your knees, and always take it easy. To give your lower back relief, raise the handlebars so you're not so hunched over.

In the earlier months of pregnancy, some women like the recumbent stationary bike because it takes pressure off the back. And some women can still tolerate the padded seats of ordinary stationary cycles throughout their pregnancies. Suzanne rode her Spin bike throughout most of her pregnancy and highly recommends buying padded bike shorts designed for pregnant bodies.

Using Wii Fit, online videos, and other media

Nintendo's Wii Fit video games involve using a balance board to control onscreen action with your body movements. The yoga, cardio, and strength-training games are easily adaptable for pregnancy simply by using common sense, but we advise skipping the balance games, because your sense of balance is off-kilter during pregnancy.

To make the workouts easier, enter an age older than you are, and wear sturdy athletic shoes instead of going barefoot. Check the available titles frequently for available pregnancy workouts.

And don't overlook many of the free and low-cost options you have for pregnancy workouts. Cruise through iTunes podcasts, both audio and video, to see what's available, as well as YouTube and other video sites. ExerciseTV (www.exercisetv.tv) has some terrific content geared toward pregnancy at a super-low cost (how does $2 strike you?), and many local cable providers offer on-demand pregnancy workouts. Of course, DVDs are a great choice, too, because they're inexpensive and the workouts can be done again and again. Generally, titles cost between $5 and $20; if you're a member of a service like Netflix, you can rent them in DVD or instant digital download format.

In the past few years, some excellent instructors have focused their efforts on pregnancy titles. Tracey Mallett has a fit-for-pregnancy series she is frequently updating, and Ellen Barrett is another great instructor in this genre.

Avoiding Risky Exercises

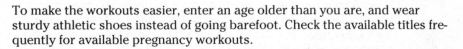

Certain activities just don't mix with pregnancy, and that list usually includes the following:

- ✔ Scuba diving, because of the intense underwater pressure, which is harmful to your baby
- ✔ Waterskiing, during which you may fall; in addition, if less-than-clean lake or ocean water enters your vagina, you risk getting an infection
- ✔ Contact sports, such as soccer, volleyball, basketball, and hockey, which introduce a major risk of falls and contact injuries
- ✔ Downhill skiing, figure skating, horseback riding, and mountain biking, all because of the risk of falling

✔ Rowing and (sometimes) cross-country skiing and running, because these can be very strenuous activities that can overtax your body; if you're a cross-country skier, consider switching to snowshoeing

Check with your healthcare provider for the final word.

Don't lie on your back after the first trimester. Starting around the fourth month, you may feel dizzy when you lie on your back. This means that your little one is pressing on your *inferior vena cava,* a major vein that carries blood to your heart. *Tip:* You can modify exercises in a number of ways to avoid this dizziness. For example, if you want to do abdominal exercises on your back, place a folded towel or small blanket underneath one hip. This shifts your body slightly, rolling the baby off the vein. Also, you can do several pregnancy exercises with your back against the wall or while standing or sitting in a chair. In addition, you can do gentle exercises with a *physioball* — a large, inflated ball that looks like a sturdy beach ball.

One friend of ours took a physioball with her into the delivery room. When she went into *back labor* (when the baby presses heavily against the spine, creating agonizing back pain), she placed the ball against the wall and pressed her back against it. By rolling the ball around on the wall and allowing it to massage her back, she was able to work through most of the pain. She did get some funny looks from the nurses, but when they saw it was working, they thought it was a great idea.

Overcoming the Obstacles to Prenatal Exercise

Right about now you may be thinking, "Okay, I'm convinced I need to exercise, but how am I supposed to go for a power walk when I have to stop every five minutes to pee?" Or, "Can I possibly make it to a prenatal yoga class when I barely have the energy to make it to the refrigerator?" Here are some ideas for working around pregnancy's most annoying symptoms so that you can stay active even when you're uncomfortable and as big as a firehouse.

✔ **Nausea:** Find a time of day that you're less prone to feeling ill, and do a less strenuous activity. Instead of taking an early-morning spinning class, try yoga in the late afternoon. A half-hour before exercising, eat some bland crackers. Motion-sickness bracelets, available at drugstores, also can help, as can ginger and high-starch foods.

Liz really struggled with nausea during her pregnancy, and on her doctor's suggestion, found relief in — no kidding — yellow cake with no frosting. (Actually, in spite of being a regular exerciser, Liz struggled with almost every symptom; her doctor says she'd have felt much worse if she didn't exercise.)

✔ **Backache or hip pain:** Stick to low-impact exercise with fluid movements, such as swimming, pool walking, or using the elliptical machine or recumbent bike. Sometimes all the back and hips need is a little blood flow to the area.

Light stretching after a light cardio warm-up may also do the trick by loosening up your hips, lower back, and hamstrings. Sit on the floor with your legs out straight, gently lean forward from your hips, and sit with your legs in a butterfly position (feet together, knees out).

Consider getting a prenatal massage by a specialist. Many specialists have special tables with cutouts for pregnant bellies, or they perform pregnancy-specific techniques with you lying on your side.

✔ **Exhaustion:** Dial down your intensity, and break up your workout into 10-minute sessions, either resting or stretching in between. Choose an activity that's enjoyable and social, like taking a walk with a friend, so you're distracted and not focusing on your low energy. If you feel particularly tired, listen to your body and take the day off. You may try experimenting with the timing of your meals and exercise sessions.

✔ **Frequent peeing:** Exercise at the gym so you're never more than a few steps from a toilet. If you prefer walking in the fresh air, plan your route in a neighborhood that has a coffee house on every block, or locate the bathroom at a local park and stay close. For trail hiking, carry toilet paper — and make sure you're still able to squat down — and then get back up!

✔ **Swollen feet and ankles:** Skip the treadmill and elliptical trainer and join a water aerobics class or go for a swim. Or simply immerse yourself in the pool and hang onto a foam noodle; you'll feel instant relief. The recumbent bike places much less pressure on your ankles than other cardio equipment, but your belly may interfere with your pedal stroke in the later stages of pregnancy. Wear athletic shoes ½ to 1 size bigger than normal so you have plenty of wiggle room, and take the laces out of the top holes. Try pointing and flexing your feet and rolling them in circles.

✔ **Achy or numb wrists:** Your wrists can get sore when fluid retention compresses the nerves in your forearms. Try doing wrist circles and using your opposite hand to guide each wrist through 15 to 30 seconds of gentle flexion and extension. Limit upper-body strength exercises, especially those that involve bending your wrists. Don't grasp the rails of the treadmill or elliptical machine. Or try putting a towel or some other padding on the rails directly underneath your hands to soak up some of the discomfort.

Monitoring Your Prenatal Workout Routine: Watching for Danger Signs

Until 1994, the American College of Obstetricians and Gynecologists (ACOG) insisted that a pregnant woman should not let her heart rate exceed 140 beats per minute. Many fit women found this guideline too restrictive; well-trained athletes have exercised during pregnancy with heart rates as high as 190 without complications. In 1994, ACOG eliminated the heart-rate limitation, making many pregnant jocks happy.

This doesn't mean it's okay to work out at your maximum heart rate. In fact, when you're pregnant, heart rate is a lousy indicator of how hard you're pushing yourself. This is because your resting and exercise heart rates are higher than normal because of increased body temperature and a flood of hormones.

The simplest option is to use the "talk test": Don't exercise so hard that you can't hold up your end of a conversation about hemorrhoids and heartburn. Stop immediately if you feel dizzy, fatigued, or experience vaginal bleeding.

A more precise way to assess your prenatal exercise intensity is to use the RPE (rate of perceived exertion) scale: Rate your effort on a scale of 1 to 10, 10 being a gangbusters effort you can't maintain. Shoot for an RPE of 5 to 8. A 5 feels like you're working moderately hard but could keep up the pace for quite a while without pooping out; at an 8, you feel like you could keep going for a few minutes without having to slow down or bail.

It's fine to push through a little nausea; it's not fine to keep walking on the treadmill when you're experiencing pain, dizziness, or any of the other symptoms that follow, which may indicate overexhaustion or, more seriously, pre-term labor or preeclampsia (a dangerous condition involving high blood pressure and excess protein in the urine). You need to stop and report your symptoms to your healthcare provider.

- ✔ **Pain:** If exercise hurts in any way, stop exercising ASAP.

- ✔ **Excessive fatigue:** If you find yourself feeling overly fatigued throughout the day — and not just when you're exercising — take a day off and relay this information to your healthcare provider at your next appointment.

- ✔ **Overheating:** If you find yourself sweating a great deal, getting excessively hot, feeling faint, getting nauseated while working out, and/or becoming lightheaded, stop exercising, drink plenty of fluids, rest, and call your healthcare provider.

- ✔ **Dehydration:** Getting dehydrated is bad for you — and your baby. Keep a water bottle with you throughout much of the day, and check the color of your urine — the lighter and clearer the better — each time you go to the bathroom. If your urine looks gold-colored or orangey, drink more fluids. If adding more water to your daily routine doesn't help, ask your healthcare provider for advice.

✔ **Contractions:** If you're not within a week or two of your due date, contractions may indicate premature labor.

✔ **Dizziness:** This could be a sign of *anemia* (low red-blood-cell count that results in weakness and fatigue) or other conditions.

✔ **Dyspnea:** If you're experiencing *dyspnea,* you may have shortness of breath or rapid and shallow breathing.

✔ **Headache:** Although many pregnant women report an increase in headaches during their pregnancies (often brought on by fatigue and stress), if you experience a severe headache or a less severe one that doesn't seem to go away, contact your healthcare provider. Headaches can be an early sign of *preeclampsia* (pregnancy-induced high blood pressure).

✔ **Increased swelling in your legs:** This could be a sign of preeclampsia, which is characterized by high blood pressure and fluid retention and can be quite serious. It could also indicate *deep-vein thrombosis,* a blood clot that develops in a vein.

✔ **Muscle weakness:** Muscle weakness can take a couple of different forms: total-body weakness (in which you feel weak all over) or specific muscle weakness (such as your right arm or the left side of your body). Either of these may indicate circulation problems or that you've simply pushed yourself too hard.

✔ **Vaginal bleeding and/or leaking of amniotic fluid:** Leaking blood or other fluids can be the result of several complications, including *placenta previa* (in which the *placenta,* the organ that grows in your uterus to provide nutrients for the fetus and eliminate its waste, blocks all or part of the cervix), *placenta abruption* (separation of the placenta from the uterus before delivering your baby), premature labor, and miscarriage.

✔ **You can't feel your baby moving:** If your baby's normal movements (that you usually begin feeling between the 18th and 22nd weeks) have diminished or stopped, your baby may be experiencing problems. Keep in mind that your baby will probably be calm during exercise, but you should start to feel several movements again within 20 to 30 minutes after you stop.

Exercising After the Baby Arrives

Working out may seem like a pretty tall order when you're getting two hours of sleep a night and your body feels like it's been through the spin cycle. But even short, easy workouts like a 10-minute walk help you sustain energy (at a time when you really need it), and exercise may help you sleep better at night. Exercise also can help you cope with the depression that sometimes results from sleep deprivation.

Don't rush back into exercise after you deliver your baby. There's no need to force yourself into anything at a time when a walk to the bathroom may seem like a feat worthy of an Olympic medal. As soon as you feel ready (a few days or weeks after delivery and only after checking with your doctor), try to start a simple routine, such as daily walking. Gradually work up to brisk walks with your baby in the stroller or a home workout while the baby sleeps. Consider buying a baby jogger or a special cart that attaches to your bicycle so you can safely take your little one along for the ride.

Six weeks after an uncomplicated birth — or sooner if your doctor okays it — you can begin more vigorous activity, such as swimming, running, or lifting weights. Just make sure you start back slowly. Your abdominal muscles have been stretched, which means they aren't supporting your back as much as they were before you got pregnant. Check with your doctor before you begin your routine again.

Postpartum exercise makes you feel better, but don't expect it to be an express ticket to weight loss. Some research suggests that if you eat regularly and exercise after giving birth, you go through approximately the same weight-loss patterns as women who don't exercise. In other words, it still takes about six months to a year to return to your pre-pregnancy weight and body composition.

But other studies suggest that exercise can help. For example, a Harvard study of postpartum moms found that for every hour the women walked each day, they had a 34 percent lower chance of retaining a significant amount of weight — defined as 11 pounds — at one year postpartum. Exercise appears to be most useful for postpartum weight loss when it's combined with other healthy behaviors. The same study found that women who watched fewer than two hours of TV daily, walked 30 or more minutes daily, and ate fewer trans fats had a 77 percent lower chance of significant weight retention than women who did none of these beneficial behaviors.

If you're breastfeeding, don't worry that exercise will compromise your milk supply or cause your baby to reject your milk. Research shows that babies nurse just fine after their moms work out, even vigorously, a finding that both Liz and Suzanne can personally vouch for.

Chapter 23

Getting Kids Fit

It used to be that a chubby kid stood out from the crowd. Nowadays, a child — even a preschooler — carrying a spare tire is a common sight. While the percentage of obese adults in the United States has doubled since 1980, the prevalence of obese kids has quadrupled. About 30 percent of kids ages 10 to 17 are overweight or obese; in some areas, as many as half of all kids are packing extra pounds. Like their parents, these kids are eating too much and not moving enough; as a result, they're developing serious diseases, including high blood pressure and type 2 diabetes, that used to be found only in adults.

The best way to prevent poor fitness in kids is to take a dual approach: Tap into your children's innate love of activity, and turn them on to healthy foods. Of course, in an era when playing tag is a lot less popular than a Sony PlayStation and Fruit Roll-Ups are more popular than actual fruit, a parent's job isn't easy. This chapter offers ideas for getting your tykes and tweens on the road to an active lifestyle.

Looking at How Exercise Helps Your Child

Being active and remaining at a healthy weight is just as important for your kids' long-term well-being as learning how to read, memorizing their times tables, and understanding how to cross the street safely. Even if your children are skinny as a Q-tip, they still benefit in countless ways from staying active. Fit kids do better in many, many aspects of life, and research shows that getting a healthy start in life sets them up for lifelong good habits. Here are just some of the ways that kids benefit from being fit:

✔ **Active kids are more resilient.** Research suggests that compared to sedentary kids, children who participate in sports are more likely to rebound from disappointment, have better self-esteem, and are less likely to feel stressed out.

✔ **Active kids often do better in school.** A recent study found that children who play vigorously for 20 to 40 minutes a day — whether it's jumping rope, playing tag, or running relays — are better able to focus on schoolwork, control their impulses, do class projects, and learn math. Compared to sedentary girls, active girls have better grades and a greater likelihood of attending college.

✔ **Active teens are less likely to start smoking.** Boys and girls ages 12 to 16 who spend much of their leisure time doing physical activity are significantly less likely to start smoking than low-activity groups.

✔ **Teenage female athletes are less likely to get pregnant as teenagers than teens who don't participate in sports.** They're also more likely to have their first sexual experience later in adolescence than non-athletes.

✔ **Active kids get to discover abilities they never knew they had.** Chances are, your kids have a real knack for some type of athletic endeavor — whether it's running, softball, or aerobic dance — but they won't know until they try.

Is your child overweight?

How do you know whether your child is among the nearly one in three who are considered overweight or obese? For children and teens, pediatricians typically assess their weight by body mass index for age. This height/weight ratio is similar to BMI calculated for adults, except that children are segmented into percentiles that indicate the relative position of their BMI number among children of the same sex and age. A child is classified as overweight if she falls into the 85th to 95th percentile and obese if she falls within the 95th percentile or above. You can determine your child's BMI-for-age score with the following calculator: www.bcm.edu/cnrc/bodycomp/bmiz2.html.

Being overweight can set your child up for lifelong health issues, including early heart disease, type 2 diabetes, and many other illnesses associated with poor lifestyle habits,

not to mention the social stigmas attached. And fat kids are likely to become fat adults. But that doesn't mean there's nothing you can do about it.

You can help your child start exercising and eating healthfully, but don't put her on a strict diet. Instead, aim for her to avoid gaining weight for a few months while her height catches up to her weight. Certainly, most children shouldn't try to lose more than a pound a month unless otherwise instructed by your pediatrician. As your child grows and gets taller without putting on pounds, he'll be leaner and have a lower BMI. The best way for a child to lose weight is to eat three nutritious meals a day, keep snacking to a minimum, and get at least 60 minutes of physical activity daily. And of course, it always helps to serve as a good example by living a healthy lifestyle yourself.

Getting Your Kids Moving

Kids love to play, indoors or out, and all that "playing" is really just exercise. You don't need to spend money on kiddie yoga classes or get your child a membership at a gym with pint-sized leg-press machines. (We think these activities are fine but hardly necessary.) Running around, climbing, kicking a soccer ball, skipping, dancing, running through the sprinklers, swimming at the community pool — all these activities count.

What matters most is your own attitude. Kids get cues from their parents, so if *you* think of exercise as drudgery and present exercise to your kids in this light, you'll likely turn off their natural desire to be highly active. But if you get jazzed for the nightly after-dinner family walk or weekly Sunday morning family bike ride, your kids will, too.

Aim to get outside with your kids every day, for more than a few minutes. This can be a challenge, especially if you've commuted home from an exhausting day of work. And of course, gone are the days when kids could race out of the back door and roam the neighborhood unsupervised from dawn until dusk. With kids of our own, we recognize that keeping children moving is more complicated and challenging than it used to be. Often, you must stop what you're doing and somehow create the activity or shell out some cash for the activity to take place.

Still, it's important to make the effort. Shooting hoops with your kids in the driveway or going for a bike ride before dinner is a wonderful way to get to know and connect with your child. In the process, you'll turn your child on to the routine of regular exercise. Who knows, you may get yourself into shape as part of the bargain as well! The following sections present more tips for getting kids of all ages excited to move.

Engaging the toddler and preschool set

Getting your little ones outdoors is like getting a bird to fly — it's just so natural that many kids wouldn't dream of not doing it. Yet a preschooler who is used to spending most of the day watching TV may think the outdoors is a foreign country, where she doesn't dare venture.

According to the Nielsen Company, children ages 2 to 5 spend 32 hours a week in front of a TV, watching television, DVDs, or using a game console. University of Michigan researchers found that just being awake and in the room with the TV on more than two hours a day is a risk factor for being overweight at ages 3 and 4½.

Here's how you can change your child's habits:

- ✔ Play soccer, Wiffle ball, and kickball with her.

- ✔ Take your child to the park to climb up the slides and climbing walls, explore the jungle gyms, and try out the monkey bars.

- ✔ Lead her in a game of red light/green light, Simon says, or monkey tail (shove a shirt in your pants so it hangs down like a tail, and have your child chase your tail; then switch so you chase her tail).

- ✔ Introduce her to hopscotch (buy some sidewalk chalk).

- ✔ Get her a tricycle or Strider PREbike. *Striders* (also known as LIKEaBIKEs) are small bikes without pedals — your tyke pushes along with her feet on the ground, learning to balance and coast downhill. Age 2½ is a great time to start on a Strider; chances are, your child will graduate to a pedal bike without ever having used training wheels.

- ✔ Take adventure walks in the woods or in the neighborhood.

- ✔ Set up a blow-up swimming pool or sprinklers in the yard when it's hot. Suzanne's 3-year-old twins love nothing more than chasing each other in and out of their $15 pool.

- ✔ Put on some danceable music and cut a rug with your child.

- ✔ Alternate 10 minutes of power walking with your toddler in the jog stroller with 5 minutes of strolling hand in hand with your child so that you both get a workout.

Motivating school-age kids to move

When kids enter school, they're often less active than they were previously because they spend more time sitting at a desk and more time in sedentary pursuits like watching TV, playing video games, and texting. Here are some ways to get your school-age kids more active.

Get the rest of the family involved

Make physical activity a family policy. You may have to make exercise mandatory and the Xbox a privilege, but after kids get rolling, they won't fight it anymore.

Plan new traditions. Is Saturday morning a time for sausage and pancakes? What about replacing that with a brisk walk to the local coffee shop or a bike ride around town? Instead of focusing birthdays around cake and ice cream, come up with active traditions (of course, you can still have the cake and ice cream). Instead of spending Thanksgiving or Christmas Day making cookies, eating candy, and lying on the couch watching TV, start a tradition of sledding or a pickup basketball game or ping-pong tournament. Although you may not be able to pull your family away from the traditional Thanksgiving football game, you may be able to get your kids to toss a football around with you during halftime.

Encourage participation in sports and activities

Encourage your children's participation in school, church, and community sports teams by attending as many events as possible, giving rides to and from practices, and so on.

Put fun first so kids don't feel judged by their sports performance. Instead of incessantly correcting their form or praising them for their skill on the soccer field, let them find their groove and focus on the great time they're having out there. You don't want your children to feel they have to perform well in order to please you. "Kids get a message early on that they are measured and judged by what they accomplish, so many develop an aversion to competition," says former pro triathlete Brad Kearns, a California dad of two and founder of the nonprofit Running School (www.runningschool.org), devoted to promoting cardio fitness for kids.

If your child loses interest in a particular sport or decides to try a variety of activities, allow her to enjoy that process, because along the way, she'll develop lifelong friendships and internalize valuable lessons about teamwork and etiquette. Very few kids who are forced into one particular sport stick with it very long. No matter how badly you want your child to be the next city swim champ or earn a sports scholarship to college, no amount of cajoling, pressuring, or forcing your teen through extra workouts will make that happen.

If your child opts out of school sports completely, try engaging him in a physical activity that appeals to both of you, whether it's inline skating, yoga, or cycling, and focus on having fun together. Let your child choose an activity, and go along for the ride — but have some suggestions in mind so that you don't spend half an hour trying to decide how to spend your half-hour activity time together.

Opt for active gaming

If your kid is a gamer, consider an active game like Wii Fit or Dance Dance Revolution. These games burn calories and develop coordination while providing plenty of fun and entertainment. Kids will spend hours mastering all the moves to the latest hip-hop video without once thinking they're getting a workout.

Don't rely on game consoles for all your child's physical activities. Active games may be an ideal choice for a rainy day, for when you don't have time to drive to the nearest recreation site, or for when you don't have time to spend exercising with them. Of course, if you've ever tried DDR you know how engrossing and challenging it can be. Even the lowest setting can quite literally trip up anyone over the age of 30!

Limit screen time

Today, kids ages 8 to 18 devote on average 7 hours and 38 minutes a day to using entertainment media — that's more than 53 hours a week! (And the number doesn't count the hour and a half that middle-schoolers and high-schoolers spend texting.) Kids ages 6 to 11 spend about 28 hours a week in front of the TV alone, twice as much as the maximum of 2 hours a day recommended by the American Academy of Pediatrics. In 51 percent of households, the TV is on "most" of the time.

Even good, educational shows replace physical activity in your child's life. While watching TV, the metabolic rate seems to go even lower than during rest, which means that a person would burn fewer calories while watching TV than when just sitting quietly, doing nothing. Plus, as kids sit staring at the screen, they're exposed to an endless parade of ads for chips, cookies, candy, and other junk food. In a Mayo Clinic study, kids who traded sedentary screen time for active screen time (such as playing games like the Wii Fit or Dance Dance Revolution) more than doubled their energy expenditure.

Set limits on screen time. Don't put a television in your children's bedrooms, and keep the computer in a family area. Only about 30 percent of kids say they have rules about how much time they can spend watching TV, playing video games, or using the computer. But when parents do set limits, research shows, children spend a whopping 3 fewer hours *per day* in front of a screen.

Spending hours in front of the TV is often a habit that can be broken more easily than you think, and your kids will follow your lead. Watching TV and playing video games is fun — no doubt about it — but so is playing a game of pickup basketball, taking a walk through town, playing touch football, and riding bikes.

Getting Kids to Eat Their Peas

Here's a sobering statistic: Snacking on junk food now accounts for more than 27 percent of children's daily calorie intake. Many parents believe that unless they offer their kids all the hot dogs, Teddy Grahams, and Goldfish crackers they want, their children will go hungry. Not true!

Given exposure and access to healthy foods and role modeling from Mom and Dad, most kids will snack on apples and peanut butter, nuts and raisins, even baby carrots and hummus. When you stock your fridge and cupboards with healthy, tasty foods — and eat them yourself — your child's acquired taste for fried foods and sugars will disappear.

Getting kids involved in meal-planning, shopping, and cooking makes them more likely to eat healthy foods and prepares them to make healthy food choices in the future. Here are some ways to get your children engaged:

- ✔ **Make healthy foods fun.** Have your kids layer fruit-and-yogurt parfaits, blend smoothies, or assemble mini-pizzas with English muffins, tomato sauce, veggies, and shredded cheese. Or do a sound test: Everyone closes his or her eyes; have your child sample baby carrots, sugar snap peas, and jicama slices and decide which makes the loudest crunch.

- ✔ **Offer choices — but not too many.** Ask, "Do you want yellow squash or zucchini?" or "Do you want your carrots crunchy and cold or soft and cooked?" Start by offering more foods that you know she likes and fewer new foods, and gradually reverse the ratio. Don't offer a different meal if she rejects what is served; you're not a short-order cook!

- ✔ **Give your kids a say in meal planning.** Institute a weekly vote night to come up with a shopping list, meal choices, and snacks. Ask, "Should we use the Crock-Pot this week?" or "What veggies should we have for dinner?"

- ✔ **Take your kids to the supermarket and involve them in the shopping.** Teach your children to dissect a cereal label to find high-fiber cereals. Shop your local farmer's market and let your child pick out the strawberries.

- ✔ **Let your children help in the kitchen.** Yes, it takes patience on your part and it requires more time and cleanup, but kids are more likely to eat food they've helped prepare. Even toddlers can help by, for example, stirring ingredients, tearing lettuce, shutting the microwave door, and dumping a tablespoon of olive oil or a cup of chopped veggies into a salad.

Following are tips for dealing with kids who are staging a vegetable strike or snubbing all food groups that aren't mac-and-cheese:

- ✔ **Practice what you preach.** If you're snacking on corn chips and drinking soda, you can't expect your kid to munch on cucumbers and drink milk.

- ✔ **Be persistent.** Keep offering healthy foods. You may need to put cucumbers on a plate 10 or 15 times before a child will eat it. Research shows that children like what they know and that the more often they're offered unfamiliar foods such as red peppers, the more they like and eat them.

- ✔ **Don't bribe your child with treats.** "If you eat your spinach, you can have ice cream" only makes spinach seem like a third-class citizen. And avoid using food as a reward. Don't promise a cookie tomorrow for going to bed on time tonight. Instead, reward him with special time with Mommy or a movie he can earn points toward.

✔ **Use the word *treat* instead of *dessert*.** That way, your child doesn't expect every meal to end with sweets.

✔ **Try the stealth route.** Add veggie puree to spaghetti sauce that your child likes. Eventually reveal that he's eaten the veggie and survived. Gradually make the puree chunkier.

✔ **Don't keep sweetened drinks, such as sodas, punches, and sports drinks, in the house.** Limit your child's juice intake to about 4 ounces a day.

Chapter 24

Staying Active as You Age

. . . .

In This Chapter

▶ Getting a later start with exercise

▶ Adjusting your longtime workout program as you get grayer

▶ Using some caution as you exercise

. . . .

*B*eing lumped into the "senior" or "older adult" category is unavoidable: Four months before your 50th birthday, that invitation for AARP is coming in the mail. Nonetheless, there's a big difference between being a fit older adult and a not-so-fit older adult. Staying fit as you age gives you the freedom to enjoy your life to the fullest — to keep up with your kids and grandkids, maintain an active life and sharp wit, feel youthful, and dramatically lower your risk of developing serious diseases. While many people focus on saving money for retirement, investing in mutual funds and savings bonds, they forget to invest in their health and fitness; they may wind up with the financial means to explore the world and take up new hobbies but not the drive, the mental quickness, or the physical wherewithal.

In this chapter, we explain why physical fitness is every bit as important as fiscal fitness as you age. If you're getting a late start on exercise, we offer tips to help you get started safely. If you've already been exercising, we give you advice on how to reset your routine and rethink your goals. Though after you hit the age of 50 you can still accomplish great physical feats, you sometimes need to give your body a little TLC to ensure you don't get sidelined by injury or get discouraged by trying to do too much. We want to make sure your workouts are successful no matter how many candles are on your next birthday cake.

Getting a Late Start: How to Begin

Even if you've never owned a gym membership or a pair of sneakers, it's never too late to begin exercising. Studies show that people of any age can benefit from getting in shape. Exercise substantially reduces your risk of developing heart disease, arthritis, colon cancer, Alzheimer's disease, lower-back pain, depression, and loss of independence. If you saw a pharmaceutical advertisement that listed even half of those benefits, you'd be lining up at your doctor's office for a prescription. So here's your exercise Rx.

Seeing your doctor for a checkup

Getting a checkup is especially important if it's been a while since your last doctor's visit, if you're overweight or have specific health issues, if you're taking any medications, or if you have chronic joint problems such as achy knees or a bad back. Your doctor can discuss limitations with you and a good starting strategy and may be able to refer you to an appropriate health club and/or a personal trainer who specializes in working with older exercisers.

Your doctor may even write a prescription for physical therapy (PT). A physical therapist is trained to help you correct muscle imbalances, rehabilitate injuries, and move correctly. In fact, if you start exercising and find yourself struggling, go back to your doctor and request a prescription for physical therapy. In most states, PT is covered by insurance for at least several sessions and can be just what you need to get your program off on the right foot.

Starting cardio exercise

Be sure to proceed slowly when you start cardiovascular exercise (in Part II, we explain what counts as cardio and how to get started). No one, regardless of age, should start his first treadmill workout at an all-out sprint, but this is especially true if you're now sporting a few wrinkles. Try 10 minutes the first day, and if that goes well, do 10 minutes the next day, too. Gradually increase your workouts by no more than 5 percent (in terms of time or mileage) a week. Pay attention to what your body is telling you. If you feel a lot of creaking and groaning in your joints or if your heart and lungs have trouble keeping up, back off and wait for your body to catch up. Chances are you'll progress more slowly than someone younger, but you will progress.

Consider joint-friendly activities. Perhaps this is not the time to start with kickboxing or jump rope. Many older newbies do best with walking, the elliptical machine, a stationary bike, or swimming. These activities allow your heart and lungs to build stamina without making your body ache quite so much.

Pumping some iron

By age 50, most people have lost a lot of muscle and bone mass. You need strong muscles to prevent injury, to continue standing up straight, and to maintain the strength required to do day-to-day stuff, like carrying in your groceries and unscrewing the cap of a childproof bottle of pain reliever.

If you've never lifted weights before, consider hiring a trainer (see Chapter 20 for tips) or at least purchasing a how-to DVD or visiting "the YouTube" your grandkids are so fond of. It's fine to start with either free weights or machines; just go easy on the weight. Know that you won't progress as quickly as someone younger, and though you can gain every bit as much strength percentage-wise, you may not see as much tone. As you age, less of your strength gains will come from increases in muscle mass, and more will come from improved wiring between your brain and your muscles and joints.

Concentrate on going through the full range of motion for each exercise so you take full advantage of improved strength and flexibility you can gain. Start with seated versions of moves, which require less balance and coordination than standing versions, until you build up your strength and confidence. For more info on strength training, see Part III.

Working on your flexibility and balance

Each year, one in four people over age 65 experiences a serious fall, which can lead to an injury that limits your mobility, sometimes permanently. As we explain in Chapters 14 and 15, developing both flexibility and balance reduces your chances of falling and makes you more likely to catch yourself if you do fall.

If you've never worked on flexibility, you're likely to find this area of fitness to be challenging, but you'll also notice dramatic improvements. Consider joining a beginner's yoga, stretch, or a tai chi class. Or look for a class that specializes in seated stretches so you don't have to stand for too long or keep getting up and down off the floor (something that's hard to do when you lack strength and flexibility). If you're stretching on your own, start with seated versions or hold on to a chair or a wall for support.

Like the younger set, you should always warm up before you stretch. If you're especially inflexible, add an extra few minutes of warm-up to ensure good blood flow and pliability. Stretch every single day, even twice a day.

If you have extra income, consider having a trainer lead you in a stretching session. It will make you feel great and teach you a lot. Also consider taking up meditation, which puts you in a relaxed state of mind; this, in turn, can prime your muscles to be more receptive to stretching. Plus it's soooo relaxing.

We think people of all ages should be doing balance exercises, but it's tough to convince a 20-year-old that it's worth the time. When your first forehead wrinkle hasn't even shown up, you don't really believe that by age 60, you may no longer bound down a flight of stairs two at a time without the risk of falling flat on your face. Older exercisers tend to take the advice more seriously. The good news about balance is that it's a skill, and like any skill, it can be improved with practice. In Chapter 15, we present a progression of balance exercises that are ideal for seniors.

Finding a senior-friendly gym

You won't find many seniors-only gyms, but with a little effort, you can likely find a gym that suits you well. Chapter 18 is all about finding the right gym, so if you're interested in joining a club, peruse that chapter. Curves clubs are especially popular with female seniors. When visiting other local gyms, ask the following questions:

✔ **Does anyone on staff carry a senior-fitness certification or other designation?** Several of the governing bodies that certify personal trainers (see Chapter 20) offer training in senior fitness, and you want to have access to a trainer who has taken advantage of these educational opportunities.

✔ **Do any of your classes specialize in senior fitness?** From water aerobics to Pilates,

yoga to marathon-training groups, some health clubs offer special classes and group activities for seniors. If your local gym doesn't offer senior classes, check with your local YMCA, community health program, running or walking specialty store, and local churches.

✔ **Do you offer senior discounts?** Hey, if you're paying 25 percent less for a movie, you should also get a discount on your gym membership, right? Don't be shy about asking for discounts. They may not be advertised, but if you ask, you may just receive a substantial discount on your membership fee.

Adjusting Your Program if You're an Experienced Older Athlete

Sports headlines still express surprise whenever anyone over the age of 30 manages to win an important bike race, cross the finish line of a marathon, or make it on to an Olympic team. But the truth is, older athletes, both the professionals and those who simply exercise for the pleasure of staying in shape, are becoming smarter about how they train their bodies. Today's veteran athlete has access to more supportive shoes, more ergonomically designed equipment, better protective gear, and solid, research-based training advice on how to prevent injury, eat for peak performance, and pack more quality training into less time.

What's more, many experienced athletes have been training since youth, so they're in tune with how their bodies should feel. For example, a seasoned 50+ runner knows the difference between a tweaked knee that should be rested for a few days and one that's simply a little sore from running extra hills. And regular exercise can certainly slow the aging process vastly.

That said, athletes in aging bodies, no matter how experienced, still need to treat their bodies differently than their younger counterparts. As you get older, you don't snap back quite as quickly from hard workouts or injuries, and you can't race as hard or as often as you used to. This is because — even in the best-case scenario — you lose muscle mass, your bones thin out, your hormone levels change, you gain fat, and your tendons shorten so you lose flexibility. So it makes sense that you may have to rethink your training priorities and your goals.

Here are some considerations for adjusting your fitness program:

- ✔ **Cardio exercise and competition:** The good news is that slow-twitch muscle fiber, the kind used for endurance, doesn't decline until you're in the age range of the average *60 Minutes* host. With training you can even continue to make gains in this type of fiber well into your sixties. If you've been racing sprints, you might consider moving up your distances as you age, since your speed will inevitably decline, up to about 7 percent per decade after age 30.

  Older athletes routinely win endurance events. It's not uncommon to see a competitor over 40 break the tape of a major marathon. Ultra-endurance races are routinely won by older women. (In extreme endurance races, women's higher body-fat percentage becomes a slight advantage; at mega distances, women have a few other advantages, too.) Even if you have no intention of going past the 5K mark, many competitions — walking, running, cycling, swimming, and skating — hand out age-group prizes, so you can compete against people your own age instead of having to be lumped in with the whippersnappers.

  Listen closely to your body, which may get tired more easily and require more rest days or shorter or less intense workouts. Consider a cross-training routine, if you haven't in the past, to help keep your body sharp.

- ✔ **Strength:** If you didn't spend much time in the weight room during your younger days, head there now. Stronger muscles not only help preserve your joints and prevent injury, they also help you maintain balance, coordination, bone density, and a healthy ratio of muscle to fat. You'll also stand up straighter, have better posture, and look more youthful.

  If you're an old-time lifter, be sure to add one or two warm-up sets into the equation to ensure your muscles are ready to move in the right pathways. As you age, your muscles are a bit slower to react. Warm-up sets help you avoid injury and post-workout achiness. Be sure to give extra attention to the joints that tend to fail as people age and become prone to arthritis. Add extra sets for your thigh muscles (to protect your knees), your glutes (to protect your hips), your core (to protect your spine), and your shoulder muscles (to protect your shoulder joints). Make sure to do "functional" type exercises that mimic and support activities you do every day so you don't lose the ability to do them.

- ✔ **Flexibility:** Maybe you're accustomed to doing your cardio and then hitting the showers, never spending a single minute on stretching. As you get older, this is a habit to reconsider if you want to keep active. Having flexibility will keep your movements more fluid. So if you're a runner, you'll still be able to stretch out your legs and maintain a normal-length stride rather than do the tight little shuffle recognizable in some older runners.

Yoga is an excellent activity to add to your repertoire, especially if you find you don't have the springiness you used to. Consider taking a class that combines flexibility, balance, and agility, three skills that often require attention as the years click by. Look for classes with names such as On the Ball or Get in Balance; read the class descriptions, because names vary. Your gym may offer 15-minute stretch classes, a good entry point. You can find loads of worthwhile DVDs for "inflexible stretchers."

Exercising your brain

Exercise is so good for your brain that it almost makes the advantages to the heart, lungs, and muscles seem secondary. The brain uses the oxygen that is delivered through the bloodstream to fuel its various functions. During a session of cardiovascular exercise, such as running, swimming, or cycling, blood circulation speeds up and your lungs soak up a higher volume of oxygen from the air, which allows them to deliver significantly more oxygen to your brain. Working out on a regular basis improves blood flow all the time so the brain constantly receives more blood and oxygen. Research shows that exercise is one of the few activities that actually results in the adult brain growing new connections, and exercise has been shown to be more effective at keeping your brain young than expensive brain-training games.

Even if you don't begin exercising until middle age, you can significantly reduce your risk of memory faliure and Alzheimer's disease. Researchers at the University of Washington found, for instance, that seniors who exercised at least three times a week diminished their risk of dementia by up to 32 percent. Also, by improving cardiovascular health, exercise prevents heart attacks and strokes, which are a common cause of brain damage.

How much exercise you need to keep your brain fit isn't clear, but some researchers speculate that working out three times a week for 30 minutes will deliver significant benefits. And by "exercise," we mean any physical activity, so walking the dog and painting the house count every bit as much as a machine circuit at the gym or a jog around the neighborhood.

Part VII
The Part of Tens

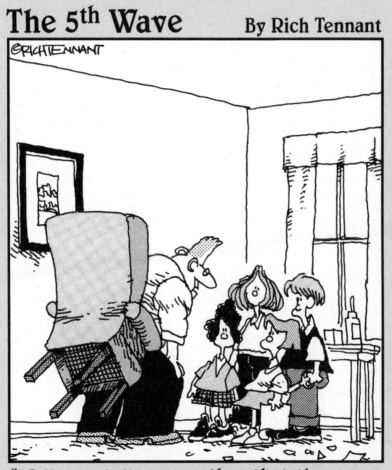

The 5th Wave   By Rich Tennant

"Well, you tell your mother that there are no indications that I need to lose weight."

In this part . . .

We carry on the *For Dummies* tradition of grouping key information in fun, easy-to-skim lists of ten. Just in case you're not sure why exercise is worth your time, Chapter 25 presents ten (well, actually far more than ten) reasons to break a sweat, and Chapter 26 fills you in on the best ways to spend your fitness dollars.

Chapter 25

Ten Great Reasons
to Break a Sweat

*Y*ou already know that exercise is important; otherwise, you would have spent your money on Oreos instead of this book. But when you start a workout program, it's always helpful to remind yourself why you're investing this effort — why you're hoisting hunks of steel instead of soda cans, why you're huffing and puffing when you could be sinking into your sofa, why you're creating more laundry for yourself by sweating up your gym clothes.

Even if you're already a committed exerciser, you probably have moments when your best intentions are stifled by excuses not to work out. You're too tired or too busy, or the dog ate your treadmill — we've heard 'em all (and used a few ourselves). Any time you experience one of these moments, flip to this chapter. Better yet, make a copy and tape it to your fridge. One glance at this list will snap you right out of your funk. Here are ten great reasons to work out.

You're Less Prone to Illness

The health advantages of exercise are reason enough to lace up your shoes and head out the door. For instance, working out lowers your risk of coronary heart disease — America's number-one killer — and you're less likely to have high blood pressure or a stroke. Research also suggests that staying active helps prevent cancers of the prostate, breast, colon, lung, and uterine lining.

In fact, you'll probably live longer. Highly active people live about 3.5 years longer than inactive people. Here's another way of putting it: People who are physically active for about 7 hours a week have a 40 percent lower risk of dying early than those who are active for less than 30 minutes a week.

Not only do you increase your lifespan, but you also improve your quality of life. By exercising, you can avoid osteoporosis, you're less likely to become diabetic, you're less likely to need gallbladder surgery, and you'll have fewer colds, because moderate exercise strengthens your immune system. Exercise is good for the mind, too. In fact, exercise may be the single most important way to prevent memory loss and dementia into old age.

You Keep Your Weight in Check

Eating less is the key to losing weight, but exercise is critical to keeping the pounds off. Plus, working out helps ensure that you're losing primarily fat rather than muscle. Check out the other weight-related benefits of exercise:

- ✔ **You keep your metabolism humming.** For every pound of muscle you pack on, your body burns an extra 10 to 15 calories per day — not a huge figure, but perhaps enough to help prevent weight gain as you age.

- ✔ **You can eat more without gaining weight.** When you burn an extra 2,000 calories a week on the elliptical, you can afford to indulge in that extra helping of Thanksgiving stuffing.

- ✔ **You have dramatically fewer medical problems.** You can reap many health benefits — including a lower risk of diabetes, high blood pressure, and heart disease — simply by losing weight, regardless of how much you exercise.

- ✔ **You can minimize, or even prevent, weight gain related to quitting smoking.** Most smokers gain 5 to 10 pounds when they kick the habit, partly because nicotine speeds up metabolism and suppresses appetite. But working out can counteract this tendency to gain weight by burning calories and reducing stress.

You Look Marvelous

Were you the nerd in high school everyone ignored? Were you the captain of the Latin club and second tuba in the marching band? Well, get on a fitness program and *you'll* be the popular one at your next high-school reunion. Though no amount of exercise can transform John Goodman into David Beckham, with the right workout program, you can shape a rounder derriere, firm up your arms, tone your legs, and thin out the jiggly layer obscuring these muscles. Say *au revoir* to speed-bag arm fat, cankles, or overbaked-bread fat hanging out of your bra. Firming up and losing weight through exercise means you'll look better in sleeveless shirts and short shorts. Long shorts, too. You can take your new body into any clothing store that your budget can handle.

You're Less Prone to Injuries and Aches

Exercisers simply feel better than people who sit on their duff. This applies even to folks with arthritis, back pain, and other conditions that may seem to preclude exercise. Here are several ways that exercise can help you prevent or cope with life's aches and pains:

- **You're less likely to injure your muscles or joints.** When your muscles are strong and flexible, they offer more support to your bones and joints. So, you're less apt to twist an ankle stepping off a curb or tweak your elbow by carrying a heavy briefcase. And when you join an impromptu game of ultimate Frisbee, you can avoid that nasty hamstring pull or sore shoulder that sends you back to the couch with a bag of ice.

- **You can relieve arthritis pain.** Not only can arthritis patients safely participate in exercise programs, but they're also rewarded for their efforts with pain relief and increased mobility.

- **You're less likely to get a stress fracture.** A study of military recruits found that those with below-average leg strength were five times likelier to develop *stress fractures* (tiny bone fractures) and other overuse injuries during nine weeks of basic training.

- **You're less susceptible to carpal tunnel syndrome.** Strong wrist and arm muscles help protect against this condition, common among folks who do repetitive-motion tasks such as typing and scanning items at the grocery checkout stand.

- **You're likely to recover faster from an accident.** If, heaven forbid, you get into a car wreck or other serious accident, your fitness will serve you well. Frail and weak people have lower survival rates and take longer to recover.

We know a woman who was in her mid-60s when she got hit by a car while riding her bike in Nebraska. Though she broke her pelvis and numerous other bones and suffered severe internal injuries, she recovered extremely well and went on to ride her bike across Nebraska. Her doctors said that had she not been so fit at the time of the accident, she likely would not have survived her injuries.

✔ **You lessen the symptoms of PMS.** Exercise may reduce the bloating, lower-back pain, headaches, and anxiety that often accompany premenstrual syndrome. And regular exercisers may be less likely to experience PMS in the first place.

✔ **You can ease the pain of varicose veins.** The walls of varicose veins have been stretched, allowing blood to pool in the legs. Exercise helps relieve the resulting swelling and aching because the contraction of calf muscles causes blood to shoot upward.

✔ **You can ease or avoid lower-back pain.** People who strengthen their abdominal and lower-back muscles are less likely to utter the words, "Oh, my aching back." In one study, most of the back-pain patients who had been recommended for spinal surgery by a physician were able to avoid surgery by following an aggressive strengthening program. Sixteen months after completing the exercise program, only 3 of the 38 patients required surgery.

You Feel Happier, Calmer, and Better about Yourself

A truckload of research shows that you have a better sense of well-being, also known as *runner's high,* following a workout. Both cardio and weight-training sessions seem to offer this boost, as well as a number of other psychological benefits:

✔ **You experience less stress.** More than 150 studies prove it: Regular exercise makes you less tense. Activities such as yoga and Pilates provide the perfect antidote to life in the era of constant texting, Tweeting, managing call-waiting interruptions on your cell — or doing all these at once.

✔ **You may become less depressed.** Research clearly shows that exercise can help clinically depressed men and women of all ages. A review of 80 studies found that depression appears to diminish after 4 weeks of regular exercise; the greatest improvements were found after 17 weeks.

✔ **You gain confidence that spills over to the rest of your life.** The sense of accomplishment that comes from being able to run 2 miles just may give you the self-assurance to make that presentation to your most important client or to ask that cute bank teller out on a date.

We know a 26-year-old schoolteacher who joined a health club, lost 85 pounds, and went from being painfully shy to having, in her words, a "bubbly personality" and taking up belly dancing.

✔ **You won't have to count sheep.** After a 12-week cardio and strength-training regimen, research subjects reported falling asleep faster and sleeping longer than before they'd started exercising, probably because of hormonal changes. Sedentary folks who start exercising regularly boost the amount of time spent in *slow-wave sleep,* the phase of sleep believed to be the most restorative. They also report waking up less often during the night.

✔ **You have a healthy outlet for your anger.** Instead of yelling at your boss, you can get your aggressions out during a kickboxing class — burning calories and improving your health at the same time.

✔ **You're more likely to visit a nude beach.** Okay, maybe not, but research does show that exercisers report having more confidence about their body than sedentary people do.

You Enjoy Camaraderie

Getting into a new fitness activity is a great way to widen your social circle. When you join a gym, a hiking club, or a softball team, you meet interesting people of all ages and from all walks of life whom you may not have had the pleasure of knowing otherwise.

Joining a group fitness activity also boosts your chances of finding a mate and can be a lot more fun than the bar scene or Internet dating. Suzanne once quit her job and signed up for a cross-country bicycle tour, where she was swept away by a fellow cyclist. Things went bust after three years, but it was a heck-uva ride while it lasted. (In fairness, Suzanne met her husband on an Internet dating site, so she doesn't like to make generalizations.)

Going for a bike ride or a walk with people you already know — a friend, a co-worker, your spouse — is a good way to catch up on the latest gossip, weigh in on the day's news, and stay current with each other's families, friends, and pets.

You Perform Better at Work and at Home

Whether you're a massage therapist, a trial attorney, a trombone player, or a stay-at-home mom chasing triplet toddlers, you'll benefit from the increased energy, concentration, and stamina that you get from regular exercise. Here's how:

✔ **You improve your memory.** In a six-month study of previously sedentary men and women ages 60 to 75, those who walked three times a week scored 25 percent better on memory and judgment tasks, such as recalling schedules and quickly differentiating between vowels and consonants and odd and even numbers.

✔ **You're more creative.** In one study, subjects who did aerobic exercise scored higher on creative thinking tests than did subjects who watched a video.

An artist we know in Hawaii joined a gym because she was overweight and borderline diabetic; the surprise bonus was that she became a better artist. "I have more clarity and stamina to paint, and my paintings are more free," she told us. "When your body is feeling good, more ideas come through."

✔ **You're more useful around the house.** You don't need help unscrewing that stubborn jar of pickles, hoisting that 10-gallon jug of water, or pulling apart the sofa bed for your houseguests. You can get all your errands done in one shot because you don't need to take a rest break.

✔ **You can better cope with shift work.** Working the graveyard shift at 7-Eleven? Swing-shift on patrol? Exercise can help temper the health problems, including sleep disorders, common to people whose work shifts toy with the body's natural rhythms.

✔ **You master the art of teamwork.** When you join a basketball league, cycling club, or walking group, you bond with your teammates and find out what it takes to play nicely with others. These skills may come in handy at the next office conference, PTA meeting, or neighborhood-watch meeting.

✔ **You have more job opportunities**. You can't be a firefighter, a police officer, or a lifeguard if you flunk the physical. And if you have your sights set on being a bouncer, big, strong muscles are pretty much a prerequisite.

Your Family Benefits

When you exercise, you have more options for family togetherness. Sure, you can all sit in the living room and watch *American Idol,* but a fit family can also shoot hoops on the driveway, go for a stroll in the neighborhood, or get in fun snowball fights. When you exercise, here's how you and your family benefit:

✔ **You set a good example for your kids.** Want your kids to grow up healthy and strong? You can be a great role model by exercising regularly.

When Liz's daughter, Skylar, was a baby, Liz would take her for runs in the stroller. One day, when Skylar was 2, she asked if she could get out and run with her mom. It was a proud moment for Liz. Skylar is now the only 4-year-old in her gymnastics class who can do push-ups with proper form. It's obvious Liz's love of exercise has been transferred to her daughter. Being an exercise role model is especially important in an era in which childhood obesity is at an all-time high. In Chapter 23, we detail the ways in which tots, tweens, and teens benefit from exercising.

✔ **You have more confidence if you're a new father.** In a study of 87 new dads, those who exercised expressed more confidence in their new role than fathers who didn't work out. Although studies haven't yet focused on new mothers, we suspect the benefits apply to mom, too.

✔ **You can keep up with your grandkids.** Wouldn't it be nice to kick around a soccer ball with your granddaughter without getting winded? Regular workouts can give you the strength and stamina to chase her around at the park and follow her as she learns to pedal her bike without training wheels.

✔ **Your pet can get in shape.** More than 50 percent of American dogs are overweight, including 25 percent who are considered obese. If you can't fit into your pants and your pooch can't fit into her collar, taking longer and more frequent walks will boost the odds the both of you live a long, healthy life.

You Feel Younger and Enjoy Life More

At all ages and stages, life is simply more fun when you're fit. Check out these additional benefits to working out:

✔ **You have more energy.** People who complain that they don't have enough energy to exercise don't realize that working out actually gives you energy. In one study, middle-aged women who lifted weights for a year became 27 percent more active in daily life than before.

✔ **You bounce back from childbirth more quickly.** Not only do active women have a lower risk of postpartum depression, but they also tend to get back in the swing of things faster. When Mom is happier and feeling good, she's better able to cope with the middle-of-the-night scream-a-thons and the mounting piles of laundry and enjoy those precious early months.

✔ **You stay lithe and limber.** As little as 5 minutes of stretching a day helps keep your muscles mobile and helps you stay agile.

✔ **Your balance improves.** In just three months, 80-year-olds who performed balance exercises — like walking a straight line and standing on one foot — gained the level of body control typical of people three to ten years younger.

✔ **You enjoy retirement more.** Not that we don't love Scrabble and gin rummy, but fit seniors have more activity choices, from golf to gardening to world travel.

One retired professor told us that during her work years, she paid close attention to the seniors she met on her travels, noticing that some were up to the task and others were not because they had not taken care of their bodies. She made a point of walking and strength training and at age 61 was fit enough to climb Peru's Machu Picchu, a grueling trek at any age. She can outrun her husband and feels she has more stamina now than she did at 30.

You Do Good for Others and the Earth

Getting involved in fitness activities provides endless opportunities to support great causes, like finding a cure for leukemia, multiple sclerosis, or breast cancer. Nationwide, thousands of athletic events raise money for important medical research. You can run, walk, bike, swim, even snowshoe — all in the name of having fun and saving lives.

While you're at it, you can help save the earth, too. Leaving your car in the garage for short trips and hoofing it instead makes good environmental sense. Driving just 2 miles spews out 1 kilogram of air-choking carbon dioxide into the atmosphere. Walking the same distance instead burns about 150 calories and adds no carbon to the atmosphere.

Dropping a pants size is not only one of the best things you can do for your personal health, it's also one of the most effective ways to help stop global warming and the overuse of precious resources. Experts estimate that overweight individuals eat about 40 percent more calories than their lean counterparts. Because food production accounts for more than 20 percent of greenhouse gas emissions, a heavy population has a significantly heftier carbon footprint than a lighter one. Fats, red meat, and refined sugars, which tend to dominate the unhealthiest of Western diets, are particularly carbon-offensive. Greater food consumption also means more organic waste, which produces the pollutant methane as it decomposes.

Chapter 26

Ten Fantastic Fitness Investments

*M*odel boat builders require glue, tweezers, and a magnifying glass to create their mini-masterpieces. Bird watchers require an identification book, a field journal, and binoculars to identify an ivory-billed woodpecker. So it goes with fitness enthusiasts — you don't have to spend a ton, and you really don't have to go much beyond the basics, but you may want to invest in some gear and a few gadgets to boost the fun factor or give yourself a bit of an edge. We're all for that! But if you're going to part with your hard-earned cash, we think you should get your money's worth. The "stuff" in this chapter is all good stuff, and happily, nothing here will break the bank.

A Heart-Rate Monitor

With a heart-rate monitor strapped to your chest, you know how many times per minute your heart is beating, and this number provides concrete evidence that your body is becoming fitter. In Chapter 6, we explain several ways that you can use a monitor to gauge your progress. Wearing your monitor during a workout, for instance, helps ensure that you stay in your target zone.

Heart-rate monitors can be plain Jane, for about $30, or super fancy. The upscale models, which run as high as $400, offer features such as a clock, timer, calorie and mileage counter, and an alarm that you can set to beep when you wander out of your target zone. Many let you upload your information to a user site on the Web, where you can then get reports and feedback about your workouts. Some really high-tech monitors sync up with a chip in your shoe or movement sensors placed on an arm band, giving you highly accurate info on everything from body temperature to calorie count in addition, of course, to heart rate.

You can buy a monitor at a sporting-goods store or on the Web, either from a retailer or directly from the manufacturer. Polar is a well-established and respected brand, offering dozens of models to choose from, ranging from the economical to the extravagant; most heart-rate-compatible home and gym cardio machines read Polar monitors. Timex and Garmin also make excellent monitors and also have generous selections.

A Digital Tracker or Pedometer

Wearing a pedometer allows you to see how much movement you accumulate throughout the day and then inspires you to increase it.

Most pedometers, even the freebies you get for opening a bank account, are quite reliable. If you want to go hog-wild, you can spend $150 on a really fancy one that tells you, in a jaunty British accent, how far you've walked, communicates with your heart-rate monitor, and downloads your workout data into a log and analysis program. Some come with a built-in GPS, a body-fat analyzer, or a built-in MP3 player.

One device we like, the Bodybugg, goes far, far beyond counting steps. You wear it on your arm, and it measures everything from shifts of movement to changes in body temperature to give you a really accurate calorie burn count each day. Other close cousins to the pedometer include the Nike chip and the Adidas miCoach. These tiny devices are clipped to your shoe and keep track of steps, mileage, time, heart rate (tied into a heart-rate monitor), and more. All these run $150 to $300, but if you're dazzled by flashing lights and computerized reports, it's money well spent.

A Hydration System

You have two options for keeping water on your person: a water bottle or a hydration pack. We like stainless-steel bottles, which are resistant to rust and don't give you that metal aftertaste that aluminum bottles do. Get a sport cap that lets you drink straight from the lid. You don't want a bottle that you have to unscrew while you're bounding up a hill; very little will make it into your mouth. Metal sports bottles cost around $10. You can hold them in your hand, with or without a strap, or carry them in any number of hip holsters.

For long, outdoor workouts, like day hikes or lengthy bike rides, we recommend *hydration packs,* insulated pouches that you wear like a lightweight backpack or waist pack. You fill the pouch with water; to drink, you bite down on the end of a flexible tube that hangs over your shoulder or retracts from a waist pack. Hydration packs cost $30 to $100, depending on the brand, the size of the pouch, and the number of zipper pockets to store food, money, extra bike tubes, and so on. CamelBak, the company that pioneered these clever devices, offers an amazing selection, along with numerous eco-friendly water bottles.

A Stretching or Sticky Mat

A mat designed for stretching, yoga, or Pilates not only makes these activities more comfortable but also reminds you to do your exercises. For about $7, you can get a perfectly functional stretching mat made of flexible plastic. (The $7 ones are too stiff to roll up, but they fit pretty neatly in a closet or under a bed.) If you're willing to pay $30 to $100, you can get a mat that folds up and has a cloth covering.

If you do a lot of yoga or Pilates, try a "sticky" mat, which costs from $15 to $70. These mats are made of soft, thin plastic coated with a slightly sticky film that helps keep you steady during moves that require balance. At some yoga studios, you can rent a mat for a few bucks, but if you're a regular, we recommend bringing your own. Even the best studios don't wipe down the mats after every use.

Virtually any mat will get the job done, but we love the sturdy mats made by Lululemon and Gaiam, which come in a variety of gorgeous designs. Both companies offer mats made from recycled rubber and other sustainable materials. Airex makes thicker mats, which are too thick and unsteady for yoga but ideal if you prefer a lot of extra padding. You can purchase a mat at any sporting goods store, online fitness store, or discount retailer — even in the fitness section of the bookstore. Shop around for the best price. Liz recently was researching a recycled mat and found a $20 variance among sites.

A Physioball

Physioballs — also known as Swiss balls, stability balls, exercise balls, and Gymnic balls — are remarkably versatile. We mention the physioball, essentially a super-sturdy beach ball designed for exercise, in at least three other chapters in this book. You can kneel on a ball to improve your balance, lean back on it to do chest presses, or drape your back across it to stretch out your spine, to name just a few of the countless uses for a gadget.

Physioballs start at around $30. Balls that come in fancier colors or pretty designs or as part of a kit that includes a pump, an instructional DVD, and book can run you more than $100. (If you don't buy a kit, spring for the pump or make sure you already have a bike pump on hand; otherwise you may pass out blowing the thing up and never make it to the workout.) You can buy a ball from most sporting-goods stores, fitness-equipment Web sites, or even Amazon.com. We especially like the selection on Gaiam.com.

When buying a ball, size matters. Balls are typically categorized by the metric system and come in three main sizes:

- ✔ If you are shorter than 5'4", your ball should be 55 cm in diameter.
- ✔ If you're taller than 5'4" but shorter than 5'10", order a ball 65 cm in diameter.
- ✔ Anyone over 5'10" needs a 75-cm ball.

A Workout Log

A workout log (see Chapter 1) offers proof of your commitment to exercise, and seeing your accomplishments in writing — or typing! — is highly motivating.

A notebook from the drugstore will suffice, but we're partial to store-bought logs designed especially for the purpose of tracking daily workouts. They cost $10 to $15 and lend a sense of importance to what you're doing; many are filled with good training tips and inspirational quotes. It won't surprise you to learn that we recommend *The Ultimate Workout Log*, written by Suzanne and published by Houghton Mifflin Harcourt.

We also love online logs, many of which are free; you sign up for the Web site and you're good to go. You earn entry to some by buying one of their products: With the Adidas miCoach, you can upload all your walking and running mileage and data such as heart rate and speed from a chip in your shoe. Heck, if you want, you can plot your heart rate for every second of every workout for the last year. If the calculus of working out is exciting to you, the $100 to $400 will be a worthy investment.

An MP3 Player or iPhone

MP3 players have revolutionized the way people work out, offering an astonishing selection of content, and after you get past the cost of the initial device, cost is a relatively minor concern. Most gym cardio equipment and some home cardio machines come equipped with MP3 ports; you simply plug in your device and your show pops up on the display screen.

The iPod is the undisputed king of all MP3 players. We're especially big fans of podcasts and iTunes U (www.apple.com/education/itunes-u/). If you want to multitask your workout time by learning all you can about social media, you can click to the iPod section of iTunes and find dozens of excellent audio and video how-tos, lectures, and workshops. In fact, iTunes U includes lectures from top professors at Harvard, Columbia, Yale, Oxford, and Princeton. Oh, and did we mention they're all free?

If you own an iTouch, iPhone, or similar model, you can choose from among dozens of applications to help manage your health and fitness efforts. Everything from a workout log or exercise reminder service is available for little or no money. A basic MP3 player that plays music only can run as low as $40; you can spend nearly $400 for the most tricked-out iPod on the planet.

Exertainment

Exercise DVDs turn your TV into your most effective piece of workout gear. For less than $20 — sometimes less than $10 — you can get access to the world's best instructors and any type of class you can think of, from boot camp to yoga to hula hoop. Best of all, you work out in the comfort of your living room any time of the day or night. Series like the *10-Minute Solution* let you pop in one DVD for the week and do quick hits of exercise whenever you have a little free time. Many DVDs let you choose your music, workout length, exercises, and intensity.

If you have cable TV, check whether your company offers an exercise-on-demand channel. These channels run many popular exercise videos for free, and most have extensive libraries that turn over every month or so, so you never get bored. Sites such as www.exercisetv.tv also post a certain number of free workouts, a great deal if you don't mind working out in front of your computer. These sites also offer downloads to your digital recorder or iPod starting as low as $1.

When parents pry their kids away from their Wiis and Xboxes, these toys can morph into mini-gyms for Mom or Dad. Starting with Wii Fit, there has been an explosion of fitness games for these devices. You can do everything from kickboxing to a step class to snowboarding down the mountain with Olympic athletes. Most games involve using a small, low stool and a game stick that senses movement and pressure. The gizmo offers encouragement and suggestions for better form. If you already own an Xbox or Wii, consider spending $20 to $60 on a game or two.

A Personal Trainer

You can hire a trainer for a couple of sessions, either at home or at a health club, to get you started on a program tailored to your goals and your fitness level or to update your current routine. Trainers cost between $60 and $300 per session. If you buddy up with a friend or two, your sessions may cost less. If you buy a block of sessions at once, you often receive a discount.

If you plan to be a short-timer, inform your trainer of your intentions so that he can cover more in a shorter period of time. And think specifically about your goals for these few sessions. Do you want to learn a routine you can take on business trips? Do you want training advice for a summer cycling vacation? Do you want a program to help you lose fat? Act like you're taking a crash course in Italian two weeks before you move to Rome: Be prepared to soak up a lot of information. Arm yourself with questions and take notes. By the end of your sessions, make sure you know how to adjust each machine, grip each handle the right way, and perform each exercise using the correct technique. And consider scheduling follow-up sessions once a month or so to check your progress, stay up-to-date, and continue to improve your skills. Also find out whether your trainer is willing to answer quick questions via e-mail as part of the overall cost.

A Massage

Okay, you've been exercising for a solid month. You deserve a reward, and besides, your legs feel a little sore. What better way to treat yourself than with a rubdown? Massage loosens up kinks in your muscles, relieves stress, and helps you relax. Research suggests it may even speed your body's recovery from a workout or injury by increasing blood flow and, therefore, delivering more oxygen and nutrients to your muscle cells and restoring muscle and joint mobility. We like massage for another reason: It feels *soooo* good.

Depending on where you live, an hour-long massage can run you between $50 and $200. Sessions in your home usually cost a little more, to compensate for the driving time and the fact that the therapist has to lug a big, heavy table to your door.

In most states, massage therapists are required to pass a certification exam. Chances are, any therapist who works at a club or spa is fully licensed and certified, but it never hurts to ask. For a home massage, get a recommendation from a doctor, trainer, or friend you trust.

Index

• *N* •

ple & Macs

ad For Dummies
8-0-470-58027-1

hone For Dummies,
 Edition
8-0-470-87870-5

cBook For Dummies, 3rd
ition
8-0-470-76918-8

c OS X Snow Leopard For
mmies
8-0-470-43543-4

siness

okkeeping For Dummies
8-0-7645-9848-7

b Interviews
r Dummies,
d Edition
8-0-470-17748-8

sumes For Dummies,
 Edition
8-0-470-08037-5

arting an
line Business
r Dummies,
 Edition
8-0-470-60210-2

ock Investing
r Dummies,
d Edition
8-0-470-40114-9

ccessful
me Management
r Dummies
8-0-470-29034-7

Computer Hardware

BlackBerry
For Dummies,
4th Edition
978-0-470-60700-8

Computers For Seniors
For Dummies,
2nd Edition
978-0-470-53483-0

PCs For Dummies,
Windows
7 Edition
978-0-470-46542-4

Laptops For Dummies,
4th Edition
978-0-470-57829-2

Cooking & Entertaining

Cooking Basics
For Dummies,
3rd Edition
978-0-7645-7206-7

Wine For Dummies,
4th Edition
978-0-470-04579-4

Diet & Nutrition

Dieting For Dummies,
2nd Edition
978-0-7645-4149-0

Nutrition For Dummies,
4th Edition
978-0-471-79868-2

Weight Training
For Dummies,
3rd Edition
978-0-471-76845-6

Digital Photography

Digital SLR Cameras &
Photography For Dummies,
3rd Edition
978-0-470-46606-3

Photoshop Elements 8
For Dummies
978-0-470-52967-6

Gardening

Gardening Basics
For Dummies
978-0-470-03749-2

Organic Gardening
For Dummies,
2nd Edition
978-0-470-43067-5

Green/Sustainable

Raising Chickens
For Dummies
978-0-470-46544-8

Green Cleaning
For Dummies
978-0-470-39106-8

Health

Diabetes For Dummies,
3rd Edition
978-0-470-27086-8

Food Allergies
For Dummies
978-0-470-09584-3

Living Gluten-Free
For Dummies,
2nd Edition
978-0-470-58589-4

Hobbies/General

Chess For Dummies,
2nd Edition
978-0-7645-8404-6

Drawing
Cartoons & Comics
For Dummies
978-0-470-42683-8

Knitting For Dummies,
2nd Edition
978-0-470-28747-7

Organizing
For Dummies
978-0-7645-5300-4

Su Doku For Dummies
978-0-470-01892-7

Home Improvement

Home Maintenance
For Dummies,
2nd Edition
978-0-470-43063-7

Home Theater
For Dummies,
3rd Edition
978-0-470-41189-6

Living the
Country Lifestyle
All-in-One
For Dummies
978-0-470-43061-3

Solar Power Your Home
For Dummies,
2nd Edition
978-0-470-59678-4

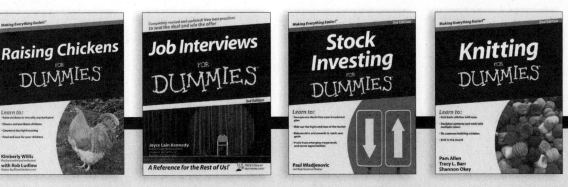

Internet

Blogging For Dummies,
3rd Edition
978-0-470-61996-4

eBay For Dummies,
6th Edition
978-0-470-49741-8

Facebook For Dummies,
3rd Edition
978-0-470-87804-0

Web Marketing
For Dummies,
2nd Edition
978-0-470-37181-7

WordPress
For Dummies,
3rd Edition
978-0-470-59274-8

Language & Foreign Language

French For Dummies
978-0-7645-5193-2

Italian Phrases
For Dummies
978-0-7645-7203-6

Spanish For Dummies,
2nd Edition
978-0-470-87855-2

Spanish
For Dummies,
Audio Set
978-0-470-09585-0

Math & Science

Algebra I
For Dummies,
2nd Edition
978-0-470-55964-2

Biology For Dummies,
2nd Edition
978-0-470-59875-7

Calculus For Dummies
978-0-7645-2498-1

Chemistry For Dummies
978-0-7645-5430-8

Microsoft Office

Excel 2010 For Dummies
978-0-470-48953-6

Office 2010 All-in-One
For Dummies
978-0-470-49748-7

Office 2010 For Dummies,
Book + DVD Bundle
978-0-470-62698-6

Word 2010 For Dummies
978-0-470-48772-3

Music

Guitar For Dummies,
2nd Edition
978-0-7645-9904-0

iPod & iTunes For
Dummies, 8th Edition
978-0-470-87871-2

Piano Exercises
For Dummies
978-0-470-38765-8

Parenting & Education

Parenting For Dummies,
2nd Edition
978-0-7645-5418-6

Type 1 Diabetes
For Dummies
978-0-470-17811-9

Pets

Cats For Dummies,
2nd Edition
978-0-7645-5275-5

Dog Training For Dummies,
3rd Edition
978-0-470-60029-0

Puppies For Dummies,
2nd Edition
978-0-470-03717-1

Religion & Inspiration

The Bible For Dummies
978-0-7645-5296-0

Catholicism For Dummies
978-0-7645-5391-2

Women in the Bible
For Dummies
978-0-7645-8475-6

Self-Help & Relationship

Anger Management
For Dummies
978-0-470-03715-7

Overcoming Anxiety
For Dummies,
2nd Edition
978-0-470-57441-6

Sports

Baseball
For Dummies,
3rd Edition
978-0-7645-7537-2

Basketball
For Dummies,
2nd Edition
978-0-7645-5248-9

Golf For Dummies,
3rd Edition
978-0-471-76871-5

Web Development

Web Design
All-in-One
For Dummies
978-0-470-41796-6

Web Sites
Do-It-Yourself
For Dummies,
2nd Edition
978-0-470-56520-9

Windows 7

Windows 7
For Dummies
978-0-470-49743-2

Windows 7
For Dummies,
Book + DVD Bundle
978-0-470-52398-8

Windows 7 All-in-One
For Dummies
978-0-470-48763-1

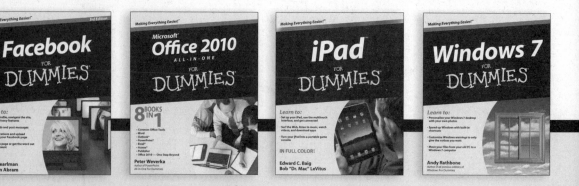